Advanced Remedial Massage and Soft Tissue Therapy

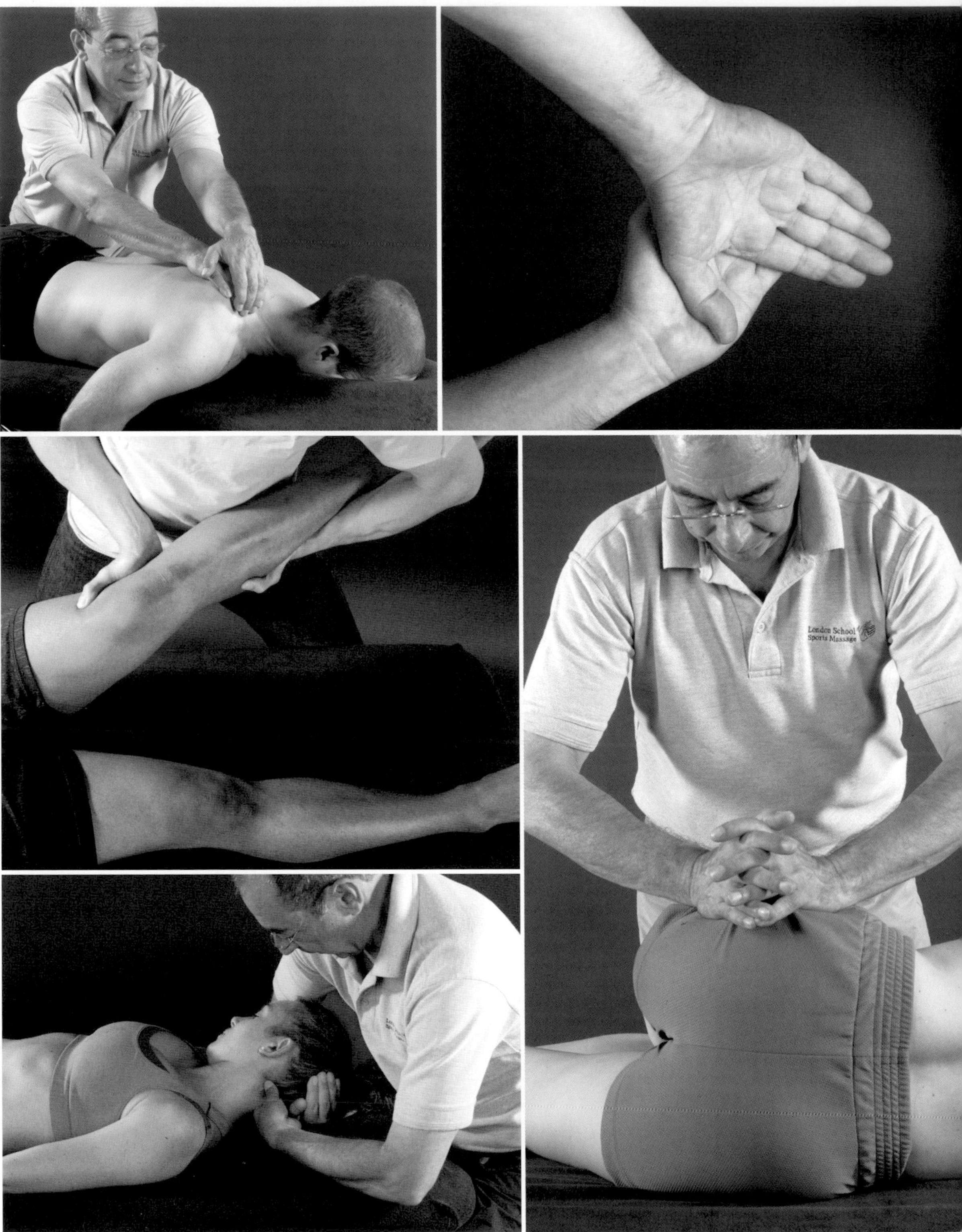
London School
Sports Massage

Advanced Remedial Massage and Soft Tissue Therapy

Mel Cash

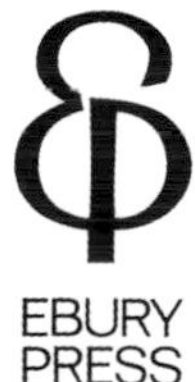

EBURY
PRESS

10 9 8 7 6 5 4 3 2 1

Published in 2012 by Ebury Press, an imprint of Ebury Publishing

A Random House Group Company

Artworks by Anne Wadmore

The Random House Group Limited Reg. No. 954009

Addresses for companies within the Random House Group can be found at www.randomhouse.co.uk

A CIP catalogue record for this book is available from the British Library

Printed and bound in China by Toppan

ISBN 9780091926700

Contents

Acknowledgements

Illustrations by Anne Wadmore
Sponsored by Institute of Sports & Remedial Massage

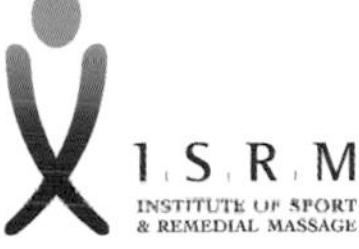

All photographs by Gavin Cottrell
Sponsored by London School of Sports Massage

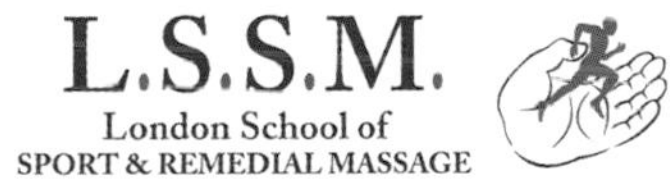

Therapists
Mel Cash
Alex Fugallo
David Katz

Models on the couch
Jonathan Arnold
Steve Barrick
Mel Cash
Stefania D'Addetta
Alison Dalziel
Alex Fugallo
David Katz
Tatiana Novaes Coelho
Morgan Harper-Brown
Glenn McFie

Cover design by Two Associates
Inside design by Lisa Pettibone

Special thanks to my friends and colleagues Alex Fugallo and David Katz who have freely shared their clinical knowledge and experience with me for many years.

Introduction

This book was intended to celebrate 25 years as a working therapist but it took longer than I expected and the anniversary passed quietly by some time before I finished it. My first book *Sports Massage* was written when I had been in practice for just a few years and it represented the level I was working at in those early days. My clinical understanding developed greatly over the next 10 years and this was reflected in the second book *Sport & Remedial Massage Therapy* in 1996. But over 15 years have now passed and, as a teacher as well as a therapist, I have not stopped discovering more. So the aim of this book is simply to try to share the knowledge and understanding I have gained through 25 years of clinical experience.

This book does not describe massage for beginners and assumes the reader is already able to do this and knows the basic anatomy and physiology necessary. Although it may be more advanced in its approach to massage therapy, it is not a heavy academic text. It had to be this way because the most talented and successful hands-on therapists are rarely great academics and they prefer clear, simple explanations. Of course it is important to understand the theories behind the techniques so they can be repeated and developed more effectively, but academic knowledge alone achieves very little and is not the main motivation behind this book.

One day early on in my career I had used Muscle Energy Technique to good effect on a wise elderly client. He was impressed and asked me how it worked but I stupidly answered, 'Oh, it's too complicated to explain.' He then looked me straight in the eye and replied, 'If you can't explain it simply then you don't understand it fully.' He was so right and his words have echoed inside my head constantly whilst writing this book.

Rather than refer directly to any of the academic texts I have read over the years I have tried to use plain language to explain things as simply as possible. It has taken far longer than I imagined to understand things fully enough to be able to explain them simply and I hope I have succeeded in this. I could probably have written twice as many words in half the time but this would have wasted a lot of the reader's time and probably bored us all.

It is the clinical experience gained beyond the classroom that makes a great therapist and the next best thing to your own experience is to share someone else's.

Writing the Book

Most of this book was written at my kitchen table overlooking the garden (*see also Appendix 4, How I Got Into Massage*). Of course this is not the best working position to be sitting in for many long hours and I suffered with quite a few aches and pains because of it. I wish I could remember to follow the advice I give to my clients! I wrote part of the book whilst working at a charity project in Pokhara, Nepal*, teaching blind people to become massage therapists. There I could look up from my laptop and see the great Himalayas which was a breathtaking distraction. But at night we constantly had power cuts so I often had to wear a head-torch to see the keyboard, which was not so glamorous.

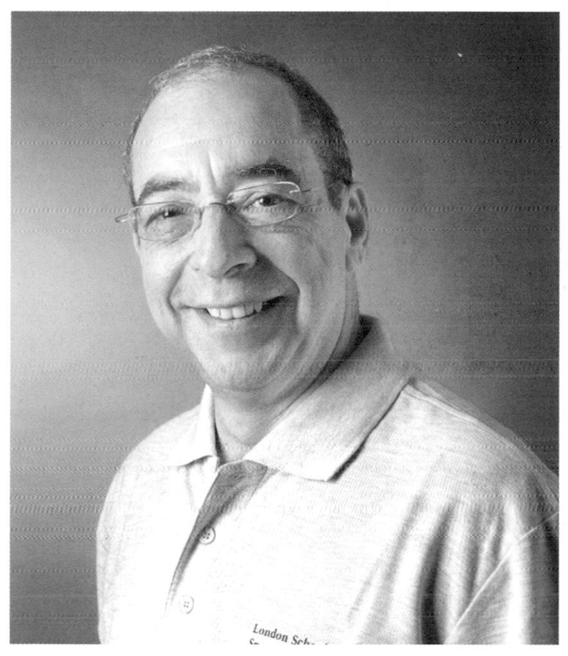

Mel Cash, Founder and Principal Tutor of the London School of Sports Massage, and Director of the Institute of Sport & Remedial Massage

The Illustrations

Massage and soft tissue therapy requires a very thorough understanding of the musculo-skeletal system and for that we need to know exactly where the muscles are. Although the best way to discover this would be by dissecting real cadavers this is something very few people have the opportunity to do, so instead we have to use visual images in books and on charts. Photographs taken of cadaver dissections cannot clearly show the multi-layers of muscles in isolation and so we must rely on the skills of the anatomical artist to do this.

Anne Wadmore is a highly experienced medical illustrator working at a London teaching hospital where she has access to cadavers when necessary. Her attention to detail and accuracy in producing the diagrams for this book has been truly outstanding and I am incredibly grateful to her.

**Seeing Hands Nepal*

1 Understanding Movement and Posture

To use massage and soft tissue techniques as a remedy for clients with pain, injury and dysfunction, therapists need to have a very thorough understanding of how the body moves and maintains posture. This has traditionally been based on a knowledge of the musculoskeletal system, which is made up of muscles that attach to bones across the joints. When the muscles contract and shorten, they pull on the bones and make the joints articulate.

From this it might be assumed that it is only necessary to know a list of muscles with their origins, insertions and actions to be able to understand movement and posture. But it is much more complex than this simple model suggests. Although the muscles and bones are the main structures we can see making the movements, other structures and systems of the body are also integrally involved.

The anatomical charts we use today have not changed in more than a century, but we can see their limitations when we consider them in their historical context. Michelangelo may have carried out dissections in the sixteenth century, but there was little scientific basis to them. It was in eighteenth-century London that a pioneering surgeon called John Hunter carried out a great many dissections using a very detailed scientific approach. It was these studies that led to the charts we are now so familiar with.

The early anatomists like Hunter wanted to look under the skin to see how the body worked, but the first thing they found there was a thick layer of fatty tissue which surrounded the whole body (the superficial fascia). This did not appear to have any obvious function and seemed to be just an insignificant outer layer of padding around the body. It obscured their view of the underlying structures, so this layer of tissue was quickly discarded.

Between this fatty layer and the muscles is another thin layer of deep fascia wrapping around the body. This also appeared to be nothing more than an insignificant layer of wrapping that stopped them seeing the muscles, bones and organs underneath, so this too was removed. We now know that, rather than being a separate outer layer, this was just the outer part of a continuous three-dimensional fascial network that runs through the entire musculoskeletal system.

Having removed these layers, they were left looking at a complex pattern of muscles and bones. They could see that the muscles pulling and shortening across the joints would create all our articulating movements. This appeared to show how the body moved, and it did not seem to need any further explanation.

As medical training became formalised in the twentieth century, this simple musculoskeletal model of movement remained unquestioned. This was because there were now skilled technicians who prepared the cadavers in the dissection room before the medical students arrived to study them. They followed the traditional model and removed these fascial layers to reveal the underlying structures, so students only saw what they expected to see, and what matched the old familiar charts. They rarely got the opportunity to examine the fascia or consider its significance, and so the misconception that they were just insignificant layers of wrapping continued.

But, from the middle of the twentieth century, manual therapists began to discover that they were achieving quite remarkable results by applying techniques specifically to these layers. This has led to a growing understanding of the importance of the fascial system. We now know that it is the key component in movement and posture because it holds the musculoskeletal system together and makes it a functioning unit.

The Fascial System

The Superficial Fascia

This layer of fatty adipose tissue forms a single continuous layer surrounding the whole body. It adheres very strongly to the inside of the skin and also binds very strongly to the layer of deep fascia along its inner surface. It is naturally thicker in some body areas like the abdomen and buttocks but much thinner in other parts like the lower arms, legs and over the skull. The thickness also varies according to the person's individual level of body fat and some genetic factors.

This layer of superficial fascia has its own nervous, vascular and lymphatic supply and can be considered as an organ itself. Although it is mostly soft fatty tissue, it has a fine matrix of stronger connective tissue running through it. This contains elastin fibres, which can stretch, and collagen fibres, which are inelastic but have great tensile strength. Together, these give it a soft and pliable texture which is also very tough and resistant to overstretching forces.

The health and condition of this superficial fascial layer is important in enabling the body to move freely. Acting like a body stocking if it is in poor condition or damaged, it could have a restricting effect on movement. This is particularly common where there are surgical scars that can leave a solid barrier of immobile scar tissue running through it. This will distort and restrict its ability to move freely and affects the body's movement. This fascia also has a very high water content, so poor nutrition and dehydration will affect its texture and ability to move.

As a sensory organ, this fatty layer works alongside the skin and is very responsive to external pressure and impact. It also appears to have the potential to contract through myofibroblasts that have been found throughout the fascial network. These specialist cells function like smooth muscle cells which can contract on an autonomic level. It is possible that on a reflex level, in response to external pressure, there could be local areas of fascial contraction, creating a tougher protective barrier when needed.

Although we talk about applying massage and soft tissue techniques to the muscles, it is impossible to do this without working through this superficial fascia in an effort to reach them. So it does get a lot of good treatment which can improve its hydration and mobility. Although therapists may think they have achieved an improvement by treating the muscles it is possible that it is the effect on the superficial fascia that can sometimes be more significant.

The Deep Fascia

The deep fascia is a single three-dimensional structure which envelops every muscle, bone, nerve, organ and cell in the body, connecting them all together and holding everything in place. It acts as both a barrier and a filtration mechanism for the various body fluids in the different organs and vessels. These can all be adversely affected if the fascia is damaged or in poor condition. It too has high water content, and if it is dehydrated this can lead to a build-up of toxins which can alter the exchange of chemicals through it.

The fascia is rich in mechanoreceptors which send sensory information to the central nervous system. It also contains myofibroblasts, which give it the potential to contract on an autonomic level, and these two connect through reflex pathways. The mechanoreceptors are particularly concentrated in the layers surrounding the muscle (epimysium), and it is possible that what we think of as muscle tone could actually be caused by an autonomic fascial contraction rather than the muscle fibres themselves contracting.

Myofascia

In terms of movement and posture, it is the part of the deep fascia that is involved directly with the musculoskeletal system, called the myofascia, which interests us most. But this is not in any way separated from the fascia that also binds around the organs, and this could explain why there can be links between organ dysfunction and musculoskeletal pain.

This fascia is made up of a polysaccharide complex called *ground substance*, which is contained within a matrix of elastin and collagen fibres. The elastin fibres can stretch and the collagen fibres have great tensile strength which together gives the fascia great physical potential. The proportion and distribution of elastin and collagen fibres varies drastically in different areas depending on the local needs.

As the human body evolved, the arrangement of the collagen and elastin fibres gradually adapted to meet the physical demands placed on the body. This has resulted in a complex network of strong collagen bands which wrap around the body in all directions, giving it its upright shape and form. The muscles are the contractile pockets along these bands, and that gives the body its ability to create movement. In between these strong and contractile bands, the fascia is very elastic so it allows the system to move freely.

Muscles, tendons, ligaments and joint capsules are not separate structures as the simple model of the musculoskeletal system may suggest. They are all just parts of this single fascial network, and the muscles are only contractile pockets along the strong fascial bands. The muscle's fascia extends to form the tendon, and the fascia spreads out to form the capsule and ligaments where this reaches a joint, becoming the periosteum at the bone.

Within the muscles, the fascia envelops every myofibril and has a high proportion of elastin, which enables it to move freely with the fibres. The force of the fibre's contraction is only turned into a functional movement through its relationship with the surrounding fascia. It may be able to contract strongly, but there will be no functional effect if the fascia is restricted.

Where the muscle fibres end the fascia continues, and it becomes mostly collagen and forms the tendon. Although this may be said to insert into a bone, it does not actually stop there because it continues on through the fascia into the next muscle. Each muscle is just part of a chain, and if there is a problem in one muscle there will be an effect on others along the chain. When one muscle contracts, other muscles along the chain have to respond and assist in the function. As a contracting muscle pulls on its attachment, there needs to be an increase in tension from the muscle on the other side to counteract the stress on the attachment point. Attachment injuries can sometimes be caused by weakness in adjacent muscles rather than strength or tightness in the primary muscle.

A muscle may appear to cross a joint in a single direction and make a movement only in that direction, but its fascial connections may also create tension and movement in other directions too. So when considering the actions of a muscle it is rarely as simple as it may appear from the charts.

The most significant feature of this incredibly

vital fascia is the way it adapts to stress and needs to keep well hydrated to function in a normal healthy way. When movement does not take place for a period of time, the fascia starts to form tiny fibrous bonds with the adjacent tissues, but these easily melt away when movement does occur. So the fascia tends to stick together when we sleep or when we are inactive for short periods, and that is why we feel stiff and naturally want to stretch to break the bonds and loosen the fascia when we get up.

Prolonged and repetitive lack of movement in local areas of the body allows these fibrous bonds to increase and strengthen. This starts to restrict movement within and between the muscles and eventually binds the tissues together. The fascial sheath around the outside of muscle (perimysium) has a smooth shiny surface which allows it to slide easily alongside other structures. It is particularly affected by this and is the most common cause of soft tissue stiffness.

The shape of the fascial network also adapts and changes in response to stress and misuse. If the fascia is held in a shortened position for prolonged periods then it will eventually become set in this position. Although we may think a muscle is short and tight, if this is a chronic situation it will be the fascia that is tight and this is far more significant. Muscle-stretching exercises alone will do very little to release the fascial tension, but manual techniques can be extremely quick and effective in doing this. Only after the fascia has been released this way will remedial exercise and postural improvement then be effective and result in a long-term improvement.

But if the fascia has been held in a lengthened position and become set that way it is much harder to deal with, because fascial release techniques cannot make the tissues any shorter. Postural improvement and a lot of strengthening/tensioning exercises are usually the best way of restoring normal length here.

The Muscular System

We have voluntary control of movement through our muscles, and so they are directly affected by the way we use, misuse and abuse the body. They are usually the starting point for students studying movement who learn lists of muscle names with their origins, insertions and actions. But this only gives a very basic level of knowledge and does not properly explain functional movement.

Muscle names can be misleading because these were mostly created more than a century ago when the system was less well understood. The group names like 'quadriceps' suggest that all four muscles in this group work together. But one, the rectus femoris, is very different in many ways from the other three. The pectoralis major and minor muscles may be found together in the chest area, but they act on different joints and have distinctly separate functions.

Standard lists of muscle actions only describe the movement that takes place if the muscle contracts concentrically (shortening), pulling bones together across a joint. But function involves more than just this action. Standing and holding something still can take considerable muscular effort, but no actual movement is taking place. This is only possible because muscles can do much more than just contract and shorten.

Descriptions of insertions and actions are also quite simplistic on muscle charts because they often ignore the many complex fascial connections. Although a muscle may appear to go neatly through a tendon to the bone, the fascial network may also connect it indirectly to other muscles and bones. So it may influence other joints and movements which do not appear to be obvious from the alignment of the muscle fibres alone. Muscles do not really have origins and insertions because they do not really stop or start anywhere. Through their fascial connections they have attachments to bones but then continue on into the next muscle. The muscles should be seen as contractile pockets along fascial chains and any deficiency in one muscle will inevitably have an effect on others along the chain.

The standard lists describe the action of muscles based on the ideal anatomical model with a well-balanced and stable posture. But with postural imbalances, which are so very common, the alignment of muscles can be quite different and so too will be their actions. Injuries often occur because the muscles are being forced to take on roles that they are not designed to do. People with good postural alignment and stability are far less likely to get injured and need treatment, so the standard lists and charts we study rarely ever match the clients we see.

For example, it appears from the charts that the sternocleidomastoid is the main muscle to rotate the neck and head. But with a forward protracted head position, it is the muscles in the back of the neck that have to take on this role and the sternocleidomastoid is almost redundant in this position.

Gravity

Perhaps the most important factor which is not considered in the basic list of muscle actions is gravity, which applies a constant downward force on the body. As we move into different positions, the angle of the body in relation to this force changes and results in significant differences in the way the muscular system has to work.

A standard list will, for example, show that the main muscle used to horizontally adduct the shoulder joint is the pectoralis major. But if you perform this movement repetitively in an upright position, it will be the deltoid and upper trapezius muscles that fatigue first. This is because they have to work harder to hold the arm up against gravity whilst the movement takes place. But do the same movement lying on your back and it will be the pectoralis major that fatigues first because this now has to work harder against gravity. The anatomical movement is just the same, but the muscle activity required to do this is very different because of the position of the body in relation to gravity.

Although gravity may be difficult, or impossible, to explain, it is one of the first things in life that we learn how to deal with. Babies quickly discover how to hold their heads upright and still so they can observe their surroundings properly. To do this they have to automatically make instant fine adjustments in the contractions of their neck muscles in response to changes in the direction of gravity as they move. Because this is learned so early on in life, however, we tend to ignore its significance.

Gravity has been fundamental in making the body the shape it is. The biceps brachii muscle that flexes the elbow, for example, is larger than the triceps brachii that extends it. This is because, in the normal upright position, elbow flexion requires more strength as it has to work against gravity when lifting things up but extending it to lower things is assisted by gravity and usually requires little or no strength.

Different Types of Skeletal Muscle Fibre

Not all muscles need to produce forces in the same way; some are used to maintain posture and work at low levels for very long periods, whilst others are used for short powerful actions whenever required. To achieve these differences, muscles are made up of different types of fibres which best suit their normal functional requirements.

- **Slow oxidative fibres (slow twitch):** These are thinner in diameter and red in colour because they carry large amounts of myoglobin. They contain a high number of mitochondria and produce adenosine triphosphate (ATP) by aerobic cellular respiration. Because of this they contract slowly but have very good endurance potential.
- **Fast glycolytic fibres (fast twitch):** These are thicker in diameter with high levels of glycogen and produce ATP through glycolysis. They can produce great speed and power but have low endurance capabilities.
- **Fast oxidative glycolytic fibres:** These fit in between the other two. They also have a lot of mitochondria and generate ATP aerobically, but also contain high levels of glycogen and produce ATP through glycolysis as well. This means they can perform with a more even balance of both speed/power and endurance.

The muscles used primarily to maintain posture have a higher proportion of slow oxidative fibres, so they can work at low levels for very long periods. Muscles in the arms, however, have a higher proportion of fast glycolytic fibres to enable the fast, strong actions they need there, but they cannot maintain this for long periods.

The proportional mix of fibre types also varies between individual people because of their genetic make-up. Although some slight adaptive changes may take place through training and lifestyle, the number of muscles fibres and the type of those fibres is set from birth. A world-class sprinter will have been born with a phenomenally high proportion of fast glycolytic fibres in the muscles used for running, and a world-class marathon runner will have been born with a high proportion of slow oxidative fibres. Although it obviously takes the right training to develop the potential, in essence world-class athletes are born that way.

At a lower level of sport, these differences can lead to problems when people take up a sport that does not ideally suit their muscle type. They may train for a marathon with high expectations because they consider themselves to be very fit. But if they were good sprinters when they were at school and keep fit now using strength-based exercises in a gym, it probably means they have a fairly high proportion of fast glycolytic fibres. In this case, they may experience greater difficulties in their training and performance in an endurance event than they might expect.

Different Types of Muscle Contraction

To create and control movement muscles have to work in different ways.

- **Concentric contraction:** This is the first type of contraction we consider when looking at how the body moves. It occurs when the force of contraction is greater than the resistance, and the muscle shortens. It pulls the bones together across the joint to create movement.

The Neuromuscular System

Without neural innervation, the muscular system on its own has no functional ability at all and it is the neuromuscular system that we should always be considering.

A muscle fibre will contract if it is stimulated by a motor nerve, but this alone would merely give us action with no functional control. For functional control, we also need to know the position our body is in so we can contract the right muscles in the right way to achieve a given task.

As with all parts of the nervous system, both motor and sensory nerve impulses are needed for it to function. The sensory information comes from several different sources, which together make up *proprioception*. This is what enables us to know where and how our body is moving without needing to be visually aware of it.

The Proprioceptors

- **Muscle spindles** run along the muscle fibres and send information about the length and rate of change in the length of the muscle.
- **Golgi organs** are found throughout the fascial system but are particularly concentrated in the tendons. They relay information on the amount of tension going through the muscle fibres.
- **Joint kinesthetic receptors, Pacini** organs in the joint capsule and **Ruffini** organs in the ligaments send information about a joint's position and the stresses on these structures.

The motor and sensory nerves are linked through connector neurons at the spinal cord where reflexes occur and automatic neural patterns are learned. All the normal daily movements we make without thinking about are created and controlled through this mechanism.

At birth we have almost no control over movement, and the neuromuscular system must develop all the neural pathways needed to do this. The system has the most incredible ability to teach itself how to create movements through practice and repetition. In just a few years, we master all of the most important and complex tasks we need for daily life such as walking, talking and tying our shoelaces.

The system's ability to self-learn does not stop there, and we continue to learn more specialist skills and refinements as our lives continue. But as well as learning through use, the system can also forget through a lack of use. Children run around and play for many hours and this constantly reinforces and develops these neuromuscular skills. But sitting behind a desk all day does not, and the efficiency of those normal everyday movement patterns can deteriorate. As well as learning to perform patterns of movement that are good, the system can also learn poor patterns if they are repeated too often, and this is why occupational factors can become so significant.

Poor, inefficient movement patterns often lead to local injury through overuse in particular muscles and joints. If just these local areas are treated, it may only alleviate the symptoms temporarily. The neuromuscular system needs to be re-educated to correct the movement pattern if there is to be a lasting improvement. To do this, functional movements with quality and control need to be the central part of rehabilitation.

Muscle Tone

No skeletal muscle is ever 100 per cent relaxed. As long as the body is conscious, there will always be some degree of contraction and tension taking place, and the neural pathways are never completely switched off. The level of tension in a muscle when it is at rest is called *muscle tone*, and this is controlled on an autonomic level through reflex actions between the motor and sensory nerves. A muscle's tone at rest is like its basic setting and if it is hypertonic at rest it will remain that way, over-contracting, throughout any activity it does.

Although it may be possible to assess the degree of muscle tone, there is no standard normal level. Therapists have to make subjective judgements on what they consider may be hypotonic (less contracted) or hypertonic (more contracted) in any given muscle on a particular individual.

Poor muscle tone (hyper or hypo) can lead to a variety of injury problems, and if only the locally affected muscles are treated the real problem may still remain. Techniques specifically aimed at influencing the neuromuscular system (Neuromuscular Technique and Positional Release in particular), are needed to restore normal muscle tone.

Psycho-emotional Factors

Many things can influence muscle tone, because no part of the nervous system works in isolation. Psycho-emotional factors seem particularly influential on the musculoskeletal system. We can often tell when someone is unhappy because their muscle tone lowers their posture, they stoop down and the muscles in their face sag. The opposite happens when someone is happy, their muscle tone increases, they stand more upright and their facial muscles go up into a smile.

Short-term changes in muscle tone caused by emotional factors are quite normal, but long-term depression or unhappiness can become a significant factor in chronic muscle / posture problems. Manual therapists naturally tend to look for musculoskeletal causes to musculoskeletal problems, but this is not always the case. If the client is being affected by more long-term emotional factors, then massage may alleviate their physical symptoms temporarily but not address the real problem.

Reciprocal Inhibition

When a muscle contracts, whichever muscle(s) work in opposition to it will automatically relax. For movement to take place freely, it is vital that any opposing muscles are relaxed so they do not restrict the action. Without this essential neural phenomenon, all movement would be stiff and require much greater effort.

Identifying the opposing muscles which can inhibit one another in the arms and legs is fairly simple. We have the quadriceps working in opposition with hamstrings when flexing and extending the knee, and the biceps and triceps doing the same at the elbow. But when muscles contract on one side of the body in sideways or twisting movements, it is much harder to recognise which muscles oppose this.

Reciprocal inhibition and muscle tone are integrally linked. If a muscle is hypertonic and is overly contracting all the time, the opposing muscle will gradually become weaker because it is being inhibited all the time. This is a very common underlying factor which should be considered in all chronic overuse conditions. A client may suffer an overuse strain in a muscle because it is being weakened through neural inhibition from an opposing muscle which is hypertonic. Treatment to the strained muscle alone may take away the painful symptoms but without dealing with the tension in the opposing muscle the injury is very likely to reoccur.

Common Examples

- Chronic overuse strain in the muscles at the back of the neck and shoulders may be, in part, due to their being weakened though inhibition coming from increased tension in the muscles across the front of the chest.
- Excessive tension in the vastus lateralis can inhibit and weaken the vastus medialis, which opposes it across the quadriceps group. The medialis is very significant in controlling the tracking of the patella and if it is weak it will allow it to be pulled laterally and rub against the lateral condyle of the femur.

It is hard for a muscle to develop strength if at the same time it is being neurologically inhibited, and strengthening exercises may have very little effect on them. If a tight opposing muscle can be identified and dealt with first, the weak muscle will then be better able to get stronger through exercise.

Because many muscles work in harmony to create movements, if we isolate and strengthen individual muscles it is very difficult to maintain the intricate balance we need. Instead, it is better to release areas of excessive tension first, in order to remove the adverse reciprocal inhibition, so the system as a whole can move more freely. Then functional exercises which replicate normal daily actions will enable the muscles to develop strength in a properly balanced way.

The Skeletal System

Massage therapists work primarily with the muscles, and so students tend to focus their initial studies on these and only learn basic lists of the bones and joints. But it requires a broader understanding of the skeletal structures to be able to work effectively on a remedial level.

The number of bones of the skeleton and their general shape are the same throughout the human race, but we do see a very wide variety in the overall shape and size of different people. The length, thickness and fine detail of a bone's shape are determined by genetics. During a lifetime, small adaptive changes can take place as the bones respond to the repetitive physical stresses put on them, as well as nutrition and other health factors. Over many generations these small changes can eventually lead to more distinct genetic differences, and over many thousands of years this has led to the wide variations we now see.

Big differences can exist within a single population and more general variations appear to be common in particular ethnic and regional groups. These genetic differences should be positive as the skeleton has gradually adapted over the generations to meet the needs of the many different environments human beings exist in. But with modern transportation and industrialisation, vast numbers of people have gone through very dramatic changes in their lifestyles in just a few decades. Having evolved through many generations of perhaps being manual/agricultural workers, they could now be sitting behind a desk all day long. People are using their bodies in ways that their skeletal structure may not be ideally adapted to, and this could be one of the more profound reasons why so many people in modern society suffer with musculoskeletal problems.

We all have the same number of joints which perform the same movements, but the range of those movements also varies between individuals. The limits of joint range depend on the unique shape of the articulating bone surfaces and the spaces between them, and this will be subject to slight genetic differences. Also the ligaments that control the end range are not equally inelastic in everyone. Although they are made up primarily of inelastic collagen fibres, here too genetic differences can result in more elastin fibres being present and will allow the joint to stretch further. People with a high elastin component in their ligaments can, with the right training, become great ballet dancers or gymnasts. But without good strength training they may suffer with structural joint injuries due to hypermobility.

Sport and exercise performance can also be influenced by these same issues. Someone who comes from a long line of heavy manual labourers may take up yoga and hope to perform the same exercises demonstrated by someone who comes from a long line of Yogis. But his skeletal structure may make such extreme positions impossible to achieve and possibly dangerous to attempt. Although a lot can be achieved through training, there are structural factors that ultimately limit what is safe and possible for each individual.

Bony Prominences

Therapists need to be very familiar with the location of the bones and their prominences because these are the landmarks which tell them exactly where on the body they are working. Many bones have large prominences on them which are important attachment points for strong muscles. *(See figs. 1 and 2 overleaf.)*

Posture

Posture is a key factor to consider with nearly all musculoskeletal problems. Poor alignment issues are endemic in modern society and are so often the root cause of painful conditions.

Gravity and Posture

The primary force influencing posture is gravity, which is constantly bearing down on the body. To hold an upright posture the muscular system has to apply equal and opposite forces up the body and hold the joints in an erect alignment. As gravity tries to push the body down, the muscular system works against this to hold it up.

Although the force of gravity remains constant, the strength and tone of the muscles are much more variable. At the start of the day, we are full of energy, the muscular system works well and we stand tall. But after a day's work, general fatigue weakens the system making it less efficient at fighting against gravity and we become shorter and more stooped. Many other factors such as injury, illness or emotional stress can also affect energy levels in a similar way, weakening the muscular system and affecting posture.

Because gravity is an invisible force, we forget to consider its effects and do not make a conscious effort to resist it. At best, when we are full of energy we apply an equal force to oppose it but when tired and fatigued gravity starts to win the battle and posture slumps downwards. The cumulative effect of this over a lifetime means that some postural deterioration is usually inevitable.

But the most significant variable factor affecting posture is lifestyle. Children normally

Main Bony Prominences that Can Be Palpated

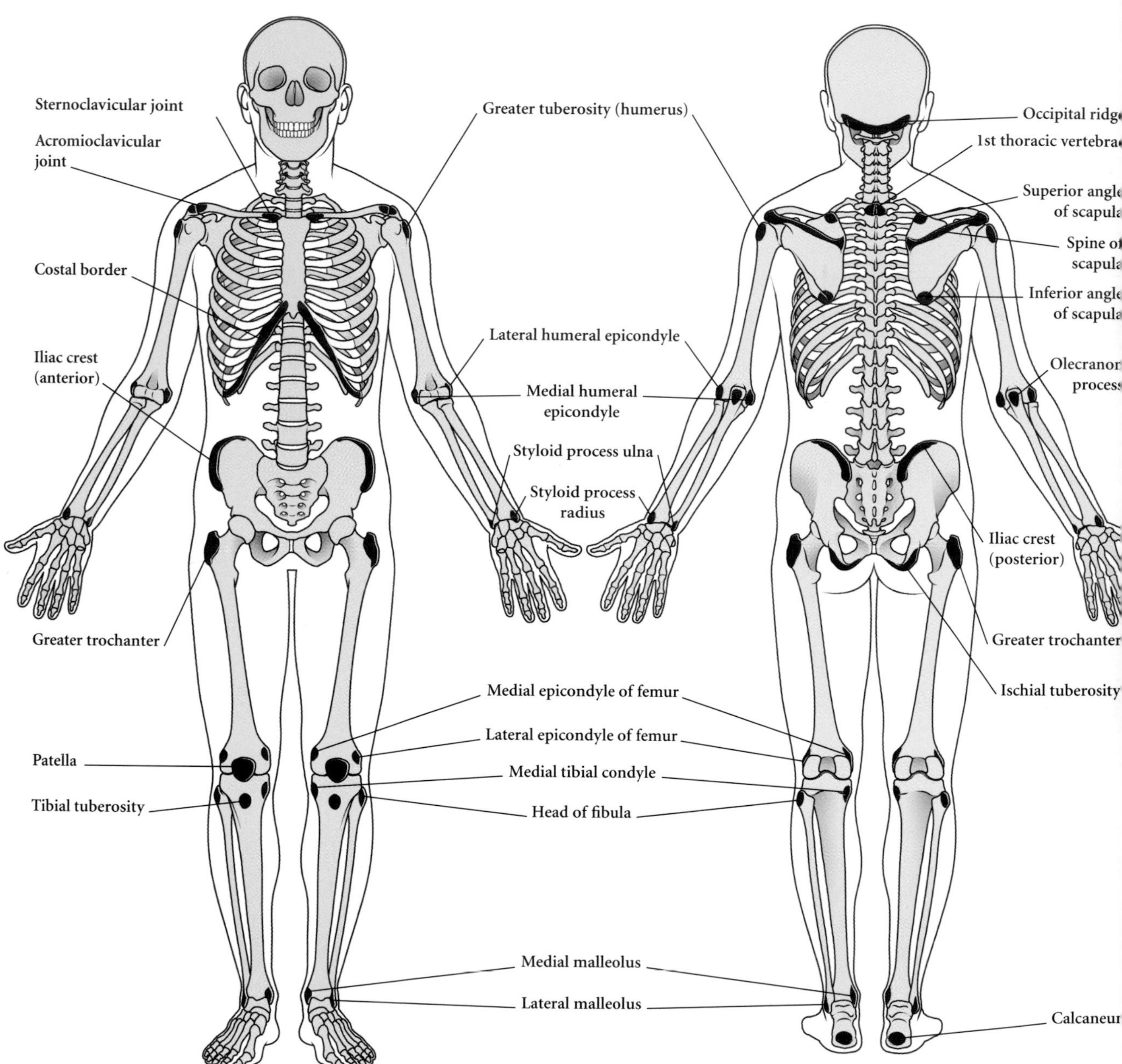

Fig. 1. Anterior

Fig. 2. Posterior

have very good postures because through play they perform a great variety of normal physical activities and spend very little time sitting still. This keeps their whole musculoskeletal system efficient and well-toned. Most adults, however, have jobs that involve many hours of physically repetitive activities such as sitting at a desk or doing a manual trade. In these situations some muscles become weak due to underuse and others may become strong and tense through overuse. Some muscles are repetitively held in shortened positions whilst others are lengthened, and they gradually become set that way.

These changes in muscle length and function mean the system cannot efficiently maintain a good upright posture so imbalances develop. Over time the fascial network gradually remodels itself to fit these changes also and the situation then becomes more permanent. In the long term the joints too can become affected by uneven stresses due to their poor alignment.

Other habitual factors also play a part in determining posture. We often see adults with identical postural deviations to one of their parents, but this was not visible when they were children. Although there may be some very slight genetic factors involved in later bone development, these postural changes must be acquired through the way they use their body. People often copy the physical mannerisms and habits of their parents and because they use their body in the same way they are also more likely to end up with the same postural tendencies.

Postural changes develop slowly over many years and may not directly cause painful chronic symptoms for a very long time. But imbalance makes the body much more vulnerable to injury in normal daily activities or sport and it does not just affect the spine and torso where the signs may be more obvious. The peripheral joints and muscles will also be misaligned and their function compromised too.

Soft tissue techniques applied to the muscles and fascia can be very effective in helping to realign posture. But these alone will only achieve temporary results unless exercise and lifestyle issues are also addressed.

Ideal Posture

In the ideal posture, the spine, pelvis and legs are all neutrally aligned through well-balanced muscle contractions throughout the whole body. *(See figs. 3, 4 and 5 overleaf.)*

Common Postural Tendencies

There are common adverse postural tendencies which are described here, but it is unlikely that a client will match any of these exactly. They will have varying degrees of excessive curvatures in different parts of their spine and pelvis. And they may even show signs of more than one of these tendencies at the same time.

Sway-back posture

This is the most common postural tendency we see in people living urban lifestyles and is most likely due to long periods of sitting. In this position, the hip flexors and abdominal muscles become weak through lack of use. Then when standing they are less able to support the front of the body so it bends and the pelvis moves forward. They then have to lean back to try to maintain balance and this creates the sway-back. *(See figs. 6, 7 and 8 overleaf.)*

The lumbar spine is usually slightly flattened, the pelvis is posteriorly tilted, and the hip joint is slightly extended. It is also common for the knees to be locked in full or hyperextension.

Ideal/Neutral Posture

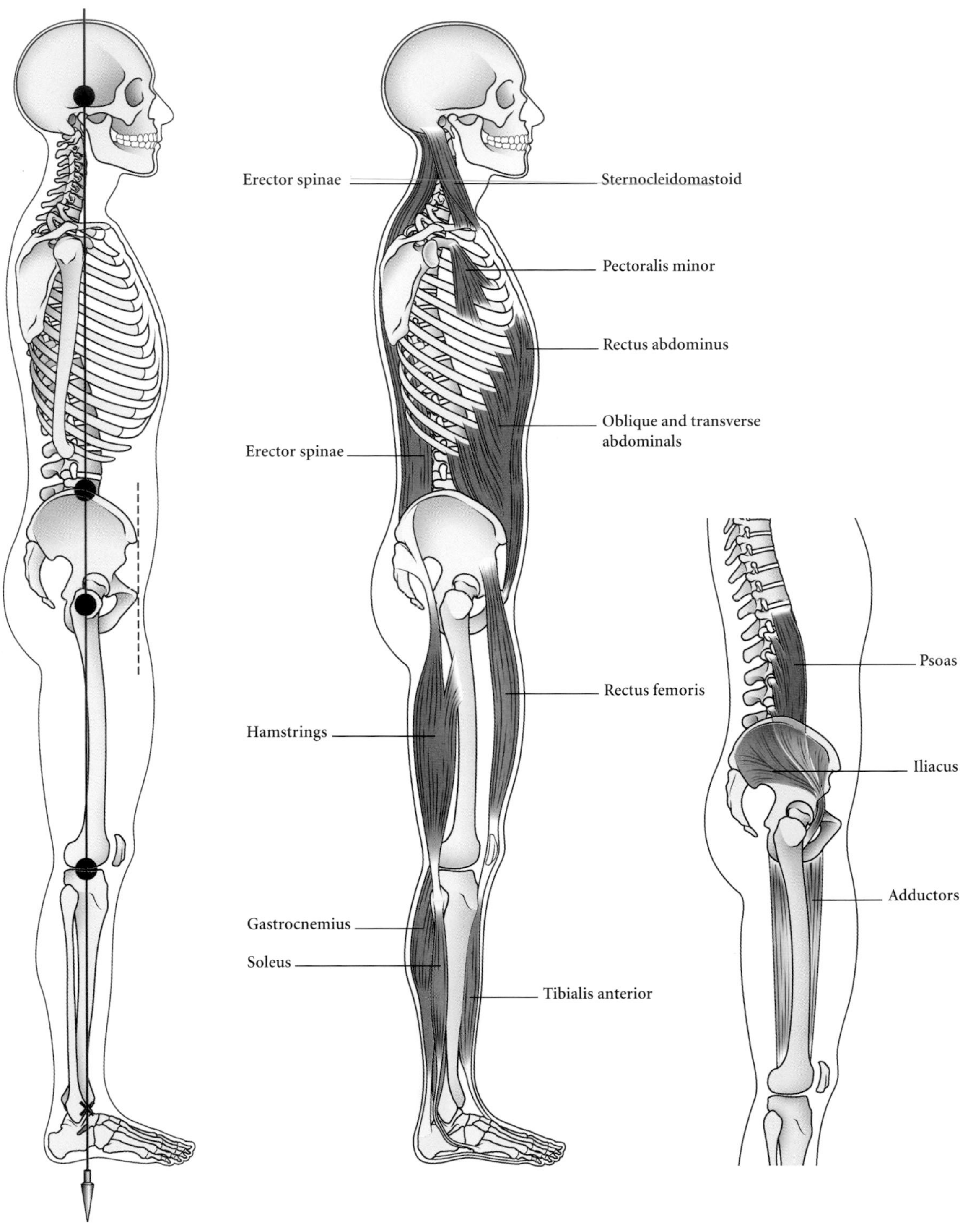

Fig. 3. Skeleton

Fig. 4. Superficial muscles

Fig. 5. Deep muscles

Sway-back Posture

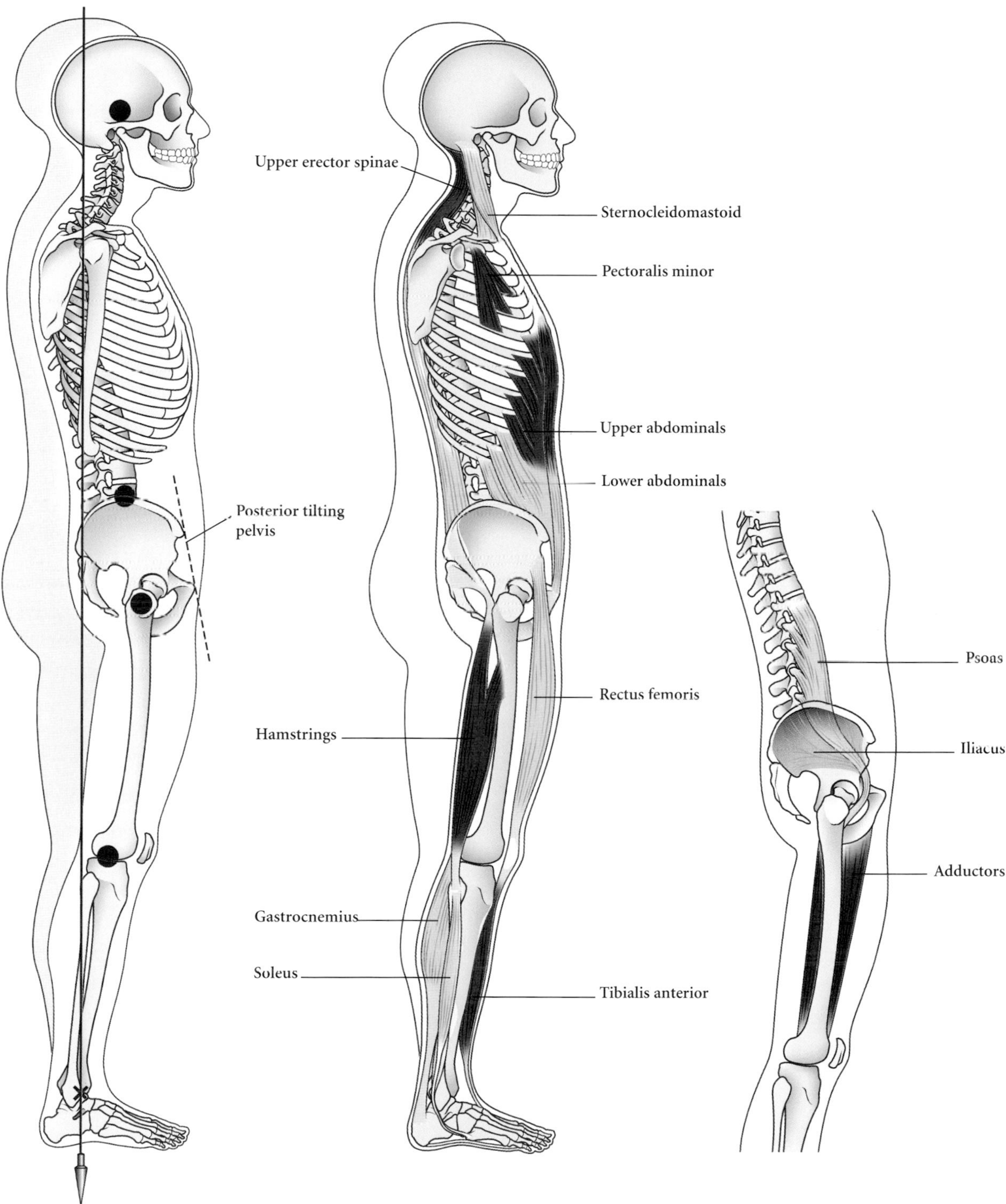

Fig. 6. Skeleton

Fig. 7. Superficial muscles

Fig. 8. Deep muscles

The muscles in the lower abdomen are lengthened and weak, but the upper abdomen and chest are usually short and tight. The upper trapezius is often tight also. The lower back muscles are short and usually strong, but if the sway-back is considerable then they become severely shortened and weak instead. The iliacus, psoas and rectus femoris are commonly lengthened, but may also be quite tense. The gluteus maximus is very often inhibited because it is held in a shortened position and so it becomes weak and dysfunctional. The adductor muscles are short and tight as a cause or consequence of the anterior shift of the pelvis.

Lordotic/kyphotic tendency

The postural tendency here shows excessive curvatures in all three main sections of the spine. Individual cases will not necessarily be the same as this, and some will have a greater curvature in just one or two sections and in various combinations. *(See figs. 9, 10 and 11.)*

Excessive lumbar lordosis

As well as the increased lordotic curvature of the spine, the pelvis tilts anteriorly and the hips are held in a slightly flexed position.

The lower back muscles are short and strong through overuse, and the hip flexors also become short as a cause or consequence of the slight hip flexion. The iliacus and psoas muscles are usually also tight in this situation. The abdominal muscles are weak and long, but sometimes the upper abdominals can be quite tight along with the upper chest muscles. The hamstrings are lengthened, but they usually remain quite strong.

Excessive thoracic kyphosis

The increased curvature also reduces the intercostal spaces which flattens the chest and can restrict breathing.

The erector spinae muscles become lengthened by the increased curve and also suffer overuse as they have to support the extra weight of the protracted head. Together this creates chronic tension in the muscles and fascia, which can become painful and further restricts movement. The middle and lower parts of the trapezius are usually overstretched and weak. Pectoralis major/minor and internal intercostals are also usually tight.

Excessive cervical lordosis

The neck extensor muscles are short and strong and the neck flexors become weak through underuse.

The common cause of the lordotic / kyphotic posture

These three excessive curvatures are very common and usually develop together due to a sedentary lifestyle. Sitting in a chair all day does not need the abdominal muscles to support the torso. Muscles are potentially very lazy; if they do not have to work then they will not bother to. So the abdominal muscles become weak, inefficient and slow to react.

Then, when standing, the weak rectus abdominis is unable to maintain the correct height of the pubis and it tilts down anteriorly. This pushes the lumbar spine into an increased lordosis.

In addition to this, the weakened abdominal muscles are less able to support the viscera and so the stomach bulges forward. The viscera is heavy, and this moves the body's centre of gravity forward so it is necessary to lean backwards from the waist to stay in balance. But this would leave the person leaning back so they have to push their head forward to see where they are going. This increases the kyphotic curve in the thoracic spine and the lordotic curve in the cervical spine.

Lordotic/kyphotic Posture

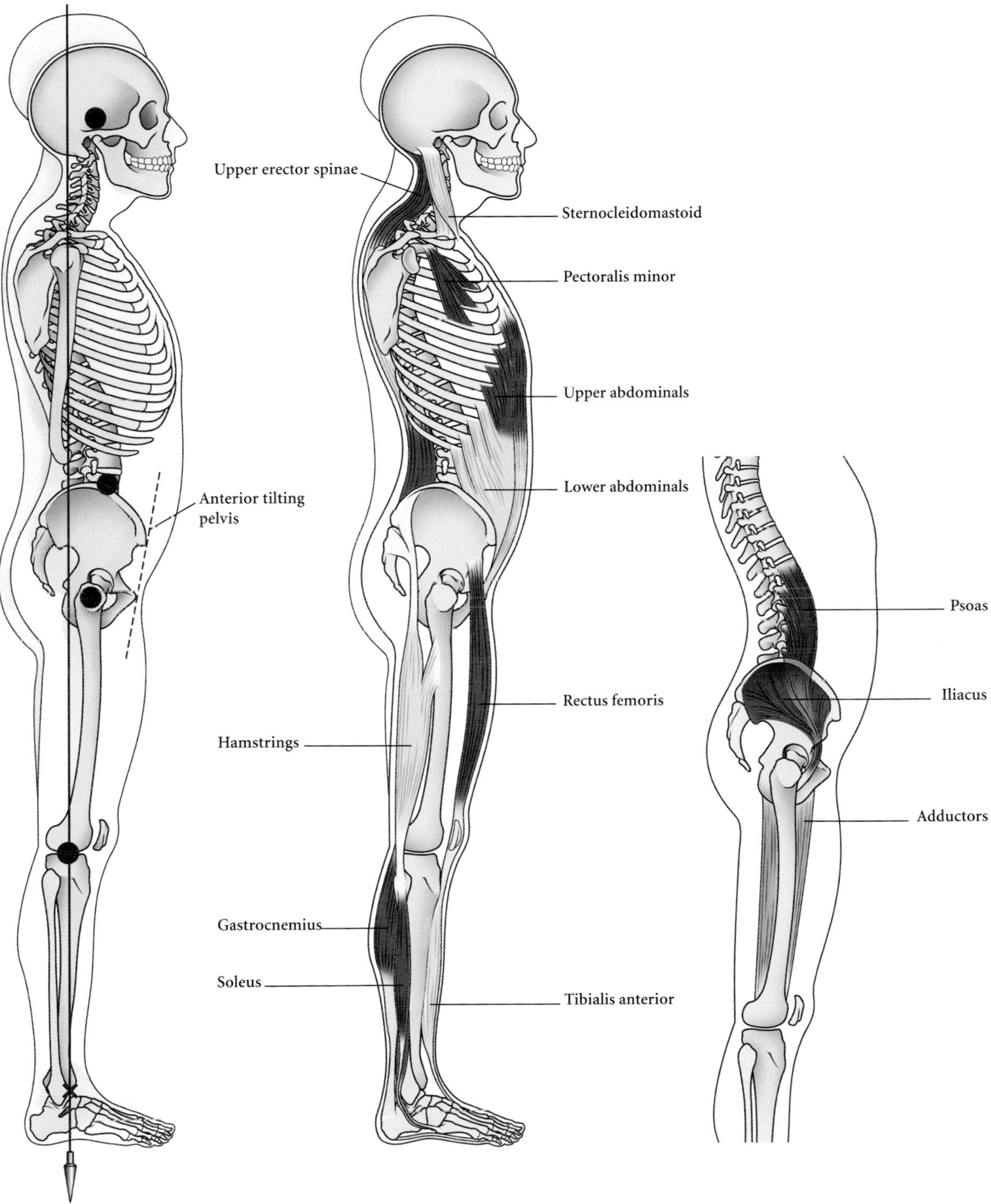

Fig. 9. Skeleton

Fig. 10. Superficial muscles

Fig. 11. Deep muscles

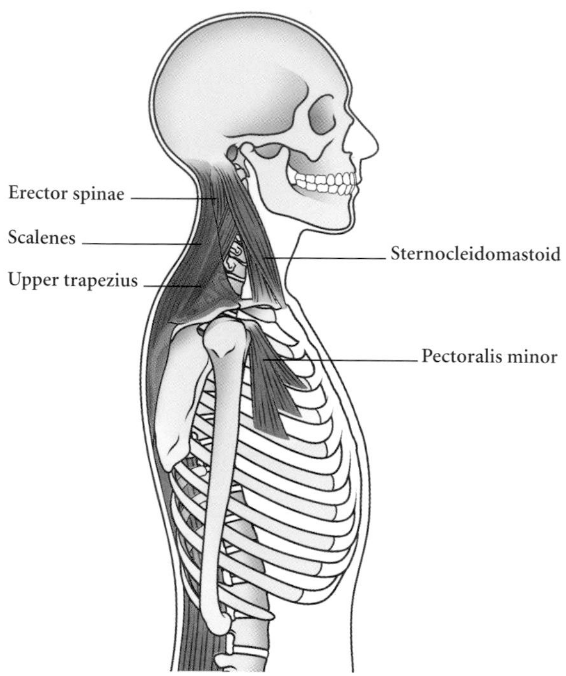

Fig. 12. Ideal neck and head posture

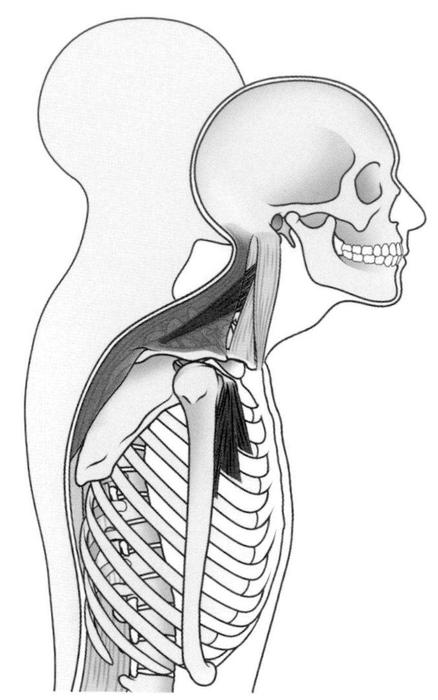

Fig. 13. Forward head posture

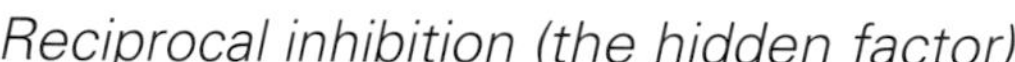

Reciprocal inhibition (the hidden factor)

As postural alignment deteriorates, some postural muscles have to work harder whilst others get underused. Those that work harder eventually become hypertonic and begin to reciprocally inhibit their opposing muscles, which are already being underused. So they become even weaker and the problem then rapidly starts to accelerate. This is why postural problems can build up without the client being aware of them until it reaches a critical level and then there is a sudden onset of pain.

Forward head posture

When sitting at a desk, many people adopt a very forward head position as they look at their computer screen. This position is much more extreme than the excessive cervical lordosis seen when standing and as many people spend so much time in this position it should be seen as another common postural tendency. *(See figs. 12 and 13.)*

Here all the posterior neck muscles get greatly overloaded by the weight of the head extending so far in front of the body and suffer overuse problems as a consequence. The anterior muscles are underused, so they become weak and can be easily strained.

Flat-back posture

The lumbar and thoracic spine are flattened and the pelvis has a posterior tilt. Knees are often locked in full or hyperextension, but sometimes there may be slight knee flexion instead. *(See figs. 14, 15 and 16.)*

The abdomen and chest muscles are all short and tight. The iliacus is long and weak, but the upper part of the psoas can be tight. The back muscles are lengthened but usually still quite strong. The hamstrings are short and tight,

Flat-back Posture

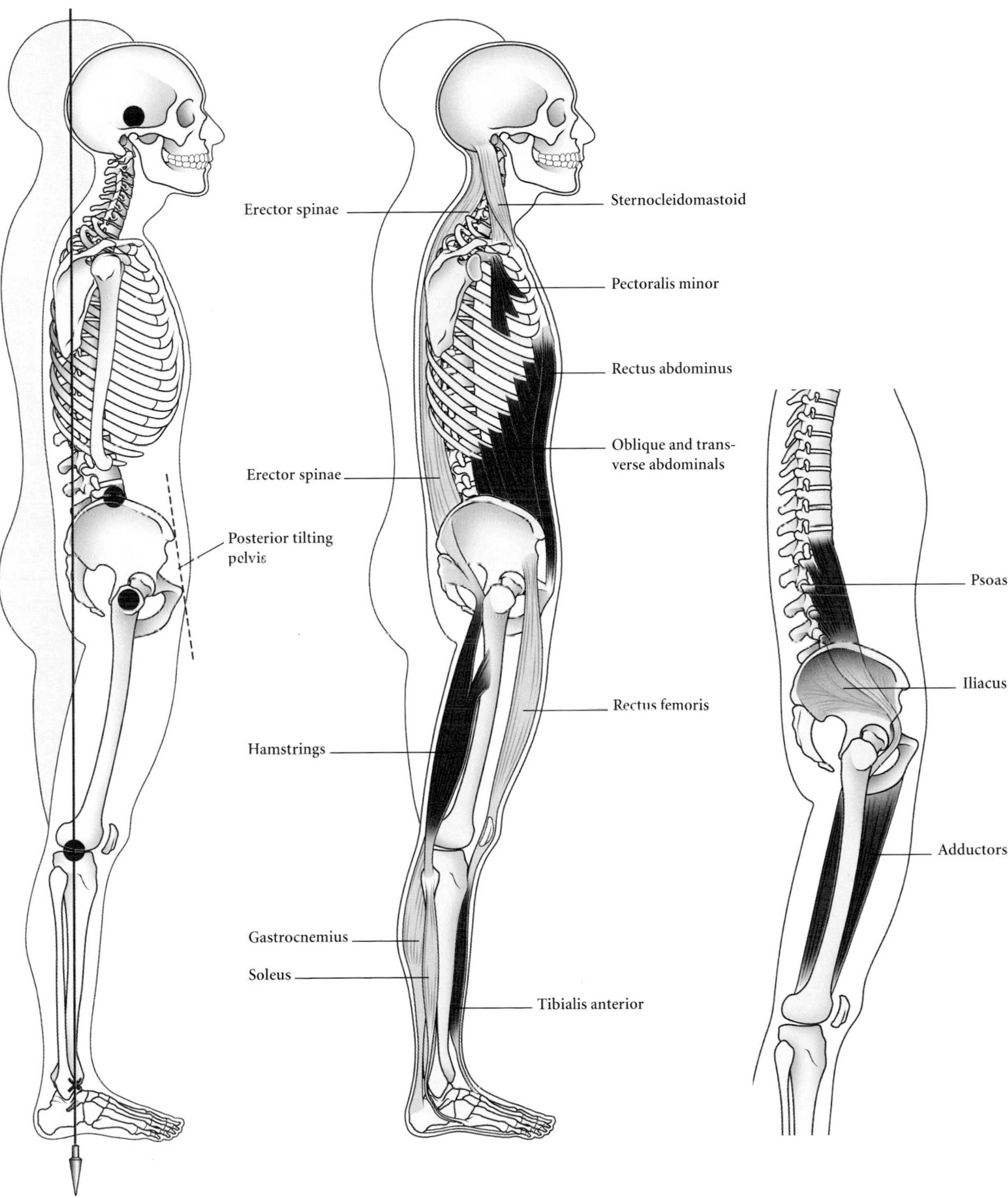

Fig. 14. Skeleton

Fig. 15. Superficial muscles

Fig. 16. Deep muscles

and the adductors are also short and tight, as a cause or consequence of the forward position of the pelvis.

Lateral deviations

Lateral deviation in spinal alignment can develop through poor postural habits, but this is often an inevitable consequence of life. We all have one dominant side (right- or left-handedness) and so will inevitably use our body asymmetrically. We naturally have a stronger side, and the muscles will develop strength and tension accordingly, especially if doing a hard manual job or powerful sport. We can cope with a degree of asymmetry, and these deviations often do not cause painful symptoms until later in life when it may be too late to correct. So even if they may seem to be natural and not causing any obvious symptoms, these lateral deviations can be seen as potential problems and treated accordingly. *(See figs. 17 and 18.)*

If there is a lateral deviation at the lumbar spine it can tilt the pelvis, with one iliac crest appearing higher than on the other side. Deviations higher up the spine will cause differences in the height of the shoulders.

Lower back, hip and adductor muscles on alternate sides of the body are short and strong. The corresponding muscles on the other side are long and weak. Alternate areas of corresponding muscle weakness and strength may continue all the way up the back.

Supination

The foot is inverted and body weight is carried through the outside of the foot. This is less common than excessive pronation but can lead to similar injury problems. (*See fig. 19 overleaf.*)

Pronation

The foot is everted and the knees are usually turned inwards with slight internal hip rotation. The peroneal muscles and toe extensors are short and tight. Tibialis posterior and toe flexors are long and weak. (*See fig. 20 overleaf.*)

Excessive foot pronation is extremely common in modern society, and the problem most probably begins when children are put into shoes at a very early age. Inside a shoe, the

Common shoulder misalignments	
Hunched shoulders	Short tight rhomboids; upper trapezius is also usually short and tight
Protracted shoulders (pointing forward)	Rhomboids, lower trapezius are long and weak Pectoralis minor very short and tight; major less so
Common lower limb misalignments	
Legs turned out	Outward hip rotators are short and tight Inward rotators are weak
Legs turned in	Inward rotators are short and tight Outward rotators are weak
Hyperextended knee	Quadriceps and soleus are short and tight Popliteus and lower hamstrings are long and weak The ankle is often slightly plantarflexed

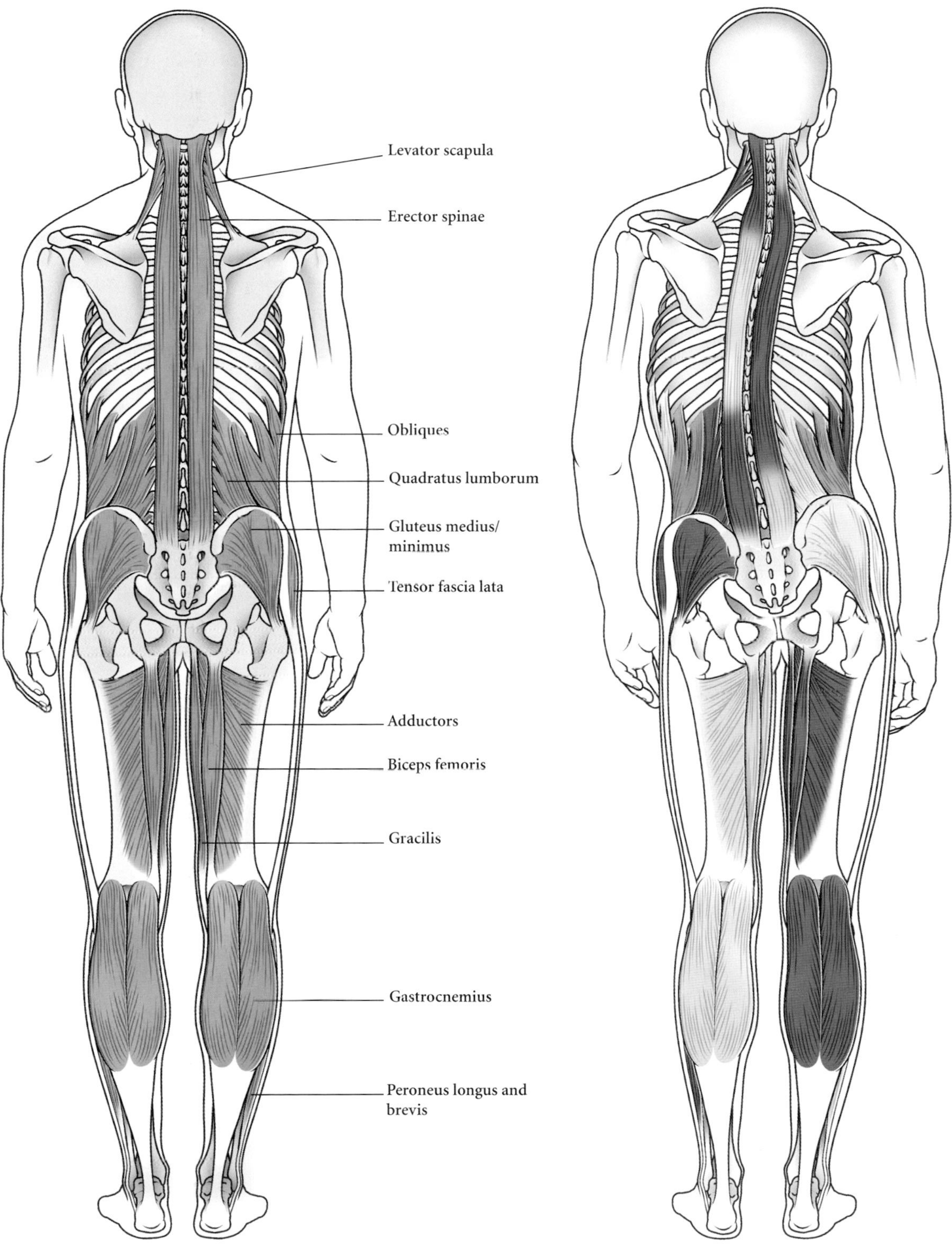

Fig. 17. Ideal posture

Fig. 18. Lateral deviations

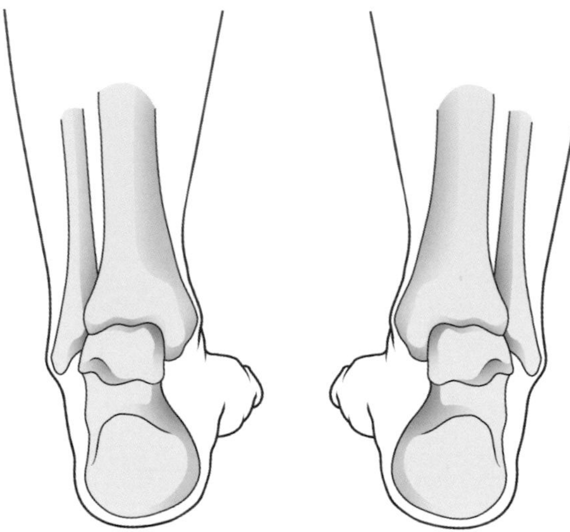

Fig. 19. Supination

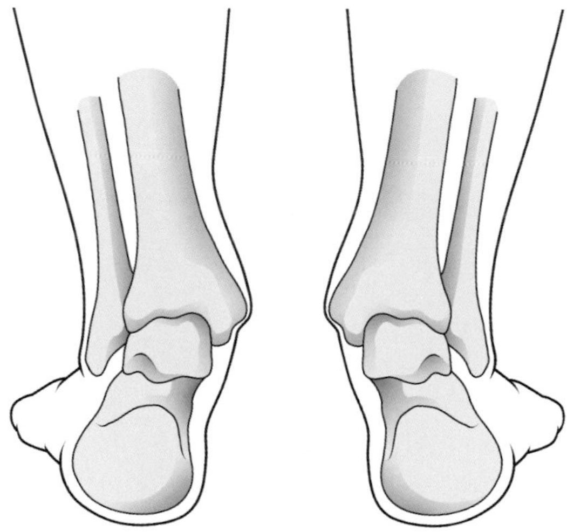

Fig. 20. Over-pronation

small muscles do not need to create the fine control movements that they do when walking barefoot, so they do not develop in the way they should. With poor muscle function, the joints in the foot get moved passively when walking or running so the stress is taken up by the ligaments and plantar fascia instead of the muscles. These structures get stretched, and eventually they permanently lengthen. The medial arch is the most significant structure to lengthen and flatten the arch which then usually causes over-pronation. *(See fig. 21.)*

In normal foot-plant during walking and running, we land more on the outside of the heel with the foot in a slightly supinated alignment. The weight is then carried through the lateral side of the foot during the mid-stride. In the final push-off phase, the foot pronates and the weight is spread inwards across the transverse arch so the weight is carried evenly through the toes.

With over-pronation, the heel-strike is still on the outside of the heel but the foot then pronates during the mid-stride, flattening the medial arch so it becomes less able to absorb shock. The foot then over-pronates in the push-off phase so all the weight goes through to the big toe.

Over-pronation causes the lower leg to inwardly rotate and this can lead to problems further up the body:

- Ankle pain due to the medial ligaments getting stretched and the lateral side of the joint being compressed.
- Deep posterior compartment syndrome or overuse strain because these muscles work harder to try to overcome the lack of foot and ankle control.
- Anterior compartment syndrome (tibialis anterior).

Loading Through the Foot

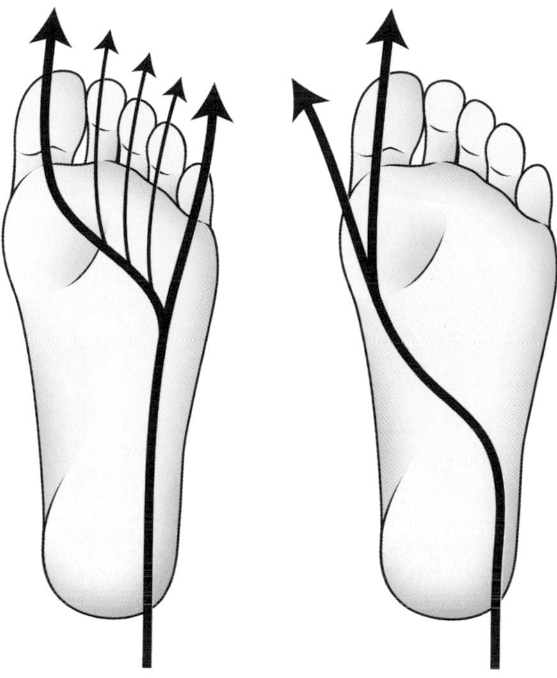

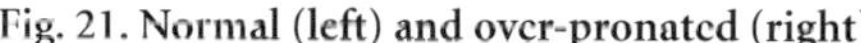

Fig. 21. Normal (left) and over-pronated (right)

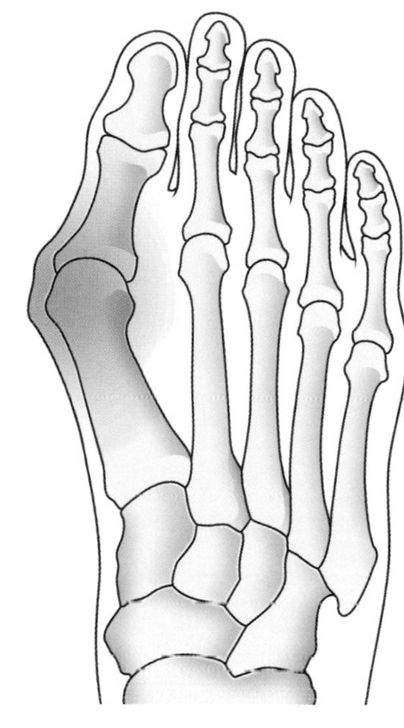

Fig. 22. Hallux valgus

- 'Shin splints': pain with fibrous adhesions along the medial tibial border.
- Uneven alignment at the knee joint leading to wear and damage to the menisci.
- Tension along the iliotibial band and into the tensor fascia lata (TFL). This commonly causes lateral knee pain but sometimes causes pain in the hip area as the TFL is affected.
- Pain in the outward rotators of the hip, particularly the piriformis as they overwork trying to correct the extra inward rotation of the leg.
- Morton's Neuroma: a nerve impingement between the toe joints causing a collapse of the transverse arch.

Although over-pronation can lead to many other musculoskeletal issues, it is surprising how often these do not actually cause painful symptoms. Many people with sedentary lifestyles do not put enough physical stress through the legs for it to cause them problems. When walking, the foot strikes the ground with a force about three times our body weight, but when running this goes up to between seven and nine times. So musculoskeletal problems caused by over-pronation only tend to become apparent in people who do high levels of these activities. A recreational runner who over-pronates may be perfectly comfortable when doing only 10 miles per week but may suffer badly if they increase this to train for a marathon.

Supination is far less common but means the person lands on the outside of the foot and carries their weight along this side to push off mostly from the small toe. This means they do not get any shock absorbance from the medial arch and there is a much heavier impact going up through the leg. This can lead to ankle, knee and hip joint issues as well as causing numerous soft tissue issues up the body.

Remedial therapists should try to find a way for the client to improve their own situation through some sort of corrective exercise and rehabilitation. But with biomechanical issues in the foot this is very difficult or impossible to achieve. People may stand for a few hours every day and take several thousand steps, which can all repeat the same negative movement pattern. Nobody living a normal life could devote enough time and attention to every footstep they make to enable them to change this. Usually the best solution is to have orthotic insoles, prescribed by a podiatrist, that will try to correct the alignment.

Hallux valgus

Over-pronation and excessive outward leg rotation often leads to hallux valgus as it forces the big toe into this position. (*See fig. 22.*)

Core Control

To maintain a good posture and move with strength and efficiency, it is essential that the central core of the body is stably controlled. Imagine trying to ride a bicycle that had a spring instead of a crossbar between the handlebars and seat. It would take a huge effort in the arms and shoulders to control the steering at the front and similar effort from the hips and legs to keep the back wheel in line. A similar thing happens if the central section of the torso is unstable, and all manner of overuse problems can occur in the upper and lower body as a consequence.

The trunk is made up of three sections: the thorax, abdomen and pelvis. The thorax (spine, ribcage and sternum) supports the shoulders and arms, and the pelvis (sacrum and ilium) supports the hips and legs. Between these two rigid skeletal structures is the abdomen, which is soft and flexible with only the lumbar spine giving it structural support. This central section needs to be able to control the position of the thorax relative to the pelvis to achieve stability.

The muscles supporting the lumbar spine are not strong enough alone to control the great forces involved in all trunk movements. To achieve the strength and stability we need, there is a set of core muscles (transverse and oblique abdominals along with the rectus abdominis) which wrap around the torso to form an abdominal wall. As well as supporting the viscera and assisting trunk movement, these muscles attach to the ribcage above and the pelvis below. When they contract, they make a strong connection between these two parts, which controls their position. (*See fig. 23.*)

This does not fully stabilise the trunk, however, as the soft abdominal section could still be compressed from above when carrying a heavy load or in high-impact activities. Within this tube-like structure, there needs to be some support from above and below to create an internal pressure which can resist a downward force. This is achieved by the diaphragm at the top and the strong pelvic floor muscles at the bottom. The fascia binds these muscles in with the abdominal wall to create a single enclosed compartment that works as a contained unit to control pressure.

We need good integrated functioning from all these muscles to control pressure and stabilise the trunk properly. But poor function is very common and is the reason behind a vast

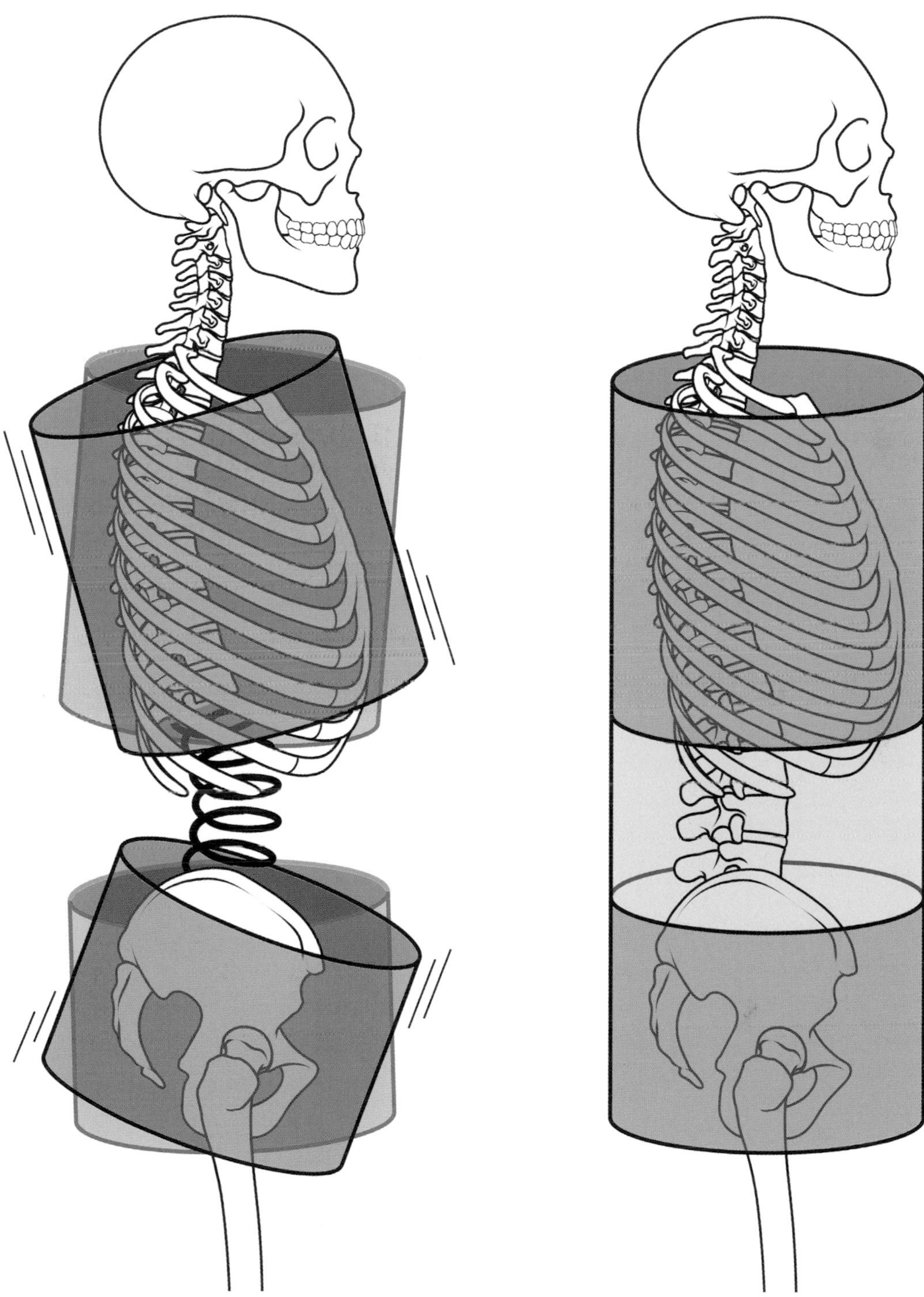

Fig. 23. Core control

number of musculoskeletal injuries. They work as *control* muscles rather than *strength* muscles, and good control requires good regular use rather than some strength exercises a few times a week. For people who have sedentary lifestyles, these muscles often do not get enough constant repetitive use to keep them as finely tuned as they should be. Long periods of sitting, which require very little activity from the abdominal and pelvic floor muscles, can make them weak and inefficient.

Poor core control can lead to a wide range of musculoskeletal problems because all the non-core muscles throughout the body are compromised and have to overwork to create some local stability. People often suffer injuries which they assume have been caused by a particular physical activity like running or swimming. But if this was true then all people who run or swim would get the same injuries, which they do not. The reason why some get injured when others do not often has to do with differences in their core control.

Considerable research has been done to try to understand the complex workings of the core control muscles, and there are many different exercise methods which aim to achieve good integrated function. There are established methods and techniques – such as the Alexander technique, the Feldenkrais method and Pilates – which all aim to do this. They may appear to be quite different in their approaches, but they are very similar in their results. Other disciplines like Yoga and Tai Chi are even more different in their underpinning concepts and philosophies, but when practised correctly they also help achieve the good core control we need.

2 Client Consultation

Telephone Contact

In private practice the first contact with the client is usually through a telephone conversation, and the therapist has to decide quickly if it is safe and correct to make the appointment. The client cannot be expected to self-diagnose their condition and know if soft tissue treatment is the right thing for it. Nor may they fully understand what the therapist can or cannot do.

The prospective client is usually quite willing and eager to describe their situation over the telephone, but it is not good for this to go on for too long and become a free consultation. It is necessary to get sufficient information to decide if it is reasonably certain that the client has a minor soft tissue problem that can be safely treated, or not. To do this over the telephone, it is better to lead the conversation by asking questions that have a simple yes or no type of answer rather than ones that allow a long descriptive reply.

If nothing at all is known about the client's needs, one could start by asking if they want a general massage or if they have a specific problem. If they have a specific problem, one must try to discover whether it may be an acute condition that would be contraindicated. If they have had a recent fall, accident or done any extreme exercise, enquire whether they have any acute symptoms (heat, redness and swelling). If they do then rest, ice, compression and elevation (RICE) (*see Appendix 2, p. 265*) procedures should be prescribed and/or they should seek medical attention. Even though a client may not be aware of any accident or overexertion, they may still have an acute condition and should be asked how severe their pain is and if they are able to stand, walk, lift, etc.

After forty-eight hours of RICE, acute symptoms should be gone if it is a minor acute injury and treatment can then begin with caution.

On Arrival

Assessment should begin as soon as the therapist greets the client. Observing the way they stand, move and sit in normal circumstances can be more revealing than how they do these when they know they are being observed in a clinical situation.

The general manner of the client – whether they seem comfortable and relaxed or anxious and nervous – can sometimes suggest possible non-musculoskeletal issues. Although it is not the role of the manual therapist to attempt to treat psycho-emotional issues, they can influence treatments and rehabilitation so they need to be considered.

Written Information

The client with musculoskeletal pain usually wants the problem taken away as quickly as possible without spending too much time answering personal questions that they may not think are relevant. To save time, it is helpful to have the client complete a basic record card that includes tick boxes which reveal whether they have any possible contraindications or cautions (*see Appendix 3*). The therapist then only has to ask further questions about any indicated conditions that may be relevant.

If the client is seeking treatment for a strained calf muscle, they may not feel inclined to tell the therapist that they also have a medical condition such as Irritable Bowel Syndrome. This may not have any significance in this particular injury, but if the client had a chronic lower-back problem it could be very relevant. If there are no obvious musculoskeletal causes to the client's condition, it may be necessary to ask further questions about their medical history.

They do not have to tell the therapist all their personal information, but the therapist should not treat a client who withholds information that they believe is necessary to determine the safety and efficacy of treatment.

Lifestyle Factors

It is not always necessary to spend too long discussing lifestyle factors in detail at the initial stage, but having basic information on their record card can be very helpful. More specific questions can then be asked about aspects of their life which seem most relevant to their problem.

Occupation

The body is very versatile and can carry out an infinite variety of tasks, but it does not like to do the same thing for eight-plus hours a day, five-plus days a week for many years. This means that occupational factors are always an important consideration. The physical stresses and the effects on posture from repetitive occupational situations are often easy to describe, but sometimes psychological stresses of the job may also be a part of the problem. So as well as finding out the active or sedentary nature of their work it can also be important to know the level of stress and job satisfaction they experience. It may indicate that deep relaxation massage could be a beneficial element in their treatment.

All occupational activities have a repetitive element, whether it is sitting for long hours behind a computer or doing a manual job. This means that some parts of the musculoskeletal system get constantly used whilst others do not, and this will cause imbalances to develop. Even though a client's injury may not appear to be directly related to their job, occupational factors must always be considered as a possible underlying factor.

A client's occupation may also be significant in how well they are able to recover from an injury. At worst, it may not allow them to stop doing the activity that caused the injury, or to rest the damaged tissues sufficiently. At best, it may be possible for them to get sufficient rest and do some sort of remedial exercise within their work situation. It is also an area where advice on postural health and well-being in the workplace can be very helpful too.

Sport and Leisure Activities

Most people who do a sport today are not trying to be great champions; instead they do it as part of a healthy lifestyle and therapists must see it in this context. Although they may want to improve their sports performance, this is not their only goal in life and the level of training and performance must balance with their other commitments.

Doing a sport or exercise is good, especially for those with sedentary occupations, but it is most important not to over-train and to recover fully between sessions. So it is necessary to find out how often they train, how hard and what methods they use to help them recover.

Family Circumstances

It can be relevant to know if the client has young children or other dependents that they care for because this may also be a source of physical stress, which could be significant.

Other Factors

Surgery

A client may not think that a surgical operation they had many years ago has any relevance to the current injury they now have, but it could. Scar tissue caused by surgery can run through the fascial layers and prevent them from moving freely, and this can affect function there and elsewhere.

Surgery can sometimes make permanent alterations to the position of bone or soft tissue structures. This can change the range of movement and function in that area leading to local chronic problems. It may also lead to overuse injuries elsewhere, as the client has to develop compensatory movement patterns.

Following surgery, people often develop dysfunctional holding patterns around the area to protect it, for example protracting the shoulders to close in on the chest following heart surgery. This is quite a normal instinct but it can develop into a more permanent postural habit, which leads to other musculoskeletal problems later on.

Previous accidents and injuries

Incomplete recovery from past incidents can be a contributing factor to current problems, and this has to be considered. The general history of injuries can also sometimes reveal a bigger picture of how the client treats their body. For example, someone with a history of overuse muscular injuries may be pushing themselves too hard for too long in their job and/or sport. In some rare cases, the history of past injuries may indicate the possibility of a more serious medical condition like multiple sclerosis.

History of serious or current/recent illness

This can be a contributing factor in musculoskeletal pain and may also affect recovery.

Specific Questions about a Client's Current Condition

- **What is the main site of pain and are there any secondary sites?**
  Clients often tend to talk only about their main area of discomfort, and it may be necessary to ask specifically if they have problems in any other parts to get a fuller understanding of the situation.

- **How did the injury occur?**
  There may be an obvious activity that caused the injury, which can make it much easier to identify the problem. A normal healthy person will not suddenly develop pain for no reason, so if they are not aware of a particular activity or incident then the cause needs to be looked for in their posture and lifestyle.

- **How long have they had the problem and has it occurred before?**
  Its history and progression over time needs to be considered. This could identify possible causes or contributing factors when viewed alongside other lifestyle factors.

- **What was the onset of the injury?**
  If it came on suddenly it suggests an acute condition, but a gradual onset would suggest a chronic overuse problem.

- **How does the client describe their pain?**
  See table.

- **What is the severity of the pain?**
  The client can rate their level of pain on a numerical scale; this can be used again later to monitor progress.

- **What activities cause pain or cannot be done?**

Description of pain	Possible meaning
Sharp (and localised)	Acute inflammation
Pain when resting the area	Acute inflammation
Aching	Chronic soft tissue
Dull, deep or boring pain	Bone issue
Crawling or burning sensation	Autonomic nerve issue
Diffused or lancing pain	Non-muscular (neural)
Radiating	Neural (entrapment)
Throbbing sensation	Vascular issue
Stinging sensation	Dermal issue

As well as indicating what tissues may be damaged, this information can be used later to monitor progress.

- **Are there activities that make the problem worse?**
  If movement increases their symptoms, this tends to suggest a muscular injury and usually highlights the tissues involved.

- **Are there any activities that relieve their symptoms?**
  If their symptoms are relieved with movement, that suggests that the soft tissues are chronically tight. But if they get relief when they rest, it is more likely to be a soft tissue strain or joint inflammation. Similarly, if they feel relief when they apply heat to the area, that suggests the tissues may be chronically tight. But if cold feels better, it is more likely to be acutely inflamed.

- **Have they had previous treatment for this problem and if so, how successful was it?**
  Information about an existing medical diagnosis – as well as what treatment has, or has not, worked in the past – can be extremely helpful. But this does depend on the client's clear understanding of the situation, and so this information should be considered but not necessarily relied upon.

- **What are the client's expectations?**
  This can give both therapist and client a positive goal to aim for.

Other Associated Factors

Symptom	Possible cause
Headaches	Caution if no obvious musculoskeletal factors are present
Numbness, pins and needles sensation	Neural or vascular issue
Palpitation	Cardiovascular issue
Dizziness	Major caution 'Red Flag'
Pain when sneezing or coughing	Spinal injury
Changes in bowel or urinary function	Major caution 'Red Flag'

Treatment Notes

Clear and accurate notes need to be kept for every treatment carried out. These should be made within 24 hours and be written in ink, initialled, dated and a line drawn underneath.

Notes should contain:

- Subjective and objective observations based on assessment.
- A treatment plan.
- Advice given.
- Progress and development in a course of treatment.

Record Keeping

Client's records should be kept for a minimum of seven years, or up to the age of 21 for children. They should be kept in a safe and secure place which can only be accessed by those directly involved in the client's care in that clinic.

Professional Care

Client's Consent

For the safety and protection of both the therapist and the client, it is essential to have the client's consent for all aspects of the treatment.

Before starting any hands-on treatment, the therapist should first explain what area(s) of the body they intend to treat, and how and why. Treatment for a back injury will almost always include the gluteal area and often the adductor muscles too, but the client may not know or expect this. So before working on these other areas the reason for doing so must be explained to gain the client's consent. The same should also be done before applying advanced remedial techniques that involve moving or stretching the client.

Removal of Clothing

The therapist should tell the client what clothing they should remove. If they seem unwilling to remove any article of clothing the therapist cannot insist that they do, and should treat them through their clothing as best as possible if necessary. If a female client is wearing a bra during back treatment, the therapist must ask permission before undoing the strap at the back and must re-fasten it afterwards (or work around it if consent is not given). The same should also be done before moving any other part of a client's clothing.

Covering

The client should always remain covered apart from the area being treated and therapists must practice a good procedure for doing this especially when moving the client into different positions. Not only does this keep the tissues warm, but more importantly it gives the client a sense of comfort and security that enables them to relax better.

In the past, it was quite normal practice to pull down the waistband of a client's underwear to expose the whole buttock area when treating the muscles there. But this is not always acceptable to the client, so it is now considered more correct to not uncover the client below the top of the buttock crease. Between here and the top of the leg, the therapist can work through the towel and/or clothing.

When treating the groin area on clients of either sex it is important to make sure there is an adequate amount of covering between their legs, especially if the hip is going to be adducted or flexed. Occasionally with some men it may be necessary to ask them to support their genitals with their own hand to prevent any accidental contact.

In remedial massage there is no clinical reason to treat breast tissue, so on female clients this area should never need to be uncovered (unless treating mastectomy scars or similar). When treating the lower intercostal area and serratus anterior, a female client can use her hand to hold her breast out of the therapist's way if required. When necessary, and with the client's consent, treatment can be given along the sternal area between the breasts by working through a towel.

Remedial therapists sometimes need to use parts of their body to support the client in different positions, so they should be suitably dressed with long trousers and short-sleeved tops that avoid skin to skin contact with the client. Place a towel in between the two if necessary.

When applying remedial techniques that involve moving and stretching the client, keeping them properly covered with towels is not always easy and adds to the task. If a client arrives wearing loose casual clothing it can be better if they get dressed first and these techniques can then be applied without the need to use any covering.

Pain

Deep techniques are often an essential part of treatment and they can cause considerable pain, but the client may not realise or expect this. So when deeper techniques are applied for the first time, the client should be warned and asked to say if it becomes too painful. And this should be done again whenever applying the very deepest pressure.

Occasionally a client may not say anything and allow the therapist to cause them an unacceptable amount of pain because they feel they have to be brave. This is not ideal because it will be hard for them to relax in this situation, so the techniques may not be as effective. But worse still, this could be a sign that it is causing a trauma. A client's facial expression or a clenched fist does not necessarily indicate that the level of pain is intolerable but it does mean that the therapist needs to check that it is still acceptable.

Treating Children

There is no minimum age limit for soft tissue treatment, but special precautions are necessary with children up to the age of 16.

- **Consent:** It is important to be sure the child wants to have the treatment and is not being forced into it by a parent or anyone else. Treatment should not be carried out if the child is not freely consenting to it.
- **Chaperone:** The therapist should never be alone in the clinical environment with a young client. Ideally, the chaperone should be the parent or guardian but if this is not possible it must be a responsible adult and not the child's friend.
- **Written consent:** If the chaperone is not the parent or guardian, written consent for the treatment must be obtained from them first.

Disclosure of Information

The therapist must get the consent of the client before referring them to another healthcare professional. This is also necessary before discussing their case with anyone else, or responding to a request for information from anyone else.

A Therapist's Reputation Is Worth Everything!

A therapist does not have to treat a client if they feel it may be in any way unsafe to do so, even if the client insists that they want to have the treatment. It is better to lose a client than lose your reputation as a good therapist.

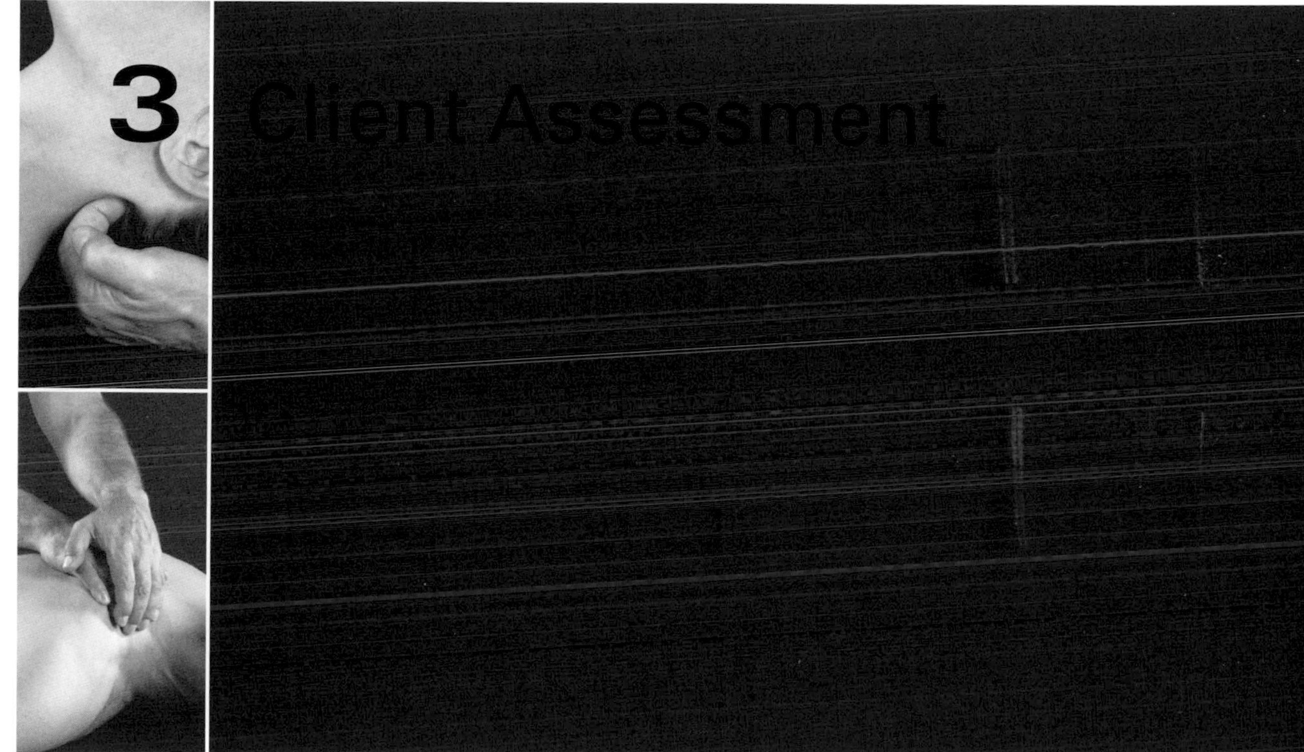

3 Client Assessment

Postural Assessment

Assessing a client's posture to identify any misalignments is essential. To get them to take up their normal posture, they should take a few steps walking on the spot first and stop in a position that feels normal and comfortable to them. As a visual guide, therapists sometimes use a suspended plumb line to see a centre line up through the body. In the side view, the bottom of the plumb line should cross just in front of the lateral malleolus, and alignment is assessed up the body from this. In the front and back views, the plumb line should be halfway between the two medial malleoli at the ankles.

A simple way to demonstrate a client's postural balance is for the therapist to stand on a chair behind them and push straight down on their shoulders. If their alignment is poor they will immediately collapse down, but with a well-balanced posture they can easily resist a considerable force.

First look at the whole body and see what general overall tendencies appear most obvious. Then look at each area in more detail to see what is happening there. It is important to see the body as a dynamic structure and identify where stronger more developed muscles are pulling the structure one way and other weaker less-developed muscles are allowing this to happen. Also visualise where the fascial network may be tight and twisted as it moulds itself to a postural misalignment. For manual therapists, a postural assessment need not be a purely visual exercise. Therapists should also palpate the boney prominences to help identify structural alignment, and feel the soft tissues to better assess postural tone.

By assessing the alignment of the body in terms of the soft tissues it is possible to determine which areas need to be stretched and released and those that should be strengthened and toned.

Side View

Compare the client's postural alignment with the 'ideal' posture to identify any of the common adverse tendencies. *(See fig. 24.)*

Pelvic alignment

Anatomically, the angle of the pelvis is measured from two points, the anterior superior iliac spine (ASIS) and the pubis, and in the ideal alignment they should be in a perpendicular line. If the ASIS is in front of the pubis the pelvis is described as being anteriorly tilted; if it is behind it is posteriorly tilted. *(See fig. 25 and photo 1 overleaf.)*

But the pubis is not a good bony prominence to observe and palpate in the clinical situation so instead it is safer to use the anterior and posterior superior iliac spines (ASIS and PSIS) to do this. But in the ideal neutral alignment of the pelvis, these two points are not exactly on the same level. On a male the ASIS should be 8–10 degrees lower than the PSIS. In females, due to a larger ilium, it is 10–12 degrees lower. If the ASIS is higher than this it is described as a posterior tilt and lower would be an anterior tilt.

Posterior Views

Observe the head and neck in terms of its perpendicular alignment and the angles made with the shoulders. Palpating the top of the shoulders helps identify any discrepancy in their level.

Observe the alignment of the spine along the

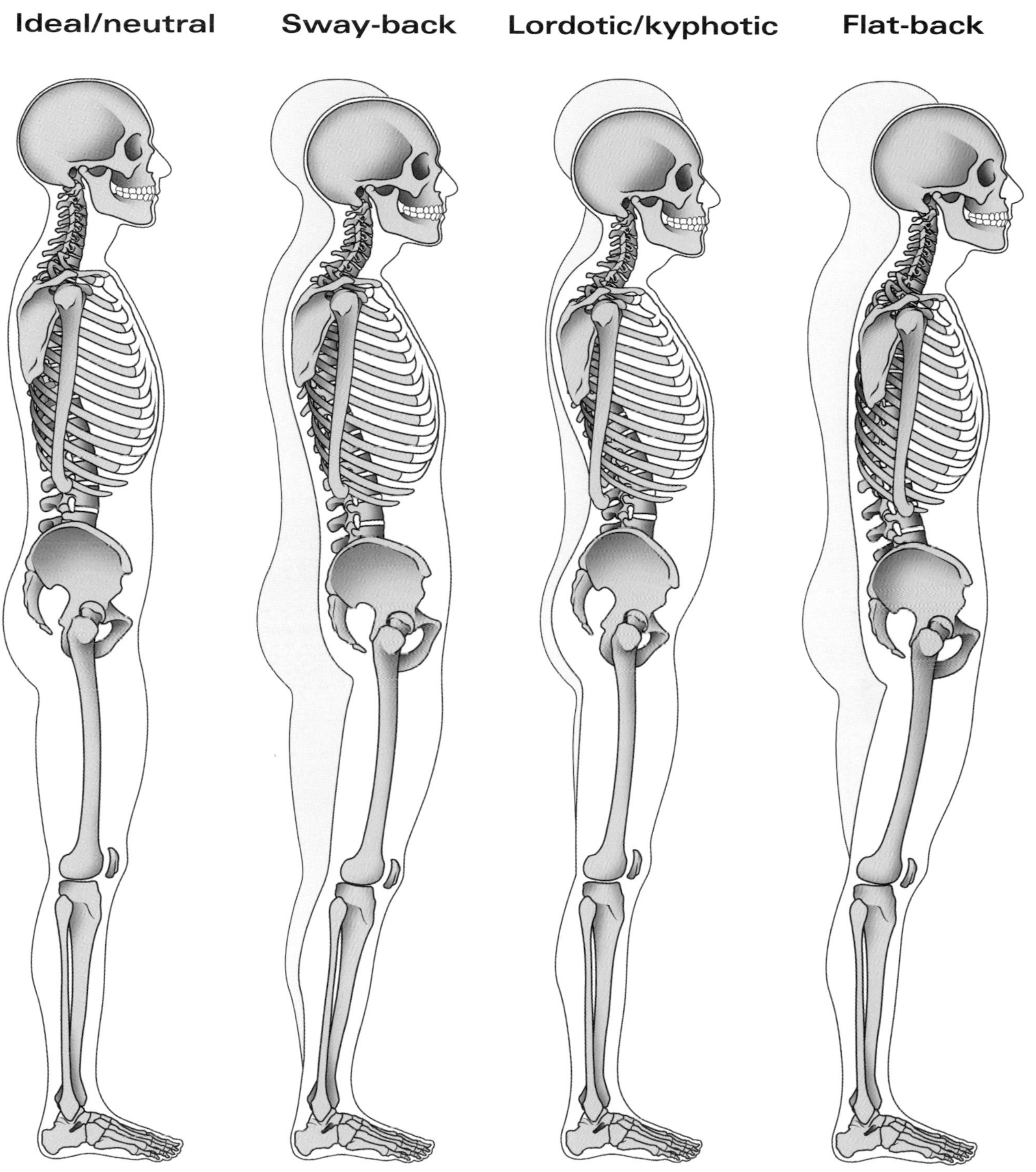

Fig. 24. Four common postural tendencies

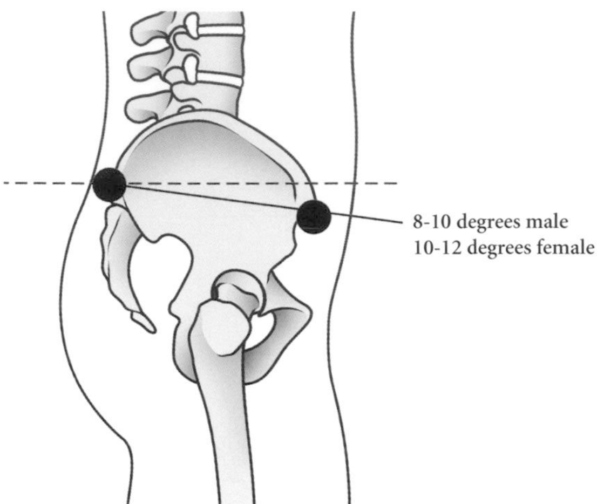

Fig. 25. Pelvic neutral

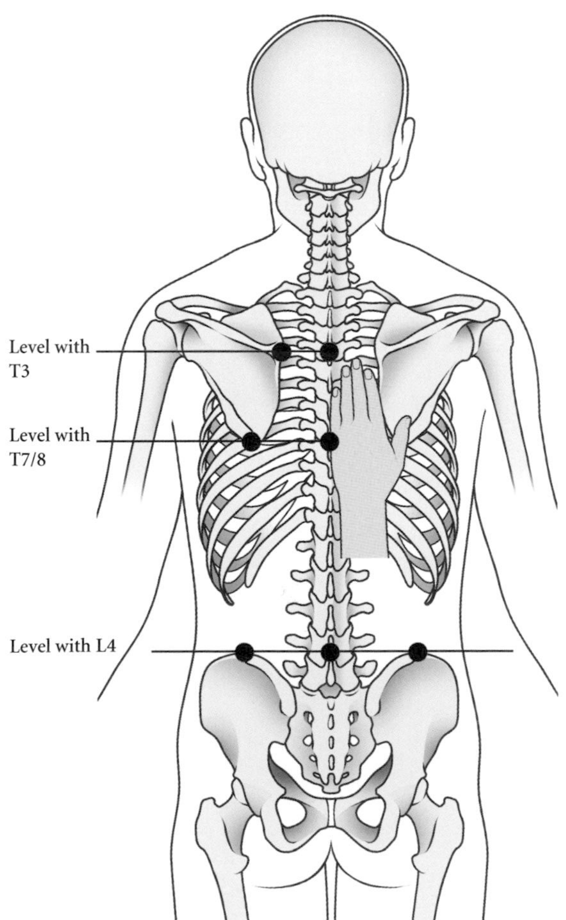

Fig. 26. Scapula and pelvic alignment

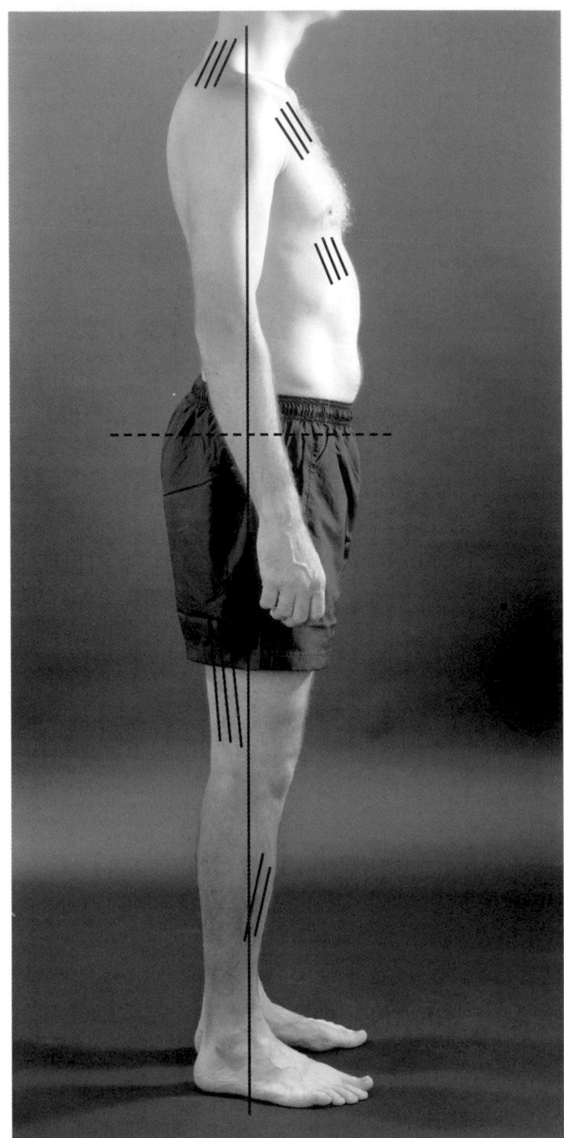

Photo 1. An example of a sway-back posture: hyperextended knees with tight tibialis anterior. Pelvis is posteriorly tilted (less than 8 degrees) and shifted forward of the midline. Lumbar spine leans back and the lower abdominal muscles are weak. Upper abdominal and upper chest muscles are tight, pulling the upper thoracic spine forward. Upper trapezius is tight, holding the neck upright.

In this and the following examples, it suggests the tight muscles are pulling on the body to cause or try to correct adverse alignments. But it can equally be the case that muscles become short and tight as they adjust to adverse alignment. Some muscle issues may be the cause of the problem and others can be the effect of it.

thoracic and lumbar sections. The indentations at the sides of the waist and the space between the body and the arms can help identify lateral deviations and rotations in the torso.

As well as observing the curvatures along the whole spine, the alignment of the individual vertebrae should also be looked at. If a vertebra is locked into a slightly rotated position, the spinous process will appear out of line with the others. And if two vertebrae are locked together this can appear as a flattened section along the curve. If these irregularities are the direct source of a client's pain, they should be referred to an orthopaedic specialist as spinal manipulation may be required to correct this. However, some abnormalities may be natural to the client, and if they are not causing any obvious symptoms they should only be noted for further consideration later if necessary.

Scapula alignment

It can be quite clearly seen when the shoulders are not at the same height, but it is necessary to determine if one is higher than it should be or if the other is lower than it should be. In the ideal posture, the medial border of the scapula should be parallel to the spine and spaced about four fingers' width from it. The spine of the scapula should be level with the third thoracic spinous process and the inferior angle with the seventh or eighth. It is better to assess this with the client seated because this will eliminate any postural issues from the lower body. *(See fig. 26.)*

Pelvic alignment

To judge the lateral alignment of the pelvis, therapists should observe and palpate the iliac crests on either side of the body. The high point on the outside of the crests should align with the fourth lumbar vertebra. *(See fig. 26.)*

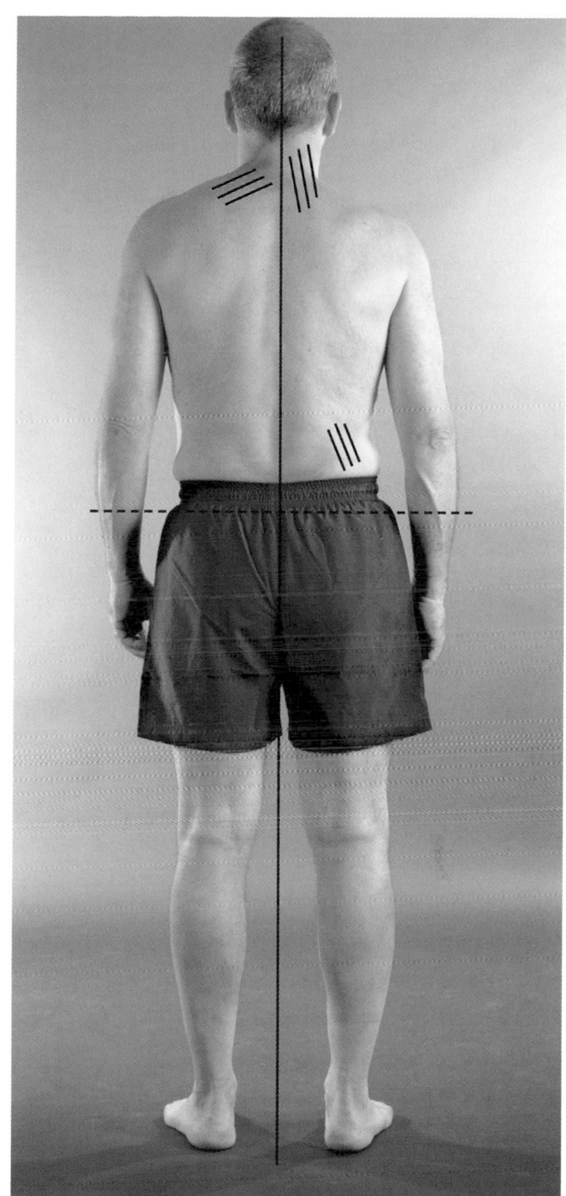

Photo 2. Example of lateral deviations (posterior view): body-weight is carried mainly through the left leg and right leg is slightly forward. Right hip is higher and forward of the left hip. Spine is fairly straight but shifting to the left of the midline. Right quadratus lumborum and obliques are short and tight, trying to pull the spine back to the midline. The neck is tilting to the right to compensate for the left shift of the torso with tightness in the right levator scapula and left upper trapezius. Right hand is resting in front of the leg and the right shoulder girdle is protracted and from the back appears to be lower. This reveals a torso rotation to the left.

Anterior View

Observe the alignment of the neck and shoulders as well as the position of the head. The ribcage should be symmetrical on both sides with the costal borders below the sternum making a 45-degree angle with the centreline of the body.

Shoulder girdle alignment

In the ideal alignment of the shoulder girdle, the clavicle should lay flat against the ribs and not be prominent, and the shoulder joint should be pointing out laterally from the body and not be tilting forward. Ideally, the arms should hang relaxed down the sides of the body with the palms resting along the outside of the thigh. But with the protracted shoulders, the arms are usually inwardly rotated and hang forward away from the body.

Hips

Compare the level of the pelvis from the front of the body in the same way as from behind, because it can appear different. Observe the general alignment of the legs in terms of their degree of rotation. Compare the alignment and degree of hip rotation through the position of the greater trochanters.

Knees

Clients may stand with their knees slightly hyperextended or the other way, slightly flexed. Particular attention should also be paid to the muscle bulk in the lower quadriceps because an imbalance of strength across this group can affect the tracking of the patella between the condyles and be a cause of knee pain.

The knees may be poorly aligned for structural reasons such as 'bow legs' or 'knocked knees'. This can put uneven pressure on the condyles and lead to arthritic problems in later life. But as this is due to the shape of the bone structure there is little that can be done to help using soft tissue techniques.

Ankle

The levels of the malleoli and alignment of the ankle joint need to be assessed to identify possible pronation/supination issues. *(See photo 3.)*

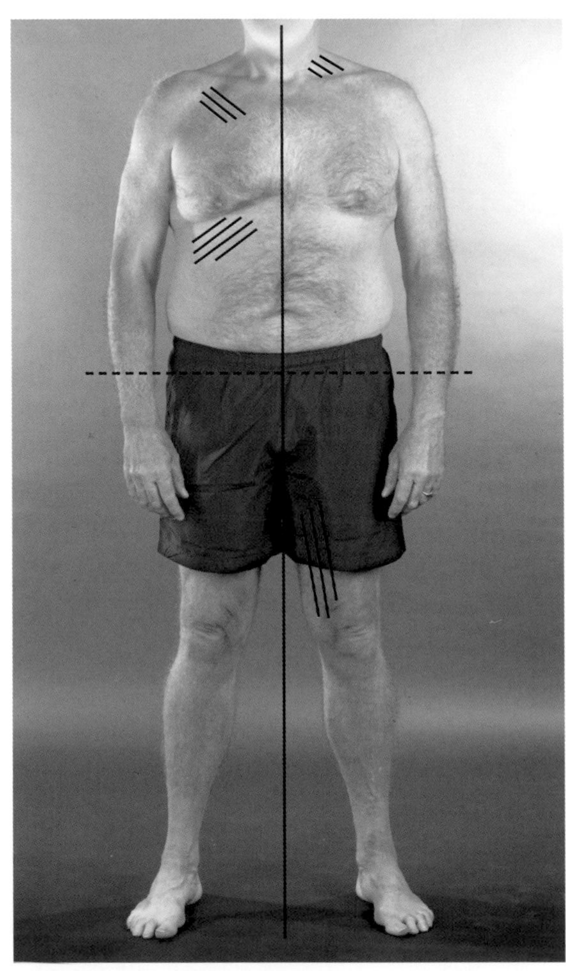

Photo 3. Example of lateral deviations (anterior view): very wide stance with body-weight carried mainly through the left leg. Pelvis is shifted to the left of the midline with tight adductors on the left leg. Right hip is slightly higher than the left. Lumbar spine tilts significantly to the left. Right upper obliques and chest muscles are short and tight, curling the thoracic spine back towards the midline. Left upper trapezius is tight, straightening the alignment of the neck.

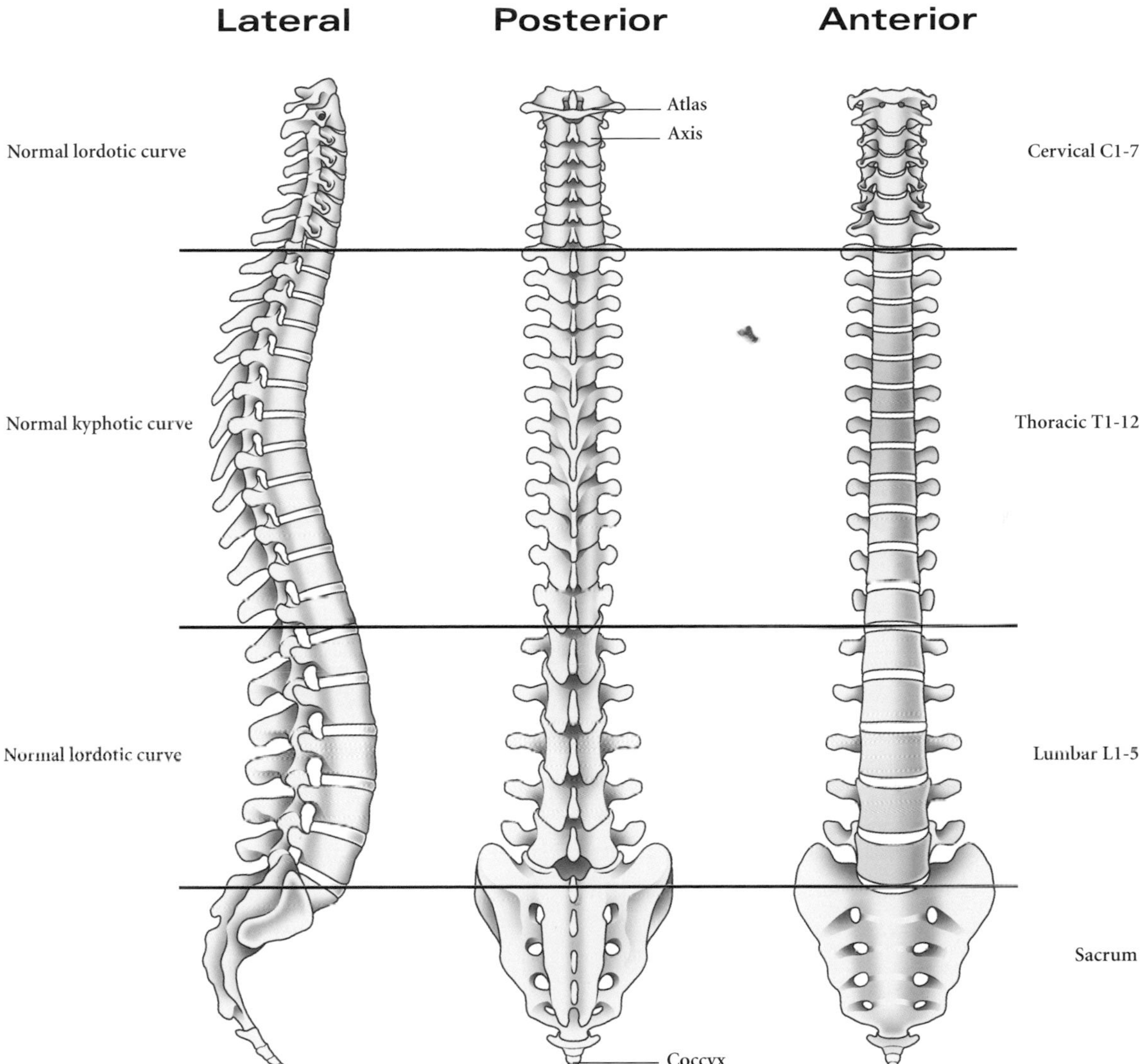

Fig. 27. The spine

The Spine

As the central structure of the skeleton, the spine needs special consideration. *(See fig. 27.)*

People are born with thirty-three vertebrae, but the five sacral bones fuse together during puberty and the four coccyx bones do the same, so as adults we have twenty-six. Between each vertebra is a fibrocartilage disc which absorbs shock and maintains the space between the bones. The transverse processes at the sides of the bones form facet joints with the adjacent vertebra. These allow a limited range of flexion/extension, rotation and side-bending at each intervertebral joint.

The spine can be divided into five sections, each of which has its own curved shape. Together they give the spine its 'S' shape, which

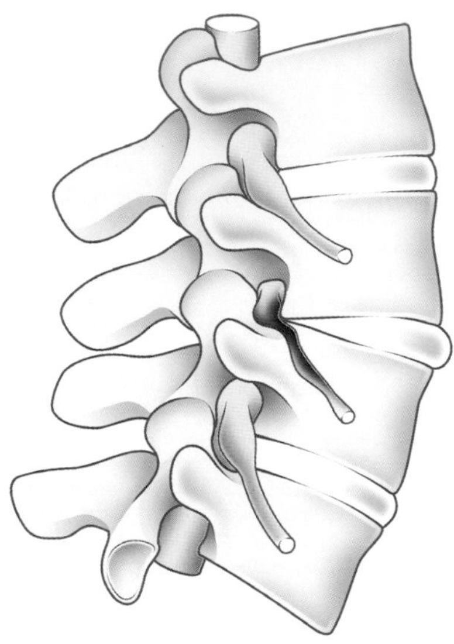

Fig. 28. Nerve impingement

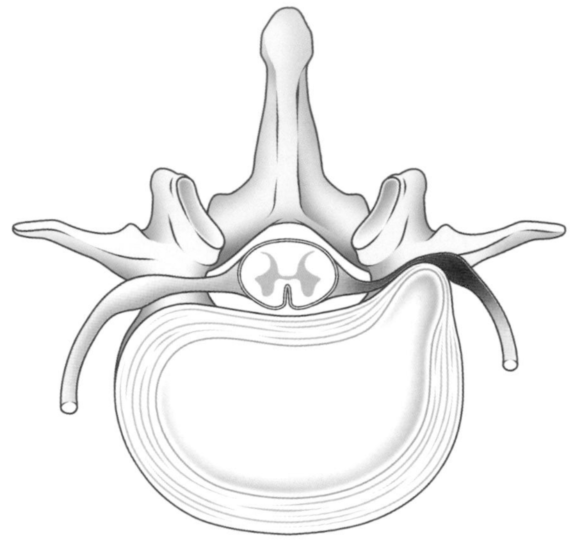

Fig. 29. Prolapsed disc

acts like a spring that can absorb downward forces. The curves are created by the shape of the vertebrae which are slightly wedge-shaped. When the spine is correctly aligned, the spaces between the vertebrae are all parallel and there is an even pressure spread across the surfaces of the fibrocartilage discs between them.

If the curvature in a section of the spine increases, it is the gap between the vertebrae that changes and the disc that gets affected. It gets compressed at one side, and this can cause excessive wear and damage to that part of the disc.

Peripheral Nerve Impingement

The peripheral nerves emerge from the spinal cord through the spaces between the vertebrae, and if this closes they can become pinched and trapped. This can lead to neural symptoms being felt further along the nerve's pathway down the limb. This can occur much more acutely if there is a sudden forced loading when carrying a heavy weight, doing high-impact activities or in traumatic accidents. *(See fig. 28.)*

Prolapsed Disc

The intervertebral discs have a soft, shock-absorbing, gel-like centre and a thick, firm outer rim. The outer part can get damaged through uneven wear or a sudden compression when the joint is misaligned. This damage makes it less able to contain the soft inner part and a bulge can develop on the outside of the disc. This bulge can press on a spinal nerve and cause extreme neural symptoms with severe pain and dysfunction. *(See fig. 29.)*

In chronic conditions which develop over time, muscular pain is usually the first sign of trouble and hopefully clients seek treatment long before it becomes a more serious neural problem. Massage and soft tissue techniques may be an effective way of alleviating the early symptoms, but without an improvement in the postural alignment of their spine they will inevitably return and worsen.

There is a danger that regular massage treatment may keep the painful symptoms away whilst a more serious disc compression is allowed to develop. Treatment alone is never the answer to this type of problem, and postural advice and remedial exercises are absolutely vital.

Although each section of the spine can be looked at separately, the relationship between them must not be ignored. Issues in one section are often compensated for in the adjacent section. Overuse problems which cause pain in one area may be caused by restrictions in another part which may not be a source of any pain.

Cervical Spine

This has a natural lordotic curve and is made up of seven vertebrae, but the atlas and axis bones at the top are distinctly different in shape as they form a pivot joint which allows the skull to rotate.

Excessive lordosis is a common postural tendency in the neck as people develop a forward, protracted head position. This closes the gap at the back of the joints, compressing the discs, and can lead to neural symptoms along the shoulder and arm. The symptoms usually begin with muscular pain in the back of the neck as these muscles suffer from overuse by supporting the extra weight of the protracted head. But at this early stage deep pressure applied between the vertebrae can cause sharp pain and show the early signs of disc damage. This is a good way of demonstrating to the client that their minor neck pain is the warning sign for a potentially more serious problem. They should start taking action to improve postural issues before it progresses further.

Thoracic Spine

The twelve thoracic vertebrae each have a pair of ribs attached and these all connect together at the sternum in the front of the body (apart from the two pairs of floating ribs). As an integral part of this cage, which protects the vital organs, it has a very limited range of movement.

Injury to the vertebral/costal joints can cause painful symptoms when breathing and coughing, and if the spinal nerves are involved then symptoms may even affect the organs. Injury to these joints can sometimes be caused by severe coughing or sneezing, especially if they are already compromised through adverse postural tendencies.

Excessive kyphosis is a common postural tendency as this spinal section often has to counterbalance an excessive cervical lordosis. The spinal muscles here lengthen as the curvature increases and they have to work harder to support the extra weight of the protracted head. And with limited movement in this section, chronic tension can easily develop here and cause quite severe muscle pain. Fascial tension across the lower chest and upper abdomen area is also usually involved in this kyphotic position.

Lumbar Spine

Although this section has more mobility than the thoracic spine, it is still fairly limited in range due to the size of the bones and their need to support such a heavy load.

Excessive lumbar lordosis is a very common problem here. This is usually because of poor tone in the abdominal muscles, which allows the pelvis to drop down at the front (anterior tilt). Through the sacroiliac joint, this pushes

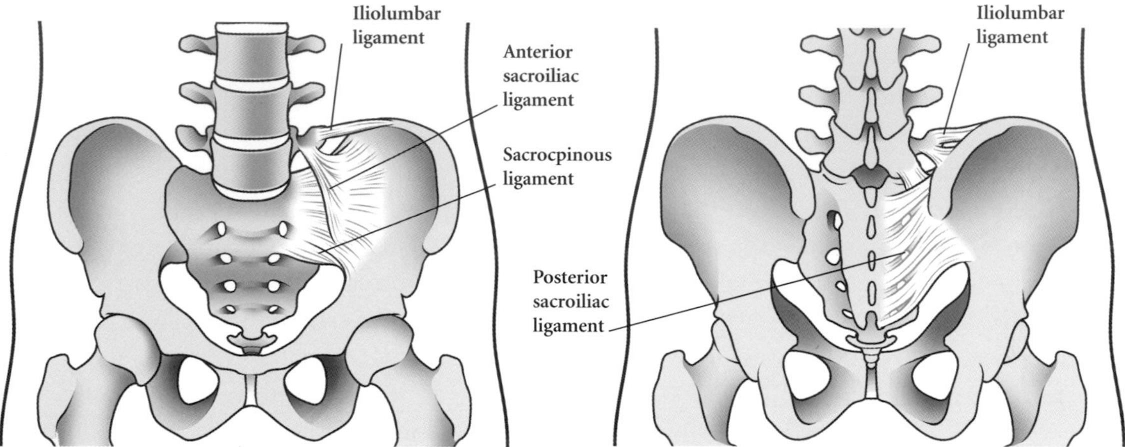

Fig. 30. Sacroiliac ligaments anterior

Fig. 31. Sacroiliac ligaments posterior

the lumbar spine into an increased lordotic position. The joint between L5 and the sacrum is usually the worst affected, and this disc is the one most commonly damaged. Muscle tension which reduces mobility in the rest of the lumbar spine can also lead to excessive wear, and the L5/S1 joint has to compensate for the restriction in the joints above. Heavy pressure applied into this joint space can produce a sharp pain, which is an early warning sign of damage to this disc.

Sacrum and Sacroiliac Joint

As well as articulating with the fifth lumbar vertebra, the sacrum connects the spine to the pelvis through the sacroiliac joint. This is a major weight-bearing joint that is bound together by incredibly strong thick ligaments which allow a very limited range of gliding movement. The joint does not really articulate but just allows enough movement to absorb the shock between the legs and the torso in weight-bearing activities. *(See figs. 30 and 31.)*

The ligaments can get overstretched and damaged in traumatic situations and are also affected by poor posture or overuse/underuse factors. Soft tissue techniques are an effective way of releasing the posterior ligaments if they are short and tight, but if they have been overstretched these techniques will not help. If the joint has become hypermobile, it may require complex rehabilitation to strengthen and stabilise the structures.

With chronic sacroiliac joint problems, pain may not be felt at the joint itself but in the hip extensors (gluteus medius and minimus) and/or rotator muscles (piriformis) instead. These tend to suffer from overuse as they attempt to compensate for the dysfunction at the joint. If these muscles are excessively tight on one side of the body but normal on the other side, the sacroiliac joint should be considered as the likely underlying issue.

Coccyx

The coccyx has only a very limited movement with the sacrum and does not have a great skeletal significance. However, the pelvic floor muscles have attachments to it and can be involved in issues affecting the muscles.

Scoliosis

Lateral curves can develop along the spine if there is uneven muscle tension on either side of it. These are most commonly caused by poor postural habits or excessive physical stress on one side of the body, usually due to occupational factors. Genetic malformation of the vertebrae can sometimes cause a severe scoliosis, and this often requires surgical procedures to correct. Lateral compression on a disc can cause nerve impingement and lead to painful symptoms along the nerve's pathway on one side of the body only.

Assessing Neck and Back Pain

Although most cases of neck and back pain are fairly minor and only affect the soft tissues, it is essential that the therapist can identify those conditions that are not. The primary concern here is the vertebral joint structures, spinal cord and peripheral nerves. Pain emanating from these joints following any traumatic incident should be seen by an orthopaedic specialist first.

The Spinal Cord

This passes down through the vertebral bodies and if it gets damaged or affected by a joint problem it can have very serious consequences. These must be referred to an orthopaedic specialist.

Symptoms that indicate serious (Red Flag) spinal cord injury:

- Significant trauma prior to the onset of neural symptoms (see below).
- Significant neural symptoms affecting both sides of the body.
- Severe symptoms at night or when resting.
- Electric-shock sensation when the cervical or lumbar spine goes into full extension.
- Dizziness or light-headedness, especially when the neck is rotated.
- Blurred vision or slurred speech.
- Feeling generally unwell since onset of symptoms.
- Bladder/bowel disturbance.

If any of these symptoms are present, then more serous spinal injury is possible and the client must be referred to an orthopaedic specialist and not treated with any soft tissue techniques at this stage.

Peripheral nerve impingement

The peripheral nerves emerge from the spinal cord and pass out of the spine through the small gaps between the vertebrae and if this gap narrows it can impinge on the nerve. Apparent musculoskeletal symptoms in a limb may be a neural sensation caused by an impingement of the nerve as it exits the spine. For this reason, clients should always be asked about any history of spinal injuries or symptoms there when assessing a limb problem.

Symptoms that indicate peripheral nerve impingement *(see figs. 32 and 33 overleaf)*:

- Pain in the neck or back which also causes referred symptoms elsewhere.
- Pain or weakness felt in areas that have no apparent soft tissue damage.
- Muscular pain is similar when the muscle is at rest as it is when active.
- Pain may be felt in different muscles along the limb at different times.

Spinal Nerves That Innervate Dermal Areas

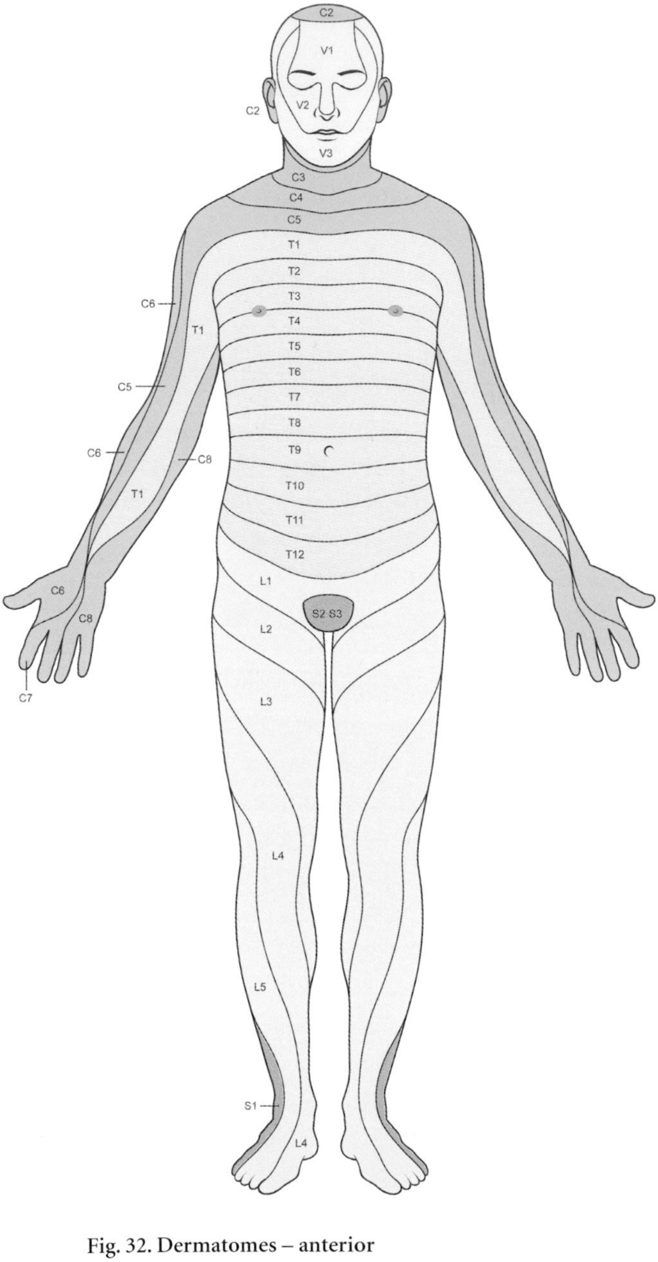

Fig. 32. Dermatomes – anterior

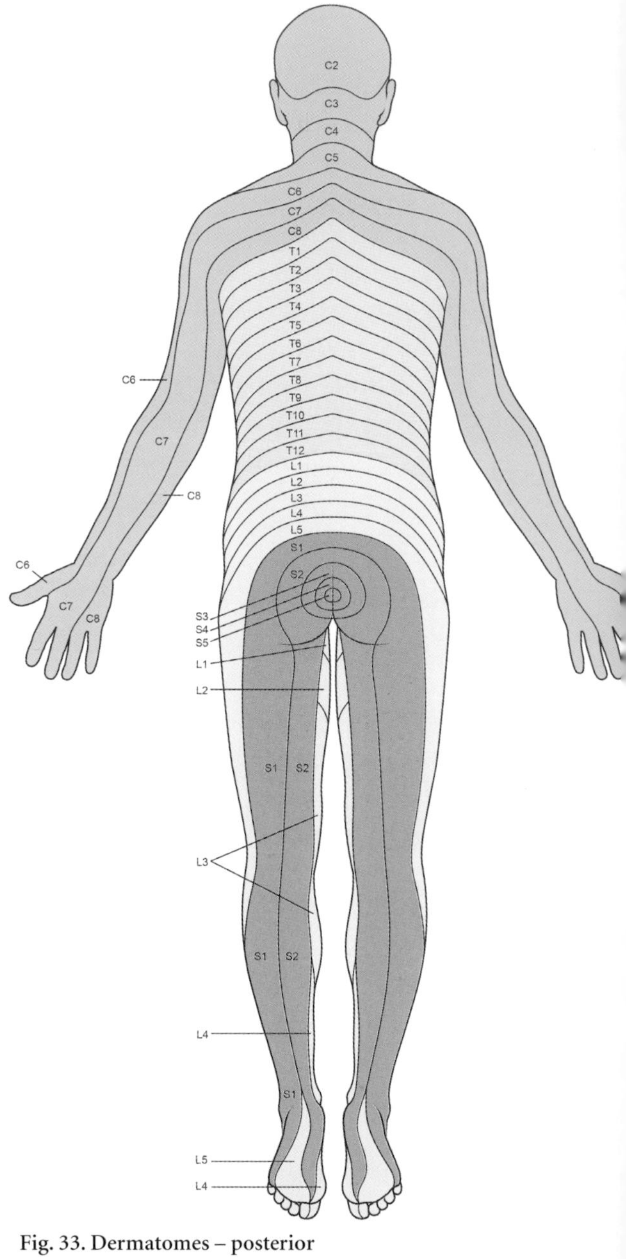

Fig. 33. Dermatomes – posterior

- Weakness or hesitance to contract a muscle.
- Numbness or pins and needles sensation
- Skin sensitivity.

With mild peripheral nerve impingement, if there are no other contraindications present, it is safe to apply soft tissue techniques, especially friction, to the relevant spinal section. But this should only be done with the client lying prone and providing they do not experience any neural symptoms in this position. Muscular tension in the back can sometimes be the sole cause of the nerve compression and in these cases soft tissue techniques can be extremely effective.

The vertebral bodies, discs and the spinal cord cannot be reached with manual techniques because the transverse processes prevent direct access to them. So if the client is lying comfortably in this neutral position, the spinal cord and discs cannot be aggravated by manually applying soft tissue techniques to the back. But this also means that it may not be of any direct benefit to these structures either so symptoms may remain just the same.

If soft tissue techniques do not resolve the problem or the symptoms soon return the client must be referred on for an orthopaedic assessment of the spine. In this case there will still be an indirect benefit from the soft tissue work that has already been done. By releasing the secondary tension around the spine first, the orthopaedic specialist may be better able to assess the situation more accurately. And if spinal manipulation is required, this will also be easier to perform if there is less secondary soft tissue resistance.

Assessing the range of movement

The ranges of movement possible in each section of the spine are flexion and extension, side-bending and rotation. The client should perform all these active movements slowly with control, describing where they experience any pain or restriction. They should attempt these movements with the whole spine as well as doing them separately with just the neck, thorax and lumbar sections. Clients are commonly unaware of their functional restrictions because they build up slowly, so they can unknowingly develop compensatory actions elsewhere. It is therefore important to observe any other body movements they may use to assist these.

Flexion should be assessed with the client both standing and also seated because this takes away any influence from fascial tension in the backs of the legs. If the client stands with their feet turned outwards, this also reduces the fascial tension through the legs. If the client has increased flexion when seated (or with their legs turned out) then it suggests that their hamstring muscles are tight and probably contributing to their back pain. Rotation movements should also be done standing as well as seated to see the influence their leg movements may be having.

Passive movements can be done by moving the client to the end of their range of movement but very great care must be taken to not stress the spinal joints. Movements can be tested this way only if the end range has a soft tissue resistance. If a hard bony resistance is felt, even if this is within a normal range, no attempt must be made to further increase this.

If the client feels pain when they make an active movement but not when they are passively moved then this clearly suggests that there is a muscular component involved. But if the client feels the same pain on active and passive movements it is more likely to be a joint/ligament issue which may not respond so well to soft tissue techniques.

Assessing the sciatic nerve

Apparent musculoskeletal symptoms in the hip and leg may be the result of sciatic nerve restriction rather than any muscle injury. Such problems are most commonly caused by lumbar spine issues which may require referral to an orthopaedic specialist. But sometimes it can be soft tissue tension compressing the vertebrae or fibrous adhesions that restrict the nerve as it passes through the soft tissues. In these cases, deep soft tissue techniques can be very effective.

It is important to first test the side of the body that does not have the injury to see the pain-free ranges that should be possible for that particular client, and then compare it with the other side.

With the client lying prone, the therapist lifts their straight leg and flexes the hip to stretch the hamstrings, stopping at the point where they feel a mild sensation of stretch or discomfort. In this position, they should only feel this in their hamstring muscles, but if they experience discomfort anywhere else this suggests a restriction within the nerve pathway.

With the leg held in this position and the hip flexed, the therapist should then dorsiflex the ankle to stretch the calf muscles and the client should then only feel additional tension through these muscles. Any significant increase of discomfort in the hamstrings or the posterior hip area would suggest that there is a sciatic issue.

With this position now fixed, the therapist then moves the leg to adduct the hip and from there inwardly rotate it. The client should feel very little difference in tension with these movements, but with sciatic restriction just small movements in these directions can cause considerable discomfort.

When one of these movements causes sciatic symptoms, the client can be asked to lift their head up to stretch the spinal cord. If this increases the symptoms, it further confirms the situation and also indicates that the spine is the more likely source of the problem.

When this test shows signs of sciatic restriction, clients may occasionally also feel a specific point of pain in the posterior hip muscles, usually the piriformis. This could be the point where soft tissue damage is causing a restriction around the nerve. Deep friction here may be able to release this and achieve an excellent result.

Common Muscle/ Tendon Conditions

Common Types of Muscle Injury

Strain (tear or rupture)

A **muscle strain** is the most common overuse trauma that occurs when muscle fibres and fascia get torn if they are subjected to a force that exceeds their tensile strength. This can happen suddenly if the muscle is overloaded by a single excessive force or more gradually if they contract against a more moderate load but too many times or for too long.

A strain can also occur in traumatic incidents if a muscle gets forcefully stretched whilst at the same time contracting. For example, when slipping sideways on a smooth surface, the hip is forced into a sudden abduction, which stretches the adductor muscles. But instinctively the person contracts these muscles to try to stop the fall. As the force of contraction cannot overcome the greater stretching force, the adductor muscle fibres get torn apart.

A mild strain will only involve a small number of fibres, which usually recover well, and the overall structure of the muscle will not be affected. But if a greater proportion of the fibres get torn, this can lead to a **partial rupture** which can cause more permanent damage. The larger area of torn fibres will recoil due to their natural elasticity, and this will create a gap in the overall muscle's structure. This can be felt as a lump of compacted muscle fibres with a hollow space immediately adjacent to it. This means there will be a very slight but permanent loss in the power of the muscle because not all the fibres are connected together. But if the rest of the muscle recovers well and is kept in good condition, this is not usually noticeable.

Whenever a tear takes place in the tissues, bleeding occurs. If the muscle then continues working, so too will the bleeding. Without immediate rest following the trauma, there will be an excessive amount of blood accumulating in the surrounding tissues. This can form into scar tissue that sticks (adheres) the fibres together and stops them gliding alongside each other to create movement. Although a period of rest alone may lead to the completed relief from painful symptoms, the scar tissue and adhesions that result may leave the muscle weak and inelastic. Not only will the muscle perform poorly but it will also be much more vulnerable to further injury.

Massage and soft tissue techniques can begin gently as soon as the condition becomes non-acute, usually after 48 hours if good RICE procedures are followed (Appendix 2). The main aim is to prevent the formation of adhesive scar tissue and so facilitate a full and speedy recovery.

Muscle Overuse Syndrome

Overuse strains can develop very slowly on a microscopic level if only a small specific area of muscle is slightly but repetitively overloaded. With very few fibres being damaged at the time, the client will feel very little discomfort and so may ignore it and continue with the same activities. This can prevent the micro-trauma from fully recovering and allows more scar tissue to build up in the area. As the dysfunction increases within the muscle, chronic pain may become more apparent and it becomes more vulnerable to an acute strain.

Incomplete recovery from past acute trauma or the build-up of micro-trauma both result in an area within the muscle that will not function because the fibres are stuck together. This can be felt as a hard lump which, if it has been there a long time, may cause little or no pain even when deep friction is applied to it. It will, however, affect the function of the whole muscle, and over time the person may alter their movement patterns to compensate for this. These changes can then lead to overuse and/or underuse issues affecting other parts of the muscular system. Injury and pain may only appear in a secondary area and it is often quite difficult to trace this type of problem back to the initial site of the overuse problem.

The muscle tissue affected by these overuse situations responds well to massage and soft tissue techniques. But the real challenge the therapist often faces is to try to identify the actual cause of the overuse so changes can be made to prevent a reoccurrence. It is easy to blame a person's occupation or sport for this, but giving these things up is rarely a viable or desirable option for the client. It is therefore necessary to look at how they do their job or sport to try to find the specific overuse factors that may be the cause, and try to change just these. Posture is also a key factor to consider here because poor alignment and stability can compromise the whole muscular system.

Delayed Onset Muscle Soreness (DOMS)

This term is commonly used in a sports context to describe the general pain commonly felt in muscles in the days following hard exercise, but it can equally apply to other aches and pains felt after any hard or unaccustomed physical exertion. DOMS is just a large amount of micro-trauma caused by overuse, which needs rest and massage to enable it to recover well.

Macro-trauma v micro-trauma

It may seem to be a contradiction that a large (macro) acute trauma is a definite contraindication for physical therapy, but massage seems to work extremely well on areas of micro-trauma. To try to explain this it is worth considering that it may be impossible to find a needle in a haystack but quite easy to find a football in it. Manual techniques will find a large area of damage and open it up to cause more damage. But they will not be able to get a fix on a microscopically small individual fibre. Because it is embedded deep within a mass of healthy fibres which can glide along with a massage stroke, an individual fibre manages to avoid being aggravated by this.

So in the early recovery stage, gentle soft tissue techniques work very well by improving local blood circulation and preventing scar-tissue formation. Deeper techniques and more advanced stretching should be introduced later as the painful symptoms disappear.

Compartment Syndrome

Muscles are contained within compartments which are bound in fascia, and if the muscle increases in size the fascia can usually stretch to accommodate this. But there are areas where the fascia needs to be thicker and stronger so it can control the shape and size of the muscle. This is particularly the case in the lower leg, where the muscles have to taper in towards the ankle. If the muscles here need to expand because of increased bulk through strength training or swelling, the naturally tight fascia prevents this happening.

If the muscle cannot expand, the pressure inside the compartment increases instead. As well as causing pain, the increased pressure can constrict the blood vessels running through the muscle. This restricts blood flow to the foot, which will feel cooler. In mild conditions, fascial release techniques should be used to try to loosen the fascia and help the release of interstitial fluids. This can reduce the pressure, but the causes of the increased muscle size must also be dealt with. Deep friction techniques should be avoided, especially if the muscle may be enlarged due to swelling from tissue damage because this could increase the swelling further and make the condition worse.

If the symptoms persist, the client should be referred to an orthopaedic specialist because in severe and chronic conditions sometimes the only solution is to surgically release the fascia.

No muscle functions in isolation

The tone and function of one muscle will influence those of other muscles which have an opposing action. If a muscle becomes hypertonic due to overuse or postural stress through reciprocal inhibition, this will cause the opposing muscle(s) to become hypotonic and weaken. These weakened muscles can easily sustain an overuse injury, but the tight opposing muscle which may be causing the weakness can remain symptom free. It is therefore important to assess and treat all the associated muscles and not just the main site of the injury.

Postural effects on muscle dysfunction

With ideal postural alignment the muscles function efficiently and the system as a whole is in balance. But with poor alignment all this can change as the muscles adapt to the situation and dysfunctional patterns become set.

Short hypertonic postural muscles

Some muscles have to hold a high level of contraction in a shortened position to maintain a postural misalignment. They become short, tight and hypertonic and the client may suffer chronic pain because of this. But the hypertonicity can also weaken opposing muscles through reciprocal inhibition and lead to injury there instead. Fascial release and stretching

exercises are needed to improve length and elasticity, and neuromuscular techniques to restore normal tone should be applied here.
Example: Muscles in the back of the neck and lower back with excessive lordotic curvatures.

Short hypotonic postural muscles

Some muscles are held in a shortened position but are underused due to postural misalignment and they become short, tight and hypotonic. But because the muscle is underused this may not lead to any painful symptoms in normal activities. However, this situation needs to be identified and treated if postural improvement is to be achieved. Fascial release and stretching techniques should be used to improve length but functional strengthening exercises are also important for these muscles.
Examples: Gluteus maximus with sway-back posture; pectoralis minor with protracted shoulders.

Long hypertonic postural muscles

Some muscles have to overwork to support a greater postural weight while in a lengthened position. These muscles can become permanently stretched but are also hypertonic through overuse with tense immobile fascia. This can cause chronic pain and discomfort and fascial release techniques are effective.
Examples: Thoracic erector spinae with excessive kyphosis; rectus femoris with sway-back posture.

Long hypotonic postural muscles

Some muscles becomes stretched and underused in postural positions. They become weak with poor neuromuscular function and are unable to give any effective postural support. Exercises to strengthen, shorten and increase muscle tone are needed here.
Example: Abdominal muscles with excessive lumbar lordosis.

Common Types of Tendon Injury

Strains

The collagen fibres making up the tendon can be torn through overuse in the same way as the muscle fibres can. As the blood supply to the tendon is less than the muscle it takes more time to heal and a longer period of rest is needed.

Complete tendon ruptures are a possibility if there is a sudden extreme overload, with the Achilles tendon at the ankle and biceps brachii tendon at the shoulder being common examples. The client typically feels a sudden sharp snapping sensation and sound but relatively little pain afterwards. This is because no further painful tissue damage can occur as there is already a complete separation. But the muscle of the tendon will recoil and bunch up away from the rupture and there will be no movement when the muscle contracts. These extreme traumas usually require immediate surgical repair and soft tissue techniques can only help recovery during rehabilitation by breaking down fibrous adhesion and helping the tissues recover.

Bone attachments

Repetitive strong contractions can put a strain on the muscle/tendon's attachment to the bone. Weakness in an adjacent muscle may be part of this problem if it does not apply enough counter-resistance across the attachment. Inflammation (tenoperiostitis) can occur at this point, and it needs rest with the muscle in a shortened relaxed position to prevent aggravating the injury.

Tendinopathies

The core of tightly packed, parallel collagen fibres of the tendon makes it a very strong structure when pulling in its correct alignment. Problems develop if the tendon gets twisted or bent during active movements because this can separate the closely compacted fibres within it. This is a common cause of pain in the Achilles tendon in people who have excessive foot pronation which makes the tendon twist and bend just above the calcaneum.

If a joint is poorly aligned then a tendon may rub hard against the bone surfaces instead of gliding smoothly around it. If a muscle is excessively tight this can also make a tendon rub against a bone as it passes around a joint. With repetitive use this will eventually cause inflammation and tendon damage and the client will feel pain in the joint.

Some large tendons, like the Achilles, run through a sheath within which a lubricant similar to synovial fluid keeps the tendon moving smoothly. If there is insufficient lubricant then friction can occur inside the sheath and inflame the tissues. In such a confined space any swelling or thickening will cause more restriction and pain.

Because these tendinopathies are often caused by friction and rubbing, deep soft tissue techniques could aggravate the situation rather than improve it. Light friction can be used with caution and only applied more deeply in following treatments if the response is positive. It is advisable to apply ice after friction techniques as a precaution against inflammation. Rest from the aggravating factors is essential for recovery and addressing any joint alignment issues may be the only way to prevent a reoccurrence.

Muscle/tendon junctions

Where the fascia continues beyond the muscle to form the tendon, it changes from being comprised mostly of elastin to being mostly inelastic collagen. The transition from elastic to inelastic makes this area more prone to strain and micro-trauma.

Attachment issues

Overdevelopment of muscle strength or sudden powerful contraction can pull too hard on its attachment point with the bone. Weakness or poor function in a muscle on the other side of the attachment can also add to the problem by not applying a counter-resistance. This can cause inflammation and damage at this critical point (tenoperiostitis) and sharp pain will be felt at the joint when the muscle contracts. Rest is essential to allow this to repair and stretching must be avoided as this could aggravate the problem in the early repair stage.

Assessing Muscle/ Tendon Function

A muscle can only contract and shorten, or relax and be lengthened. If there is no restriction in the joint, the muscles should be able to contract strongly enough to achieve the full range of movement in one direction, and stretch freely enough to allow a full range in the opposite direction.

When assessing a muscle's function, it must be compared with the same muscle on the other side of the body. But this may also be restricted so it is also sometimes necessary to consider what the normal range should be for that individual.

As well as the muscles where the client feels pain, others along the chain and working in opposition to it should be assessed because they are all functionally linked.

Active Movements

The client contracts and shortens the muscle

to assess its strength and function. If pain is felt and there is a limited range, this usually indicates an overuse strain. If there is restricted range but little or no pain, this is more likely to suggest a build-up of scar tissue through overuse micro-trauma.

The client then stretches the muscle by moving in the opposite direction, contracting and shortening the antagonist muscle(s). A short range with pain at the end suggests a strain but restriction with little or no pain indicates chronic overuse tension.

Resistive Movements

If there is only minor muscle/tendon damage, active movements alone may not be enough to identify any problem. In this situation, the therapist can apply a resistance to the movements to increase the forces needed to reproduce the symptoms. As well as feeling the strength of the muscle, the therapist should observe the quality of movement to see if there is any hesitance or weakness along the range.

Passive Movements

If there is no acute injury present, the muscle/tendon can be passively lengthened to its comfortable end of range. If this causes pain, the therapist can then add pressure to stretch the tissues to test their elasticity.

Muscle Control

Most normal daily activities involve muscle control rather than overall strength and range. They need to make fine adjustments in their length and tension and perform well at low levels of strength too.

The ability for the muscle to do this can be assessed by the client performing slow eccentric contractions and observing how smooth and controlled this is. It can either be done against the force of gravity or with the therapist applying a mild resistance. For example, sitting with the knee extended and then allowing the lower leg to slowly go down requires good eccentric contraction from the quadriceps.

Palpation

Undoubtedly the most valuable assessment tool a massage therapist has is palpation, and this is perhaps the only thing we need. Areas of tissue damage and tension can easily be felt by the skilled therapist and any pain response from the client is instant and direct from those tissues. Although a muscle may feel softer than a tendon, they should all be smooth and uniform in their texture and any irregularities in this indicate areas of damage and where treatment needs to be applied.

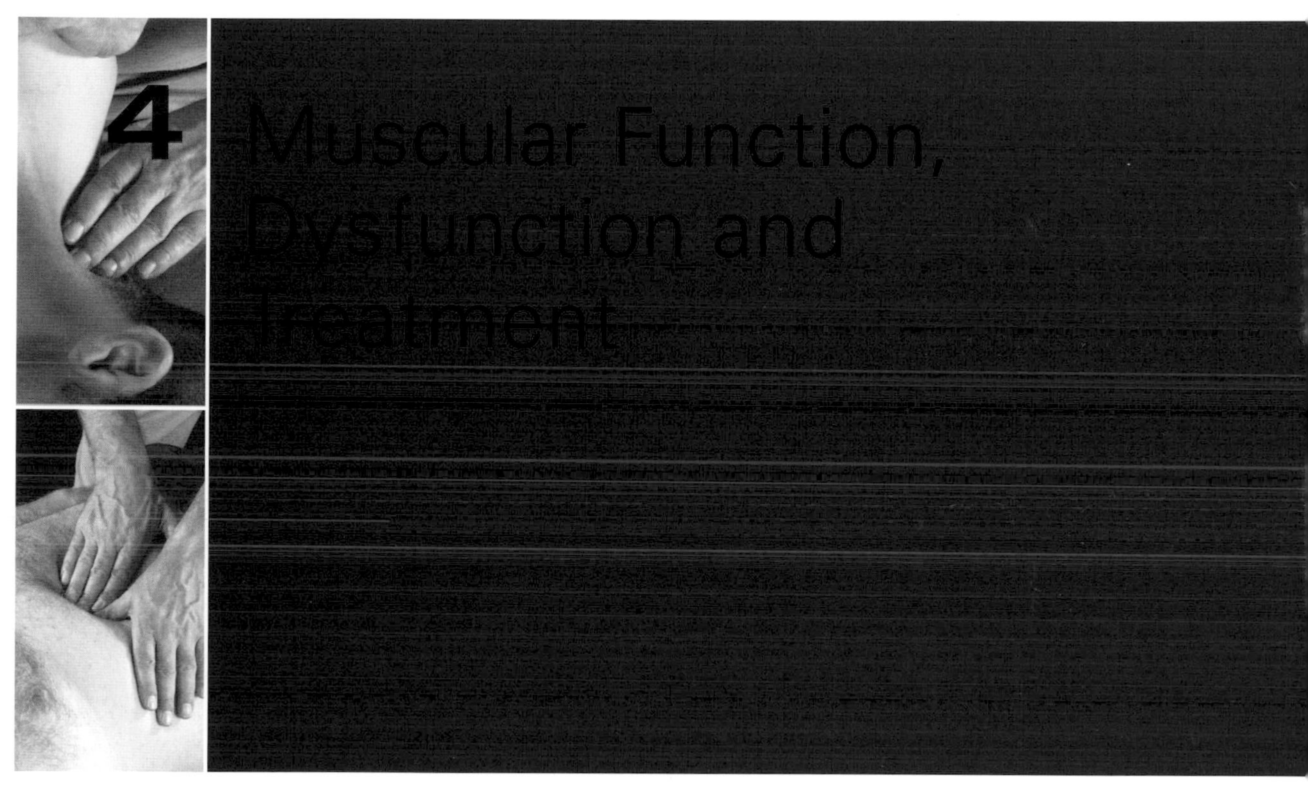

4 Muscular Function, Dysfunction and Treatment

There are limitless treatment methods and techniques that can be used to treat muscles, and the photographs in this section only show a few examples. They are not intended to be copied exactly but to show some of the possibilities. Not all the techniques described in the text are shown in the photographs.

Anterior Neck and Torso

Face

Unlike other skeletal muscles in the body, those in the face attach to skin instead of bone. Instead of moving joints they make facial movements which play a major role in how we communicate with other people. Painful overuse injuries are very rare because they have nothing more than the force of gravity to resist. But the link between emotion and facial expression is clear to see and this can mean that good deep massage of the facial muscles is very relaxing.

Muscles of the face can be affected in neural conditions such as **Bell's palsy**, and friction massage techniques along the nerve's pathway can be very beneficial. General massage techniques to help keep the muscles in good health are also worthwhile.

Jaw

The temporomandibular joint (TMJ) is a complex joint with strong muscles which pull the mandible bone up and glide it forward and back when chewing and talking. Even though they may be in almost constant use in some people, normal activity rarely leads to overuse injury. But muscular problems do result from joint misalignment, which may be caused by dental issues. Grinding teeth at night can also lead to overuse muscular problems and, although massage may help alleviate painful symptoms, it will be unlikely to affect the underlying causes of the problem. The joint and its muscles can also be vulnerable to impact trauma in some violent activities.

There can be a strong link between chronic problems around the TMJ and deep emotional issues. If there is no traumatic incident or obvious dental issue associated with the injury, this should be considered carefully before proceeding with deep soft tissue techniques.

The **masseter** and **temporalis** muscles, which raise the mandible up to the temporal bone and close the joint, can easily be seen working on the outside of the jaw. These short strong muscles can be treated quite easily and connective tissue and Soft Tissue Release (STR) techniques are particularly effective on them. *(See photo 4.)*

Inside the joint is a small group of short powerful **pterygoid** and **buccinator** muscles, which create the forward and backward chewing action. To treat these muscles, it is necessary to wear sterilised gloves and work from inside the mouth without any lubricant. Short, strong fascial strokes into and along the muscle borders can be a very effective way of releasing restrictions here. But these can be very painful techniques which should only be done once during a treatment session and should not be attempted on a normal, mobile and unrestricted joint. (If practising this technique with colleagues only use very mild pressure.) *(See figs. 34 and 35, and photo 5 and fig. 36 overleaf.)*

Because this is a very unusual technique to perform, and as emotional factors may be linked to the condition, this needs to be discussed first. It is important that both client and therapist feel comfortable with the situation before proceeding.

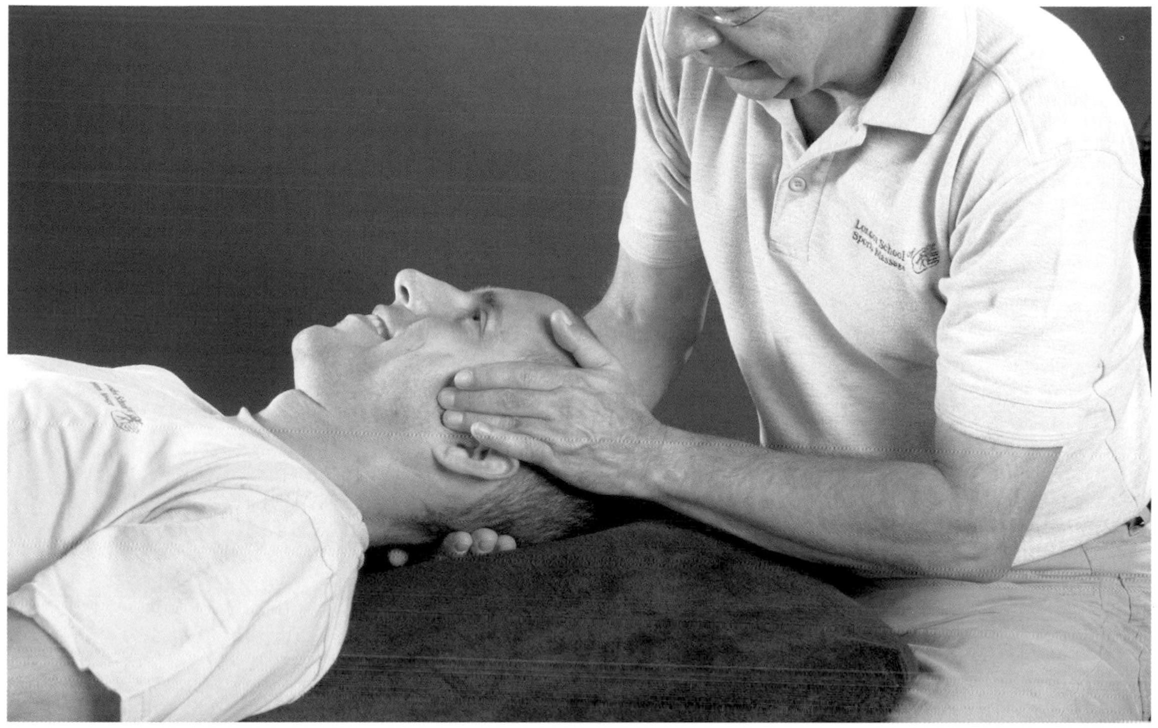

Photo 4. With the client's head comfortably supported with one hand, the other hand is used to treat the masseter and temporalis muscles. Fascial strokes can be applied, with the client opening their jaw at the same time. STR lock can be applied in a superior direction as the client opens their jaw.

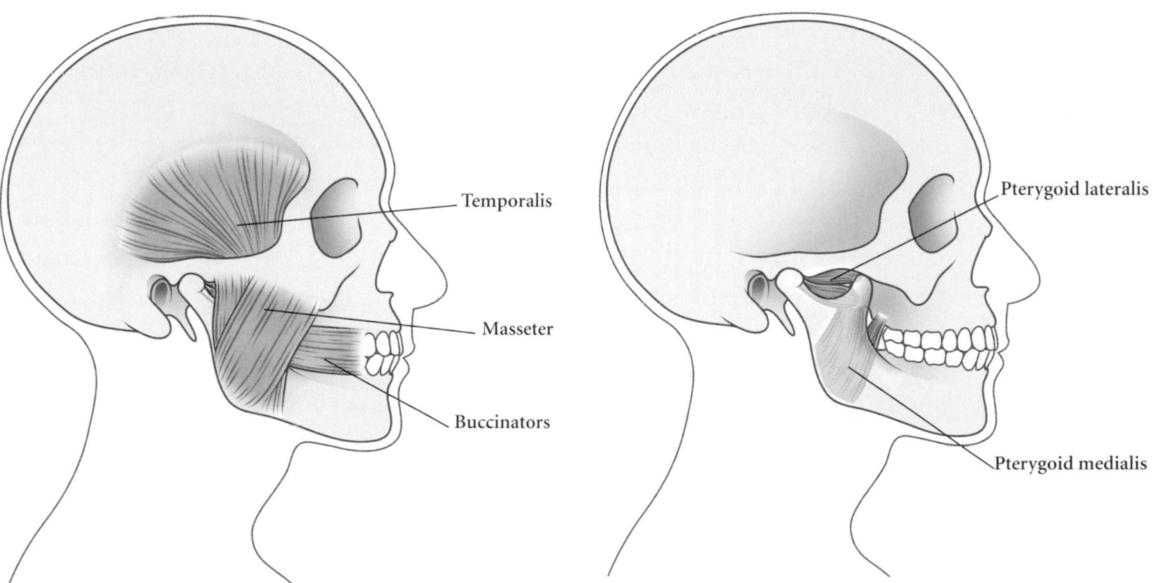

Fig. 34. Superficial jaw muscles

Fig. 35. Deep jaw muscles

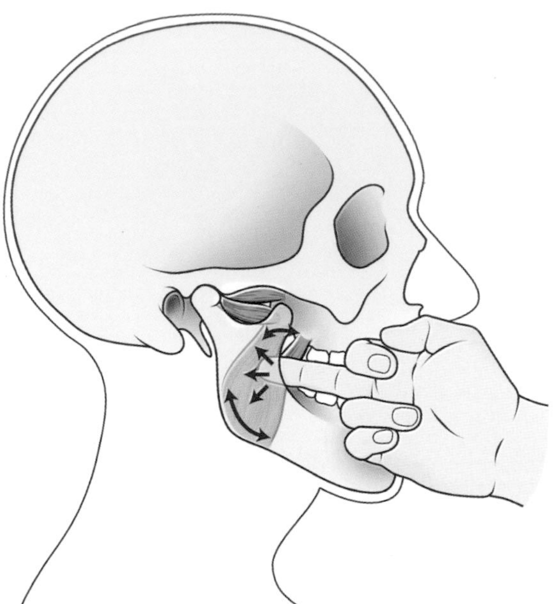

Fig. 36. Treating the deep jaw muscles

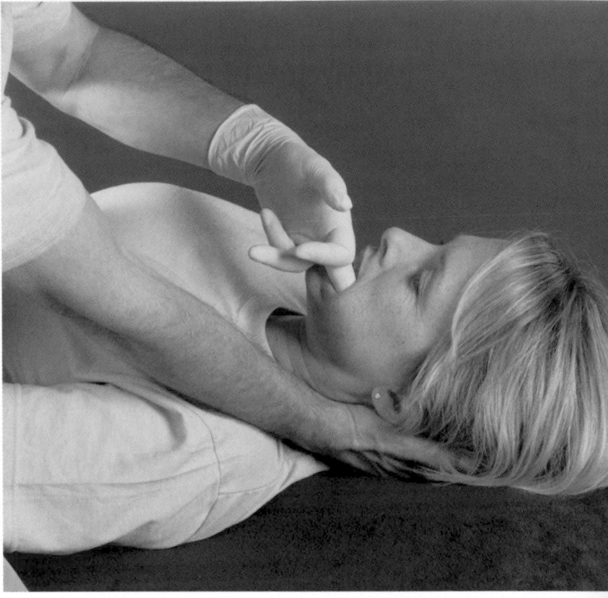

Photo 5. Supporting the client's head with one hand, a finger of the other hand can be used inside the mouth to release the pterygoid and buccinator muscles.

Neck

The muscles of the neck have to control the weight of the head, which is very dense and heavy, and they have to do this for very long periods without fatigue. With good postural alignment, the head is well balanced and needs little effort to control and move; but, with poor alignment, much greater stress is put on some of the muscles whilst others get underused. The muscles also sometimes have to deal with huge loads when sudden movements cause very strong forces of inertia on the head and neck and acute injury (whiplash) is common in these situations. *(See fig. 37.)*

The long thin **omohyoid** muscles run down the front of the neck and are the only muscles used to assist in opening the jaw through their fascial connections to the mandible bone. Opening the jaw comes mainly from gravity, so this muscle is rarely put under any strain. Although they get lengthened in people with a forward-head posture, this does not usually cause any problems to the muscle. The **sterno-hyoid** muscle runs down from the hyoid bone to the manubrium and depresses the hyoid bone as well as assisting in neck flexion.

Deep behind these muscles are the **longus capitis** and **longus colli** muscles, which run from the anterior upper cervical vertebra down to the upper thoracic vertebrae and so flex and bend the cervical spine anteriorly. But people with a forward head posture are already set in this position, so the muscles are underused and therefore injury is unlikely. Deep massage techniques are not possible on the hyoid and colli muscles because they run alongside the windpipe and any compression to this can give the client a choking sensation.

The largest muscle in the front and side of the neck is the **sternocleidomastoid** (SCM), which

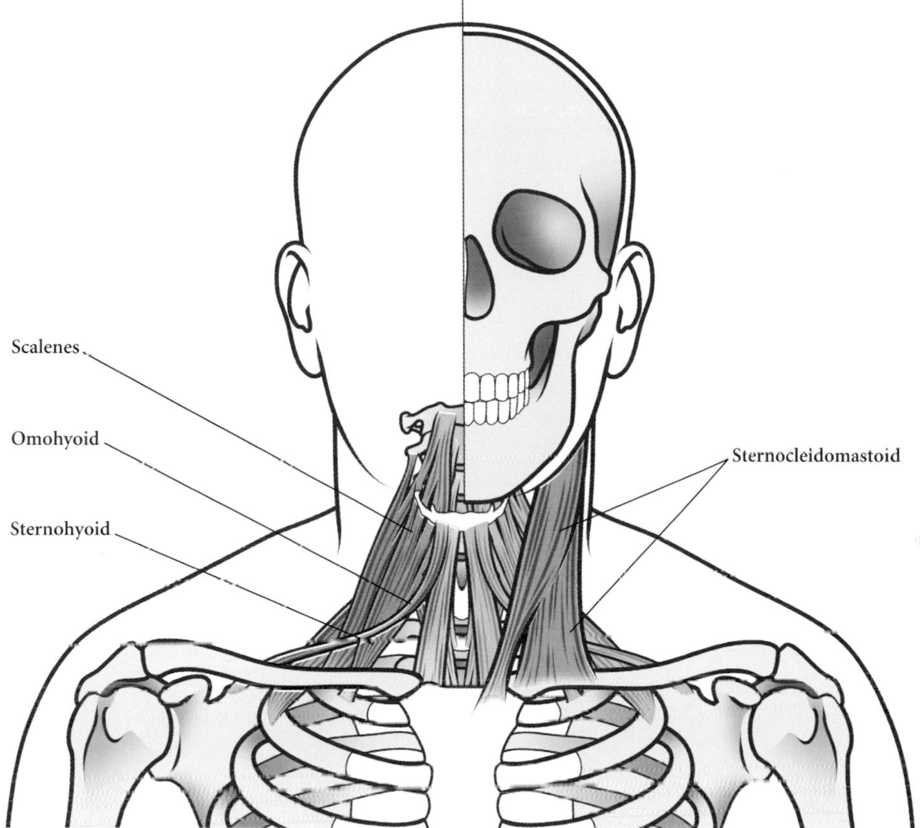

Fig. 37. Anterior neck muscles

attaches from the sternum and clavicle to the mastoid process on the skull. Its main action in the upright position should be to rotate the head, with the muscle on the left side turning the head to the right and the muscle on the right side turning it to the left.

But this only happens with a good postural alignment. People who hold their head in a very forward position will not use this muscle at all when rotating the head (see levator scapula and upper trapezius). This means that the muscle is commonly underused and becomes weak, but does not usually suffer any chronic symptoms from this. However, bilaterally these muscles have to work powerfully to lift the head when flexing the neck from a supine position. So overuse strain can easily occur in people with weakened SCM muscles who take on an activity involving this movement. *(See figs. 38 and 39.)*

The SCM cannot be treated with normal massage strokes that apply a deep pressure into the tissues because these could compress the jugular vein and windpipe beneath it. Instead, a squeezing/pinching technique across the belly of the muscle is very effective without interfering with any underlying structures. *(See photo 6 overleaf.)*

The **scalene** muscles at the side of the neck attaching from the transverse processes of the cervical vertebrae, down into the first and second ribs. With this wide insertion along the curving ribs these muscles create neck movements through a wide range of sideways directions.

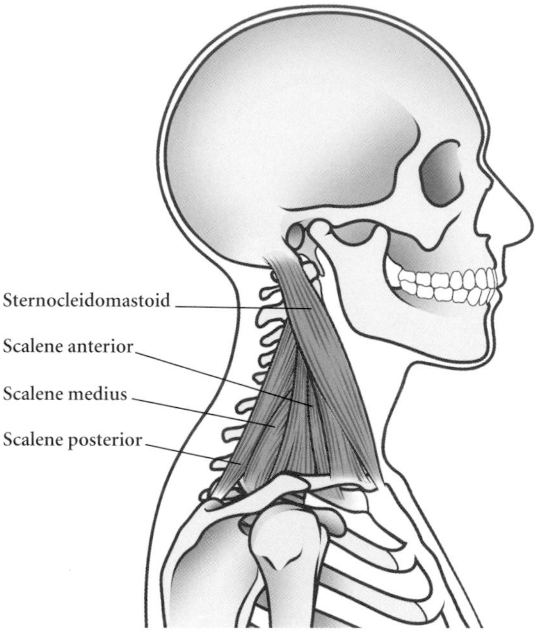

Sternocleidomastoid
Scalene anterior
Scalene medius
Scalene posterior

Fig. 38. Lateral neck muscles in ideal posture

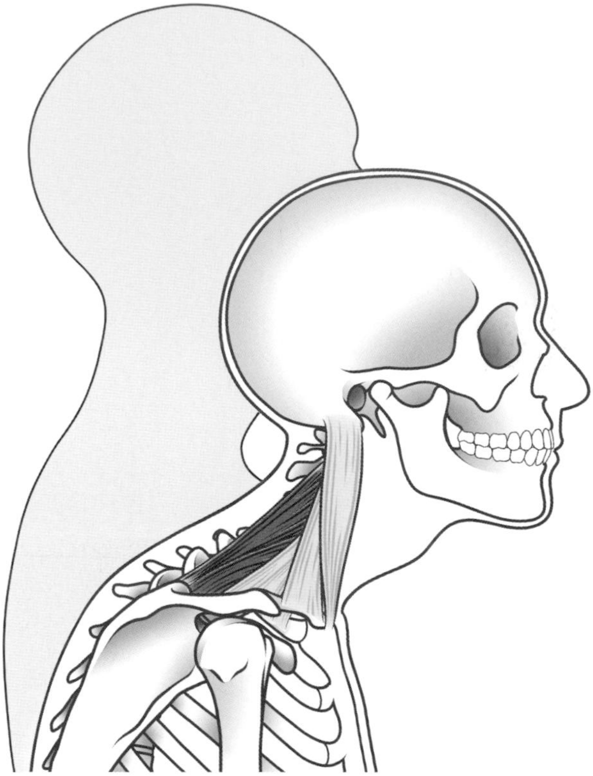

Fig. 39. Lateral neck muscles with forward head posture

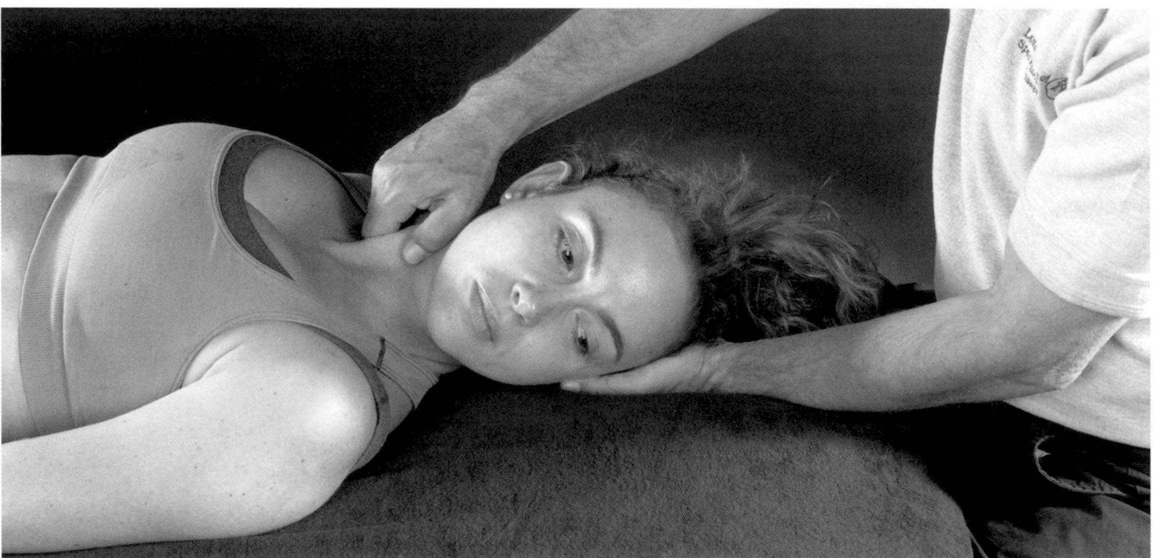

Photo 6. With the neck rotated, the client first actively lifts their head a few centimetres. This raises the sternocleidomastoid as it contracts; the therapist can now grasp the muscle between thumb and finger. The client then relaxes, and short strokes are applied along the muscle. Neuromuscular Technique can be applied by pinching the tissues at the trigger point.

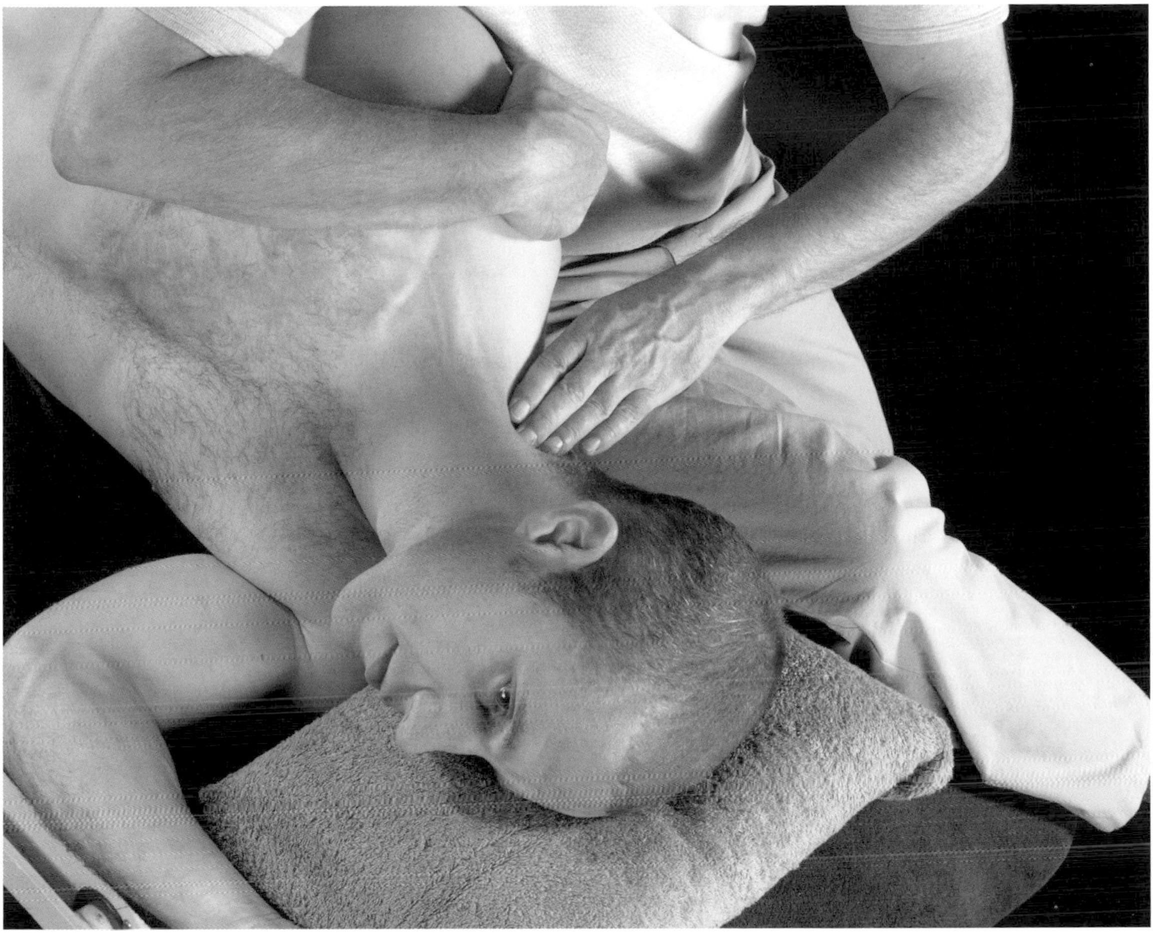

Photo 7. A side-lying position with the therapist sitting behind the client is excellent for treating the lateral neck. From here, deep strokes can be applied along the scalenes as well as friction in and around the vertebrae and along the occipital ridge. The therapist can pull back on the shoulder girdle at the same time to add a stretch to the tissues.

With a forward head position, the posterior part has to overwork to support the weight of the head and can suffer chronic overuse pain. But the anterior part can become weak through lack of use and shortening, so it becomes vulnerable to trauma with sudden head movements.

The attachments of the scalenes to the ribs are significant in respiration since they act as stabilisers, holding up the top of the ribcage, and they work concentrically to pull the ribs up in forced inhalation. They often become chronically short and tight through overuse in people suffering with respiratory conditions. Although they may not feel any muscle pain here, releasing this tension can help ease some of their symptoms.

These muscles can be most effectively treated with massage techniques when the client is in a side-lying position. *(See photo 7.)*

Chest

The **subclavius** muscle runs from the manubrium at the top of the sternum, inserts along the distal part of the clavicle and draws it

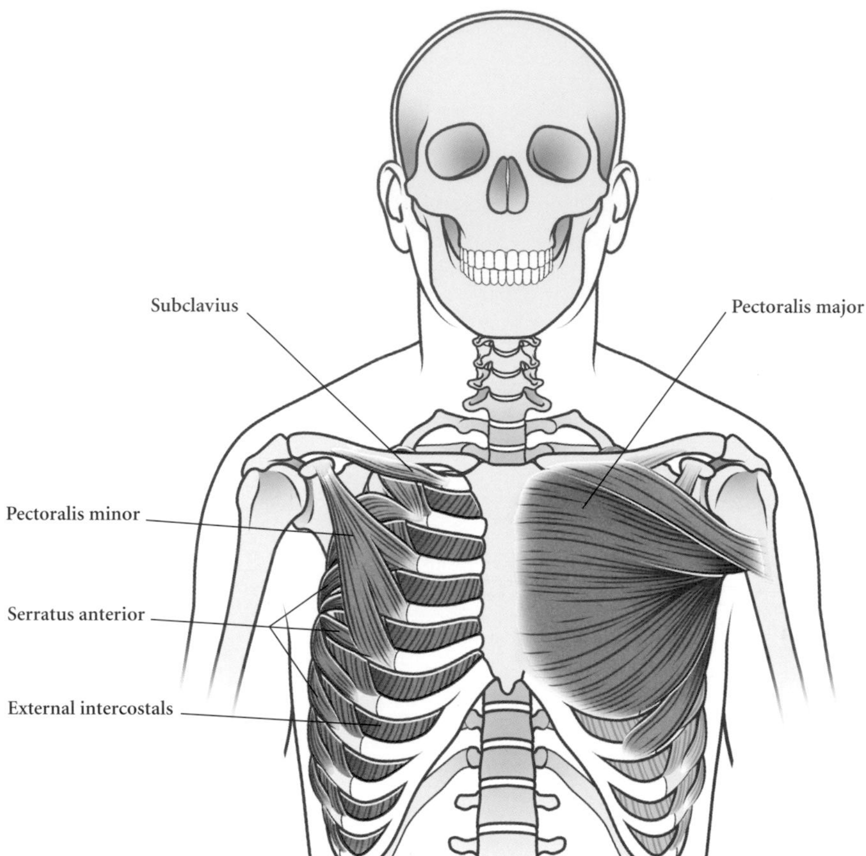

Fig. 40. Chest muscles

posteriorly. It becomes short and tight when the shoulders are protracted for long periods and can be treated with fascial techniques to restore normal length. *(See fig. 40.)*

The large superficial muscle of the chest is the **pectoralis major**, which has its origin all the way round from the clavicle, down the sternum to the lower ribs and costal cartilage. As the muscle extends out towards its insertion along the crest of the greater tubercle of the humerus, it twists around. The upper fibres coming from the clavicle insert at the bottom and the lower fibres from the costal area insert at the top. This twist makes the fibres cross the front of the shoulder joint through a very wide range of angles, and this enables it to perform a wide range of horizontal and diagonal adduction as well as internally rotating the shoulder joint.

The muscle is divided into many compartments which can each develop strength according to the demands placed on them. So the muscle is very versatile and adapts well to normal activities and tends not to suffer chronic problems in normal daily life. Overuse strains are, however, commonly caused by strength-training exercises and by working in some heavy manual trades.

People with protracted shoulders will constantly have their glenohumeral joint internally rotated and this will keep the pectoralis major in a shortened position, which eventually makes it chronically tight. In this state it can perform well within a limited range when doing weight-training exercises in a gym. This may encourage people to do more of this exercise, which could further increase the tension and shoulder protraction. This muscle commonly requires soft tissue techniques to release the tension and needs stretching exercises rather than more strengthening.

The pectoralis major is easy to treat, except where it runs beneath the breast tissue (even on men). Breast tissue is very different to muscle and does not physiologically benefit from massage in the same way. Attempting to treat the muscles through this tissue would need considerable pressure which could be harmful to it.

Although the name is similar, the **pectoralis minor** has a very different role and does not even move the same joint as the major. Running from the coracoid process down to the third, fourth and fifth ribs, it moves the shoulder girdle by pulling the scapula anteriorly and posteriorly.

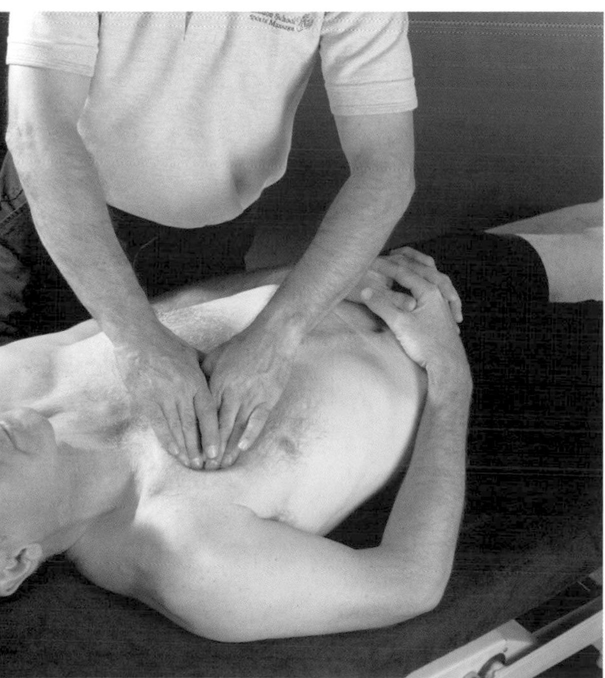

Photo 8. Friction and deep strokes can be applied to the pectoralis minor through the major muscle.

With a well-balanced posture, this muscle is mainly used from a pre-stretched, lengthened position in actions such as overarm throwing, and it is only likely to suffer injury in that way. But with protracted shoulders the pectoralis minor will become chronically short and tight because the scapula hangs in this anterior/posterior position. It is essential to apply deep fascial techniques to lengthen this muscle and allow better postural alignments. Although the client is unlikely to feel any muscle pain normally, it can be very painful when it is being treated.

The pectoralis minor can usually be treated by working through the major but if this is very well developed and tight it may be difficult. It can be reached by working under the pectoralis major with the client in a side-lying position. *(See photo 8, and photos 9 and 10 overleaf.)*

The deepest muscles of the chest are the intercostals. The **external intercostal** muscles pull on the outer surface of the ribs and cause them to be drawn outwards. This increases the volume of the ribcage, which helps suck air into the lungs. The upper ribs only move slightly but the lower ribs move out considerably more to allow the lungs to expand downwards. The internal intercostals work in the opposite way by pulling on the inner surface of the ribs and drawing them inwards to help expel air from the lungs. *(See photo 11 overleaf.)*

These muscles are only likely to get injured through a traumatic incident or through overuse as a result of excessive coughing or laboured breathing in people suffering with respiratory conditions. However, restricted breathing patterns are quite common and although there may be no muscular pain, releasing tension in these intercostal muscles can be very beneficial. The intercostal muscles can be reached quite

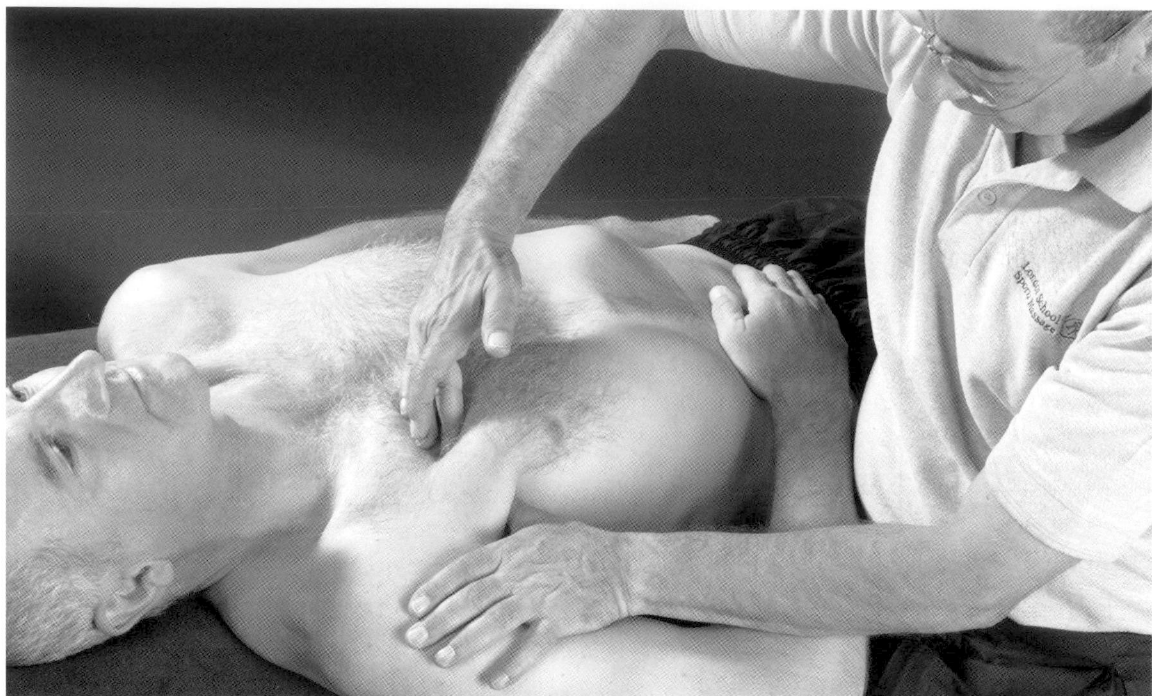

Photo 9. Use one thumb to lift the lateral border of the pectoralis major and push medially over the ribcage to reach the pectoralis minor. The other hand strokes in from the medial side to reach its other border. From this position, both hands work together to apply deep longitudinal and transverse strokes to the pectoralis minor.

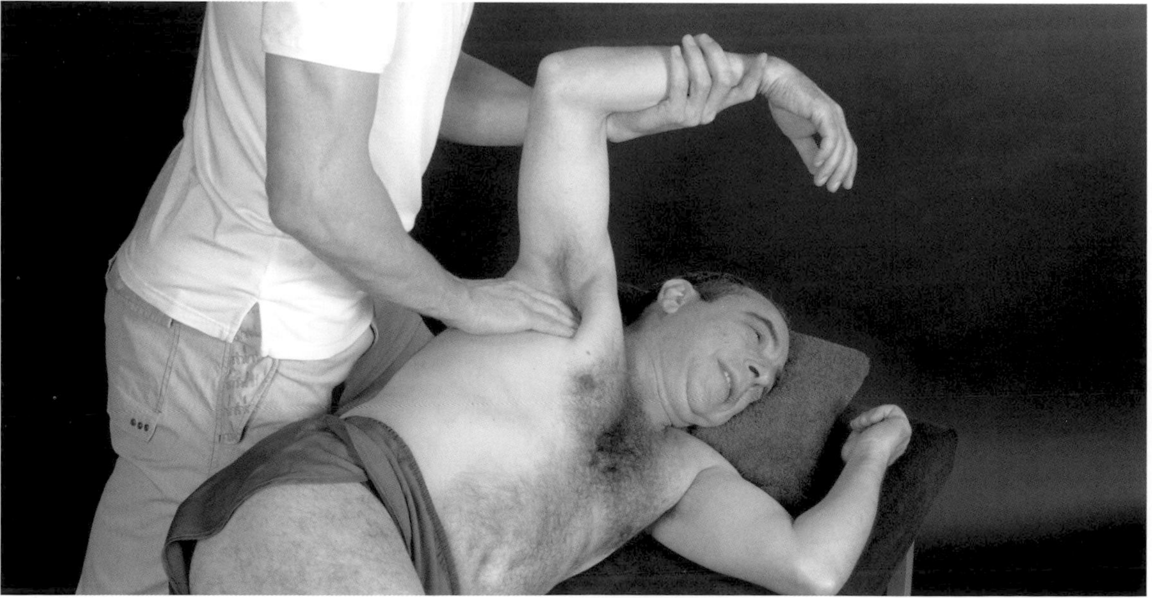

Photo 10. In the side-lying position with the arm held in abduction, deep strokes can be applied behind the pectoralis major to reach the pectoralis minor, serratus anterior and intercostal muscles.

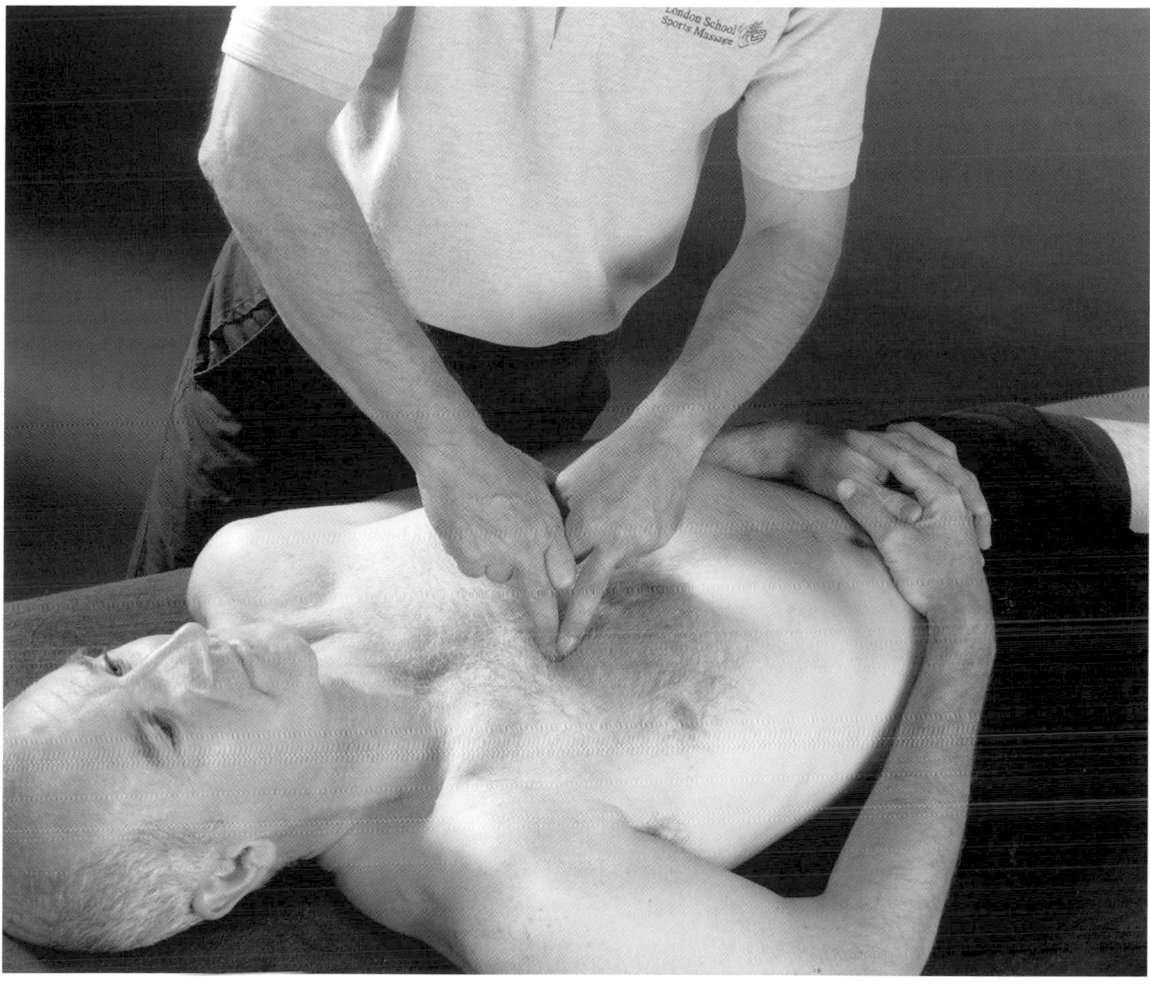

Photo 11. Deep strokes and friction can be applied to the intercostal muscles between the ribs.

easily with soft tissue techniques with the client in supine and side-lying positions.

The **serratus anterior** muscle is found around the sides of the upper chest. It is a broad, flat muscle which is made up of a number of strips that attach from the anterior medial border of the scapula to the outer borders of the first to the eighth or ninth ribs. It pulls the scapula anteriorly around the ribcage and also rotates it.

This range of movement is essential in enabling all forward-shoulder joint movements. If poor muscle function restricts this it can lead to overuse problems in the muscles of the shoulder joint, which have to overwork to compensate for it. The serratus anterior is also an important stabiliser of the scapula and the reciprocal relationship with its antagonist, the rhomboid muscles, is crucial in doing this.

The serratus anterior is commonly found to be short and tight in people who have protracted shoulders. Although rarely a source of pain, these muscles need to be treated and stretched in an effort to improve posture and this can be quite painful.

Most of the muscle can be easily treated with the client side-lying, but the proximal part is sandwiched deep between the scapula and ribcage, which is very difficult to reach with manual techniques. (*See photo 12.*)

The **diaphragm** muscle separates the chest and abdominal cavities. It is the primary muscle used for inhalation and is not directly involved in any skeletal movements. It attaches to all the bones around the lower thorax from xiphoid process at the front, round inside the lower rib to the lumbar vertebrae. Through the fascia, it is integrally connected into the abdominal wall and pelvic floor muscles.

Although it is usually described as a dome-shaped muscle, it has a central tendon which spreads out very widely and gives it a fairly flat non-contractile top. The muscle fibres mainly run down the sides, so when they contract the flat tendon head is pulled down like a piston. This action decreases the pressure in the chest cavity, causing a vacuum which sucks air into the lungs.

The muscle works automatically without voluntary control which makes it unlikely to be overused and injured in anything other than

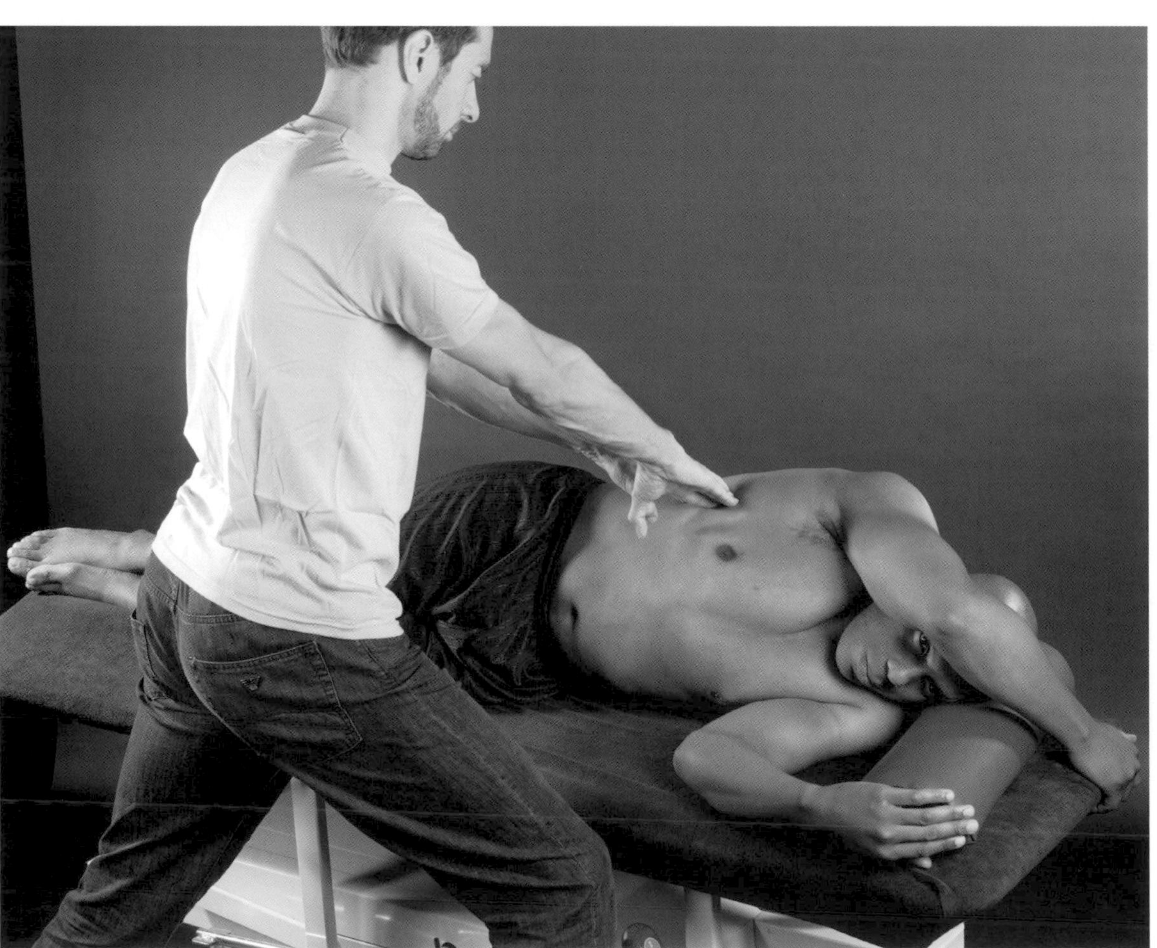

Photo 12. In the side-lying position, the serratus anterior can be treated between the ribs and the scapula.

the most extreme physical exertion. If people spend many hours lying back slumped in soft armchairs, however, they are compressing the ribcage into the abdominal cavity. This restricts the diaphragm and over time can make it weak, inefficient and lead to respiratory dysfunction.

The free movement of the diaphragm relies on good abdominal control. Excessive tension in the abdominal muscles increases abdominal pressure which acts against the diaphragm as it tries to contract downwards.

If a person is unable to use the diaphragm properly as their primary muscle of inhalation, they have to overuse the secondary muscles which open the chest cavity to draw in the vital air they need. This can lead to a range of musculoskeletal problems in the neck and shoulders, which may not obviously be related to a dysfunctional breathing pattern.

It is only possible to reach the diaphragm with manual techniques along part of its anterior border by working under the ribs and xiphoid process. This is a useful technique which can help release fascial tension here and can have a neuromuscular effect on the whole muscle. *(See photo 13.)*

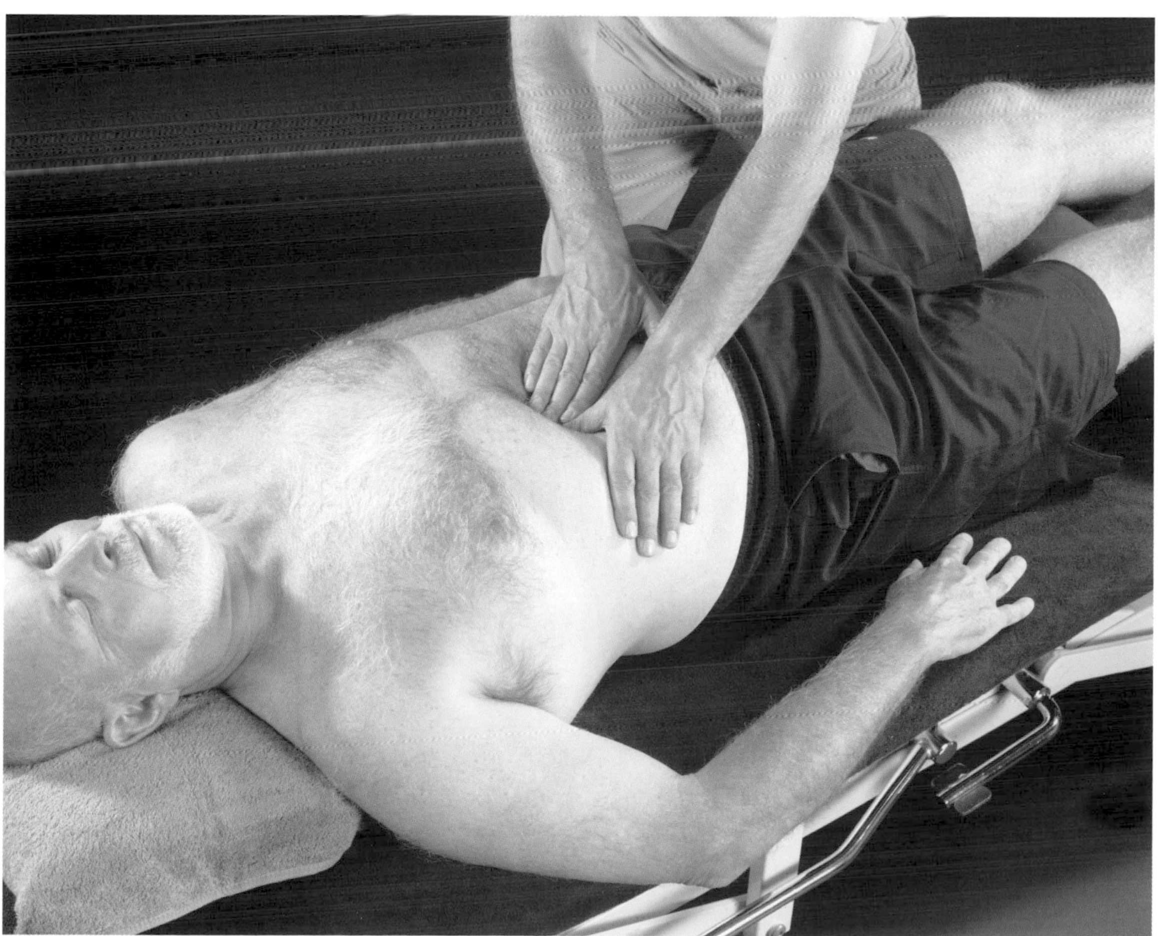

Photo 13. Using a supported thumb, work beneath the costal border to reach the anterior border of the diaphragm.

Abdomen

As well as moving and controlling trunk movement, the abdominal muscles have an important role in supporting the viscera. General muscle weakness gives poor support and allows the heavy viscera to distend, and this shifts the body's centre of gravity forward. The same thing happens with overweight people, with the increased size of the abdomen stretching and weakening the muscles. To counterbalance this they have to lean into a sway-back posture with an increased lumbar lordosis, and numerous other musculoskeletal issues can result from this.

The abdomen muscles also control the pressure in the abdominal cavity and this plays a vital part in respiration. The muscles need to relax slightly during inhalation to reduce the visceral pressure and allow the diaphragm to move down. In forced exhalation, the abdominal muscles need to contract strongly to increase the pressure and force the diaphragm upwards more quickly to expel the carbon dioxide.

These muscles need to be able to subtly control tension and they rarely need to apply high maximum strength in any normal daily activity. The common problem we often see is with overly strengthened abdominals (the 'six-pack'). Developing strength through strong exercise increases the muscle tension which can restrict the diaphragm. When this happens, breathing patterns change and more movement has to take place in the upper chest instead. Even though the client is unlikely to be aware of any respiratory dysfunction, this may contribute to musculoskeletal issues in the neck and shoulders. Of course, a restricted diaphragm will also reduce the amount of oxygen the client can take in when attempting aerobic exercise.

Weakness and poor function in the abdominal muscles are very common indeed and this is directly caused by lifestyle. The body is potentially very lazy, and if a muscle does not have to work then it won't. Sitting in a chair does not require the action of the abdominal muscles to support the torso in an upright position. Doing this for many hours every day means these muscles will eventually weaken and lose tone through lack of use. Powerful abdomen exercises may make the muscles stronger, but this will not help them perform the fine control they need for their vital postural and respiratory roles.

Although massage is generally beneficial for muscular weakness, it will not make the muscles any stronger: exercise, weight loss or breathing exercises are needed for this. But with excessive muscle tension and overuse strain, deep massage is both necessary and effective.

Pain in the abdomen could be caused by either a muscular or a visceral problem. In the case of a muscular injury the client will normally be able to report a physical incident which may have caused it, although this is not always the case.

To differentiate between the two, with the client lying supine, the therapist should carefully palpate the area to identify where the pain is and then apply a gentle pressure into it to cause a mild discomfort. Keeping this pressure constant, the client should attempt to raise and lower their head. This slightly contracts the abdominal muscles and, if the problem is muscular, the feeling of pain will increase. If they feel no change in the painful area, this suggests there may be a visceral problem and referral to a doctor may be advisable.

The abdominal muscles can be strained through overuse in heavy exercise and, in the post-acute stage, deep massage will be beneficial in improving recovery as well as preventing the formation of scar tissue and adhesions. But deep techniques are difficult to perform as the soft underlying viscera will absorb the pressure of the stroke. To overcome this, the client should lift their head slightly off the couch to mildly contract the muscles. This makes them firm so they can be more effectively treated. This should only be done for about 10 seconds at a time so the client can rest and not add any further strain.

In remedial massage therapy, the abdomen is probably not treated nearly as often as it should be. Not only does this area play an important role in posture, stability and respiration it can also help other systems of the body too. It can improve visceral motility and aid digestion. The area is very rich in blood vessels, so massage here can have a good effect on the general circulation. On a psycho-emotional level, abdomen massage can sometimes be profoundly effective also.

The abdominal muscles get severely stretched during pregnancy and need to recover carefully after childbirth, and sometimes the linea alba between the rectus abdominis on either side does not reunite fully. Severe overweight issues will also stretch these muscles and massage alone can do little to help this.

The large **rectus abdominis** muscles run down the front of the abdomen, attaching at the costal cartilages of the fifth to seventh ribs and xiphoid process and go down to insert into the pubic crest. The muscle is divided by thick bands of fascia into a series of up to six muscular pockets. These enable it to contract with an inward curl which allows the lumbar vertebral joints to flex. The pair of muscles are fixed together down the centre with a very strong band of fascia: the linea alba. On the lateral borders, it connects through strong fascia into the transverse and oblique abdominal muscles. *(See fig. 41 overleaf.)*

Although the rectus abdominis is usually described as lumbar flexor, this is not something it has to do very much of in normal daily activities. When flexing from an upright standing position, the muscle may initiate the movement but then gravity takes over the job. It does, however, have to work powerfully to flex the torso when lying in a supine position (doing a sit-up), but that is something usually only done in an exercise environment. In normal daily life, we do not need great strength from this muscle but good fine-control is vital.

The most important postural function of this muscle is to control pelvic alignment by maintaining the right distance between the ribs above and the pubic crest below. If the rectus abdominis is weak and stretched, the pelvis will drop down at the front causing an anterior pelvic tilt which also increases the lumbar lordosis. Through the sacroiliac joint, it changes the alignment of the sacrum and the fifth lumbar vertebrae above it. This compresses the posterior part of the L5/S1 disc and causes disc degeneration and sciatic nerve impingement. *(See photo 14 overleaf.)*

Abdominal wall

Wrapping around the outside of the abdomen are three very thin layers of muscle which are extremely strong due to their large surface area. They are all connected together with the rectus abdominis at the front by strong fascia to create a single continuous wall around the body. These muscles also connect to the ribcage at the top and the pelvic girdle below.

The **external obliques** run from the outer surface of the fifth to twelfth ribs, as well as the serratus anterior and part of the latissimus dorsi.

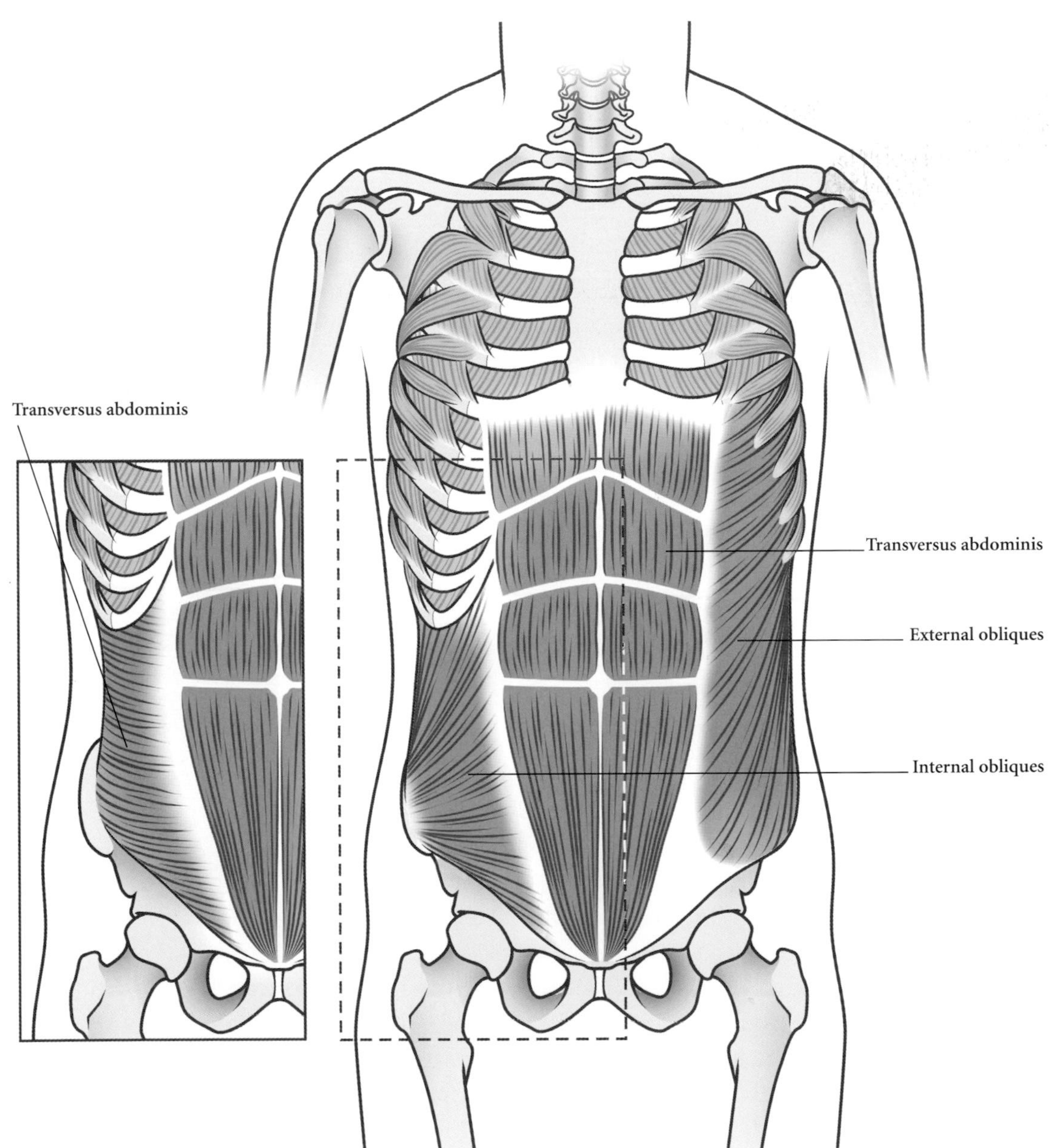

Fig. 41. Abdominal muscles

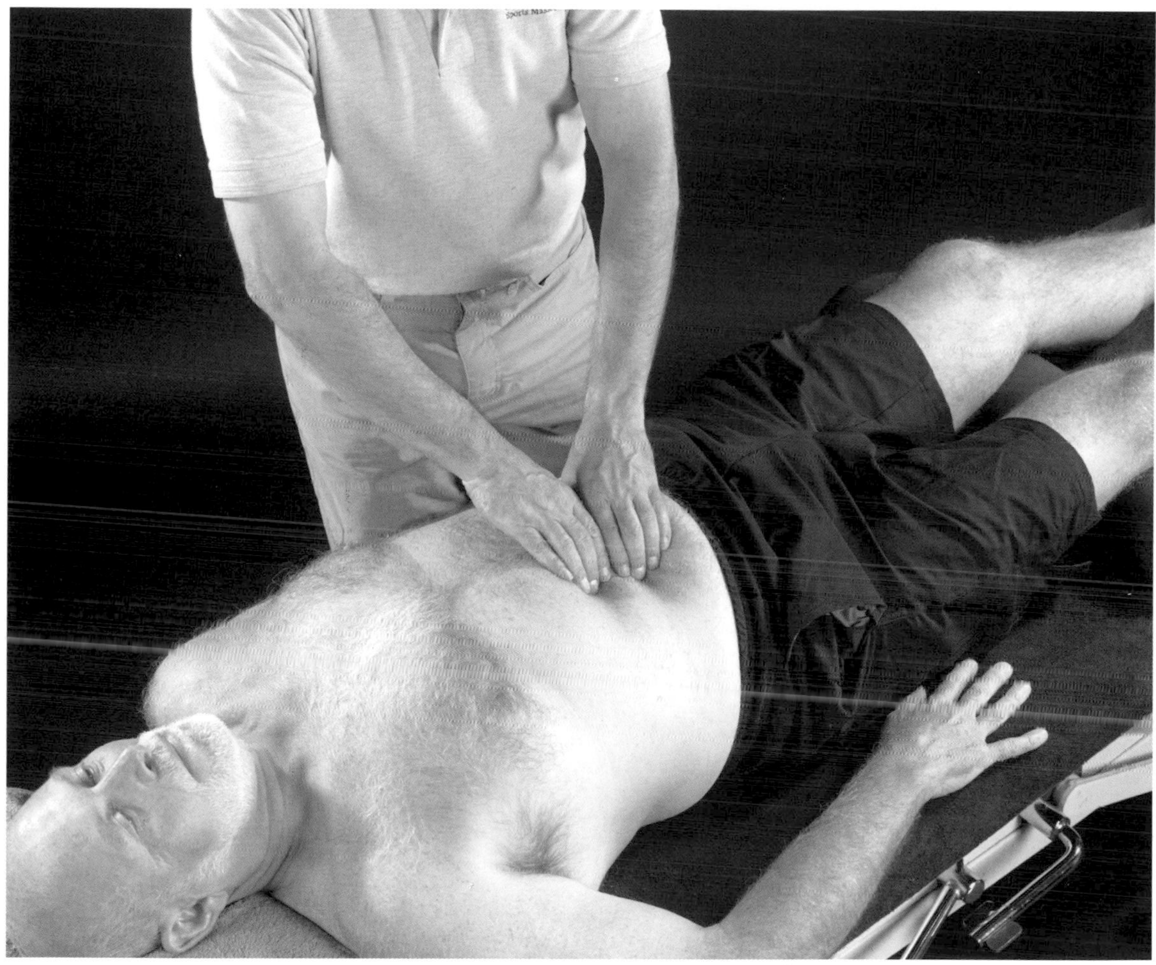

Photo 14. The rectus abdominis can be picked out from the rest of the abdominal wall and treated with a variety of massage techniques.

The fibres go diagonally downwards towards the front of the body and insert along the abdominal aponeurosis and iliac crest. These are the main muscles involved in trunk rotation.

The **internal obliques** originate from the thoracolumbar fascia and iliac crest. The lower fibres run horizontally, but the majority go diagonally upwards inserting along the abdominal aponeurosis and costal cartilage. Although these are involved in rotation, they also assist the rectus abdominis in trunk flexion.

These muscles create all ventral, flexion and rotational movements of the lower torso and are in almost constant use when standing and moving. They are very important postural muscles also, maintaining stability between the ribcage and the pelvic girdle as well as supporting the viscera.

When the client is in a supine position, the costal borders of the ribcage below the sternum should be at about a 45-degree angle with the midline of the body. If the ribcage is lower on one side and less than 45 degrees, it usually means the external obliques are short and tight on this side. If the ribcage is raised more than 45 degrees, it usually means the internal obliques are short and tight.

These are difficult muscles to treat with basic massage as the pressure of the strokes sink through them into the soft viscera beneath them. Fascial techniques are the most effective, especially when applied to the attachments along the costal borders and iliac crest.

The deepest muscle layer in the abdominal wall is the **transversus abdominis**. It emerges mainly from the thoracolumbar fascia but has upper attachments with the seventh to twelfth ribs and lower attachments along the iliac crest. All the fibres run transversely around the body towards their attachment with the abdominal aponeurosis.

The transversus does not directly make any skeletal movements, but by creating a contractile band around the torso it controls the pressure in the abdominal cavity. This plays a vital role in respiration. When breathing in, the muscle has to slightly relax to reduce the pressure and allow the diaphragm to lower. When exhaling, the transversus contracts to increase the pressure which pushes the diaphragm back up again to expel air.

Each of these abdominal muscles must be able to apply fine control, contracting and relaxing independently but in harmony with each other. It is very hard to isolate these when doing exercises, and it is too easy to develop basic strength without any real control.

When placing a very high demand on the muscles, when doing a sit-up exercise for example, all the muscles have to contract maximally together, and then they all relax together at the end. But this does nothing to develop the postural and functional fine control they need and can have an adverse effect on them.

Pelvic floor

Although quite small in size, the muscles of the **pelvic floor** are extremely important. *(See fig. 42.)* Together they attach all the way round the pelvic girdle from the coccyx and ilium to the pubis. It makes a complete seal around the bottom of the torso and acts as a sling which works statically to support the weight of all the visceral contents above it. There are sphincter muscles within the pelvic floor which control rectal and urinary functions. There are thick layers of very strong fascia across the upper and lower surfaces of the muscles which provide much of the pelvic floor's static strength.

These muscles, and more significantly the fascia, can get severely stretched during pregnancy and require good recovery afterwards. The muscles can get injured in falls and accidents, they can also be influenced by structural issues with the pelvic girdle.

Although weakness and poor tone are thought to be a common problem affecting the pelvic floor, strong exercising can lead to hypertonicity instead. If the muscle is tight and continually over-contracting, it rises up and this compresses the bladder which can lead to incontinence issues.

Deep anterior hip

The **psoas major** is a large, deep, strong muscle which runs down through the centre of the body. The upper part has its origins along the lateral part of all the vertebrae from T12 down to L4, and this helps stabilise the lumbar spine. From there, the middle section extends anteriorly to go around the front of the ilium. Although it does not directly attach to the bone here, it does bind strongly to it through the fascia, and so it does move the ilium and assists pelvic alignment. The lower part of the muscle curls back posteriorly to insert into the lesser trochanter,

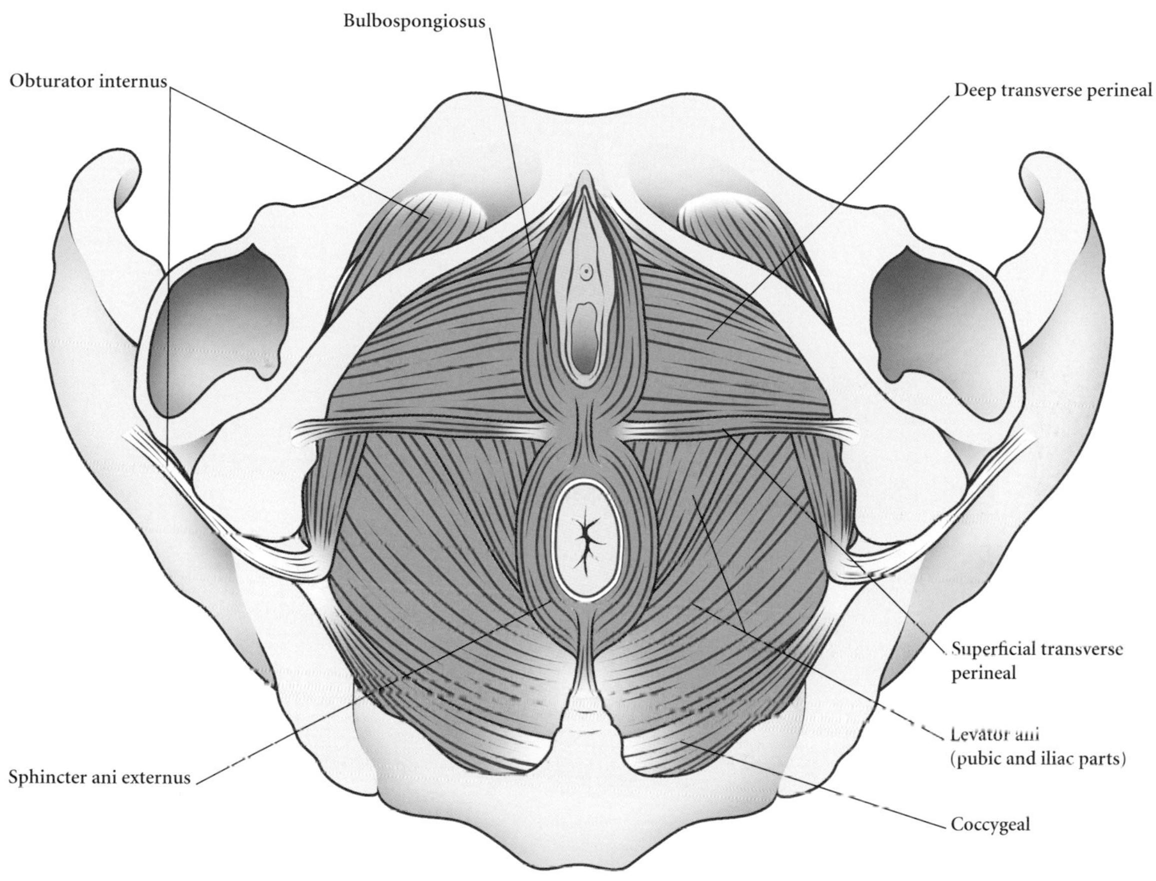

Fig. 42. Pelvic floor muscles (female)

and this is a powerful hip flexor which also assists inward rotation. It also controls the position of the head of the femur in the hip joint. The **psoas minor** is only found in about half the population, and is just a slightly separate strip of muscle along the lateral border of the major muscle. *(See figs. 43 and 44 overleaf.)*

Because it is involved in several actions, it is often affected by lower back, pelvis or hip issues. It is rarely a source of pain but commonly becomes short and hypertonic especially in people with excessive lumbar lordosis. As well as performing poorly in hip flexion, this tension can also restrict hip extension and cause the hamstrings to suffer overuse problems as they try to overcome this.

Hypertonicity in the psoas can inhibit and reduce strength in the quadratus lumborum, which can lead to back injury. Sometimes just releasing tension in the psoas can resolve back pain, so this muscle should always be considered.

Imbalance between the psoas muscles on either side of the body is quite common. This

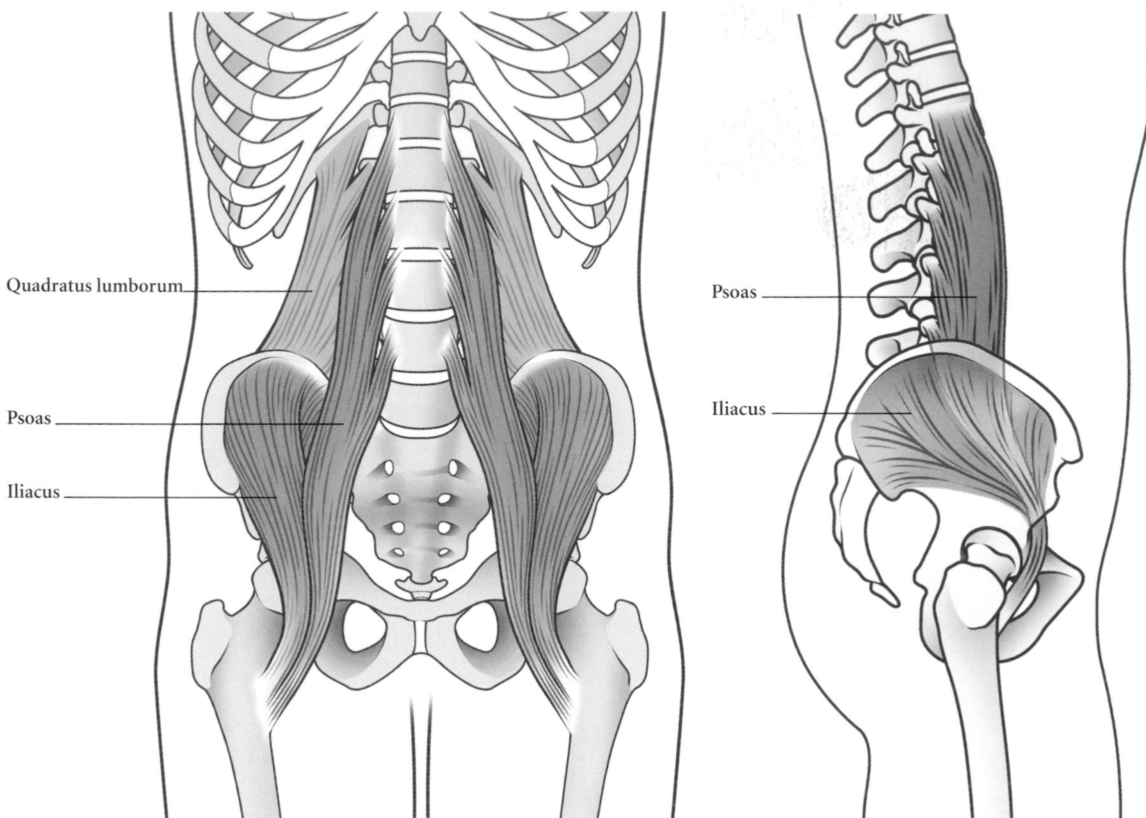

Fig. 43. Deep hip muscles – anterior view

Fig. 44. Deep hip muscles – lateral view

can cause a leg-length discrepancy and/or a postural twist through the torso.

The psoas is a difficult muscle to reach and requires great care to treat. The upper part lies deep beneath the visceral organs and is impossible to palpate safely, and the lower part going to the lesser trochanter is also too deep to reach. Only the middle part is accessible where it comes closer to the surface as it goes round the front of the ilium, but here it lies directly underneath the colon which should be avoided.

With the client supine with their hip and knee flexed, the therapist should slowly apply a downward stroke along the inside of the ilium, starting just above the anterior superior iliac spine. It requires considerable pressure to push down almost to the level of the spine to get past the colon and the client may find this difficult to receive. If they tense up in response to this, the therapist should slightly ease off the pressure and have the client take a deep breath in. When they then breathe out and relax, the pressure can be increased comfortably at the same time.

When the correct depth has been reached, the pressure should be applied inwards behind the colon to reach the psoas. To check that the muscle has been reached effectively, the client should try to lift their leg and the therapist will feel the muscle fibres contract under their fingers. If the muscle is hypertonic, this action will cause considerable pain and they may find it impossible

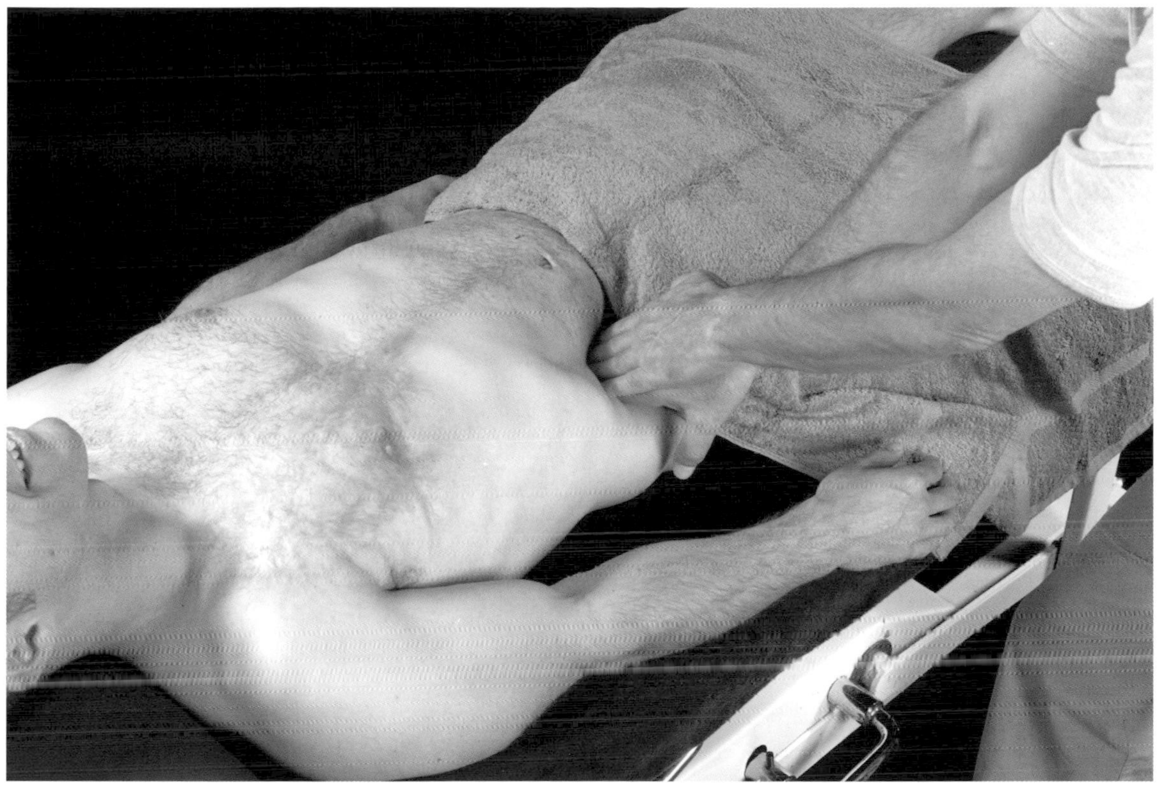

Photo 15. It is necessary to press down along the inside of the ilium to get pass the colon before pushing medially to reach the psoas. To confirm this, if the client attempts to raise their leg, the therapist should feel the muscle contract beneath their fingers.

to make any movement. (*See photo 15.*) The whole muscle cannot be treated with massage techniques because only the mid-part can be reached where it comes anterially around the front of the ilium, so neuromuscular techniques have to be used instead. To reduce hypertonicity, Positional Release is very effective, and MET is a good way of stretching it if it is tight.

The **iliacus** is a broad muscle with its origin on the anterior surface of the ilium, and it merges into a common tendon with the psoas to insert into the lesser trochanter. Crossing the front of the hip, it is a primary flexor of the joint. It is difficult to reach with massage techniques, but it is possible to treat the anterior part if done slowly and carefully.

Posterior Neck and Torso

Neck

Deep in the nape of the neck is a group of small **capitis** muscles which all attach between the occipital bone and the atlas and axis at the top of the spine. They are all bound within a thick fascia, and the muscles work together to raise and turn the head. They are very small muscles which should only be used for fine-control movements of the head. But people who hold their head in a forward potion have to maintain a strong isometric contraction with these muscles to hold the head upright. Hours of driving can add to this because it also requires constant small head rotations as well. *(See fig. 45.)*

Chronic tension, stiffness and pain can gradually build up here and may contribute to headaches. Deep fascial strokes and neuromuscular techniques may be painful here, but they are very effective. *(See photos 16, 17 and 18.)*

Back

The **deep spinal muscles** form a complex network of muscles running along the sides of the spine. At its deepest level, the **rotator longus** and **brevis** muscles cross between the spinous and transverse processes of the adjacent vertebrae. These create small extension and rotational movement between the bones. The **intertransverse** muscles are also very small and attach between the transverse processes of adjacent vertebrae. There is one set in the neck between C1 and T1 and another set in the lower back between T12 and L5. They close the gap between the transverse processes so creating side-bending. A set of very small **interspinalis** muscles link between the spinous processes from C1 to T3 and another set from T11 to L5, and they extend the spinal joints.

These are all very small muscles which create very intricate inter-vertebral movements, and they can be strained if they make these movements when carrying or moving a heavy load.

The **multifidus** muscle is made up of a large number of small parallel segments which each

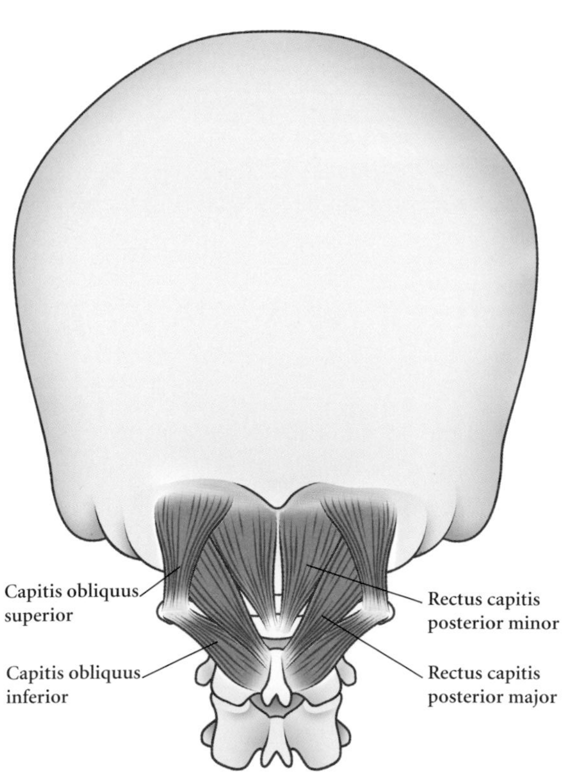

Fig. 45. Deep neck muscles

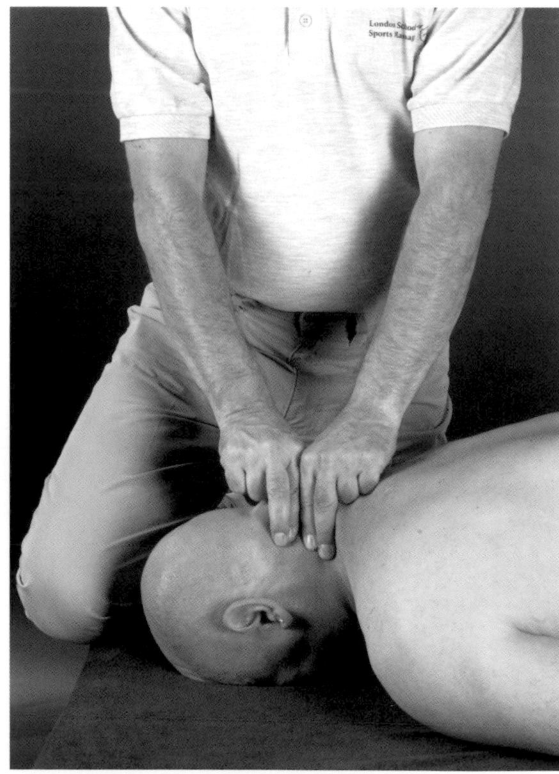

Photo 16. With one knee on the couch, the therapist's body weight is more central over the client, making it much easier to apply friction and other techniques to the posterior neck muscles.

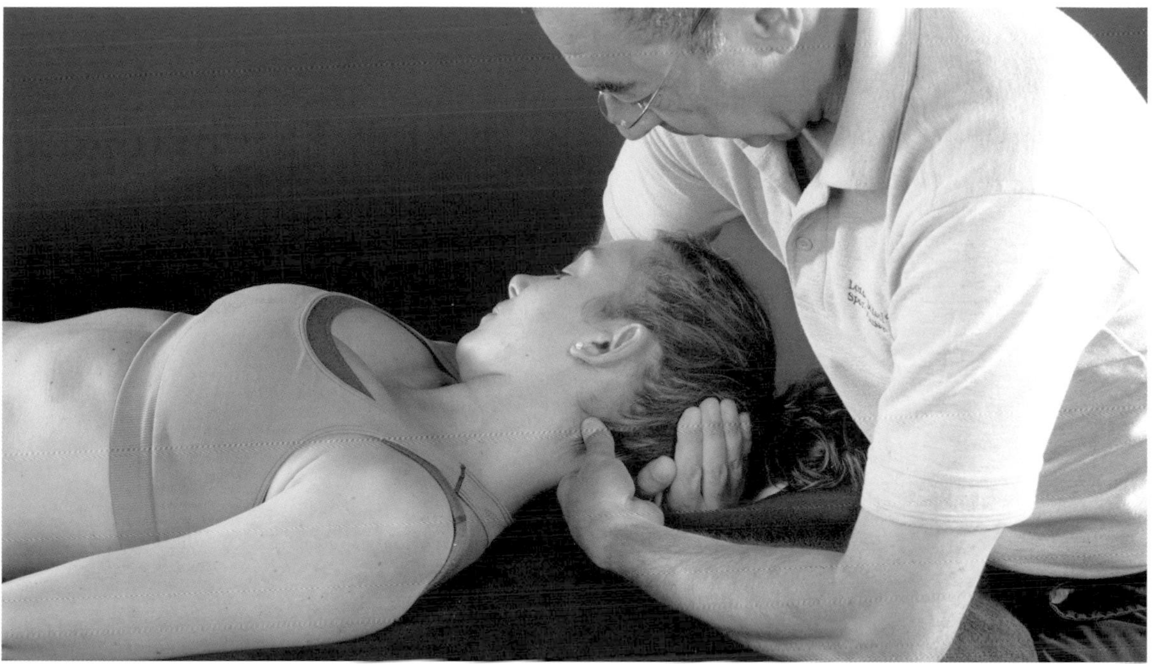

Photo 17. With the client's head firmly supported in a rotated position in the therapist's arm; friction, neuromuscular and myofascial techniques can be applied very effectively to the muscles deep in the nape of the neck.

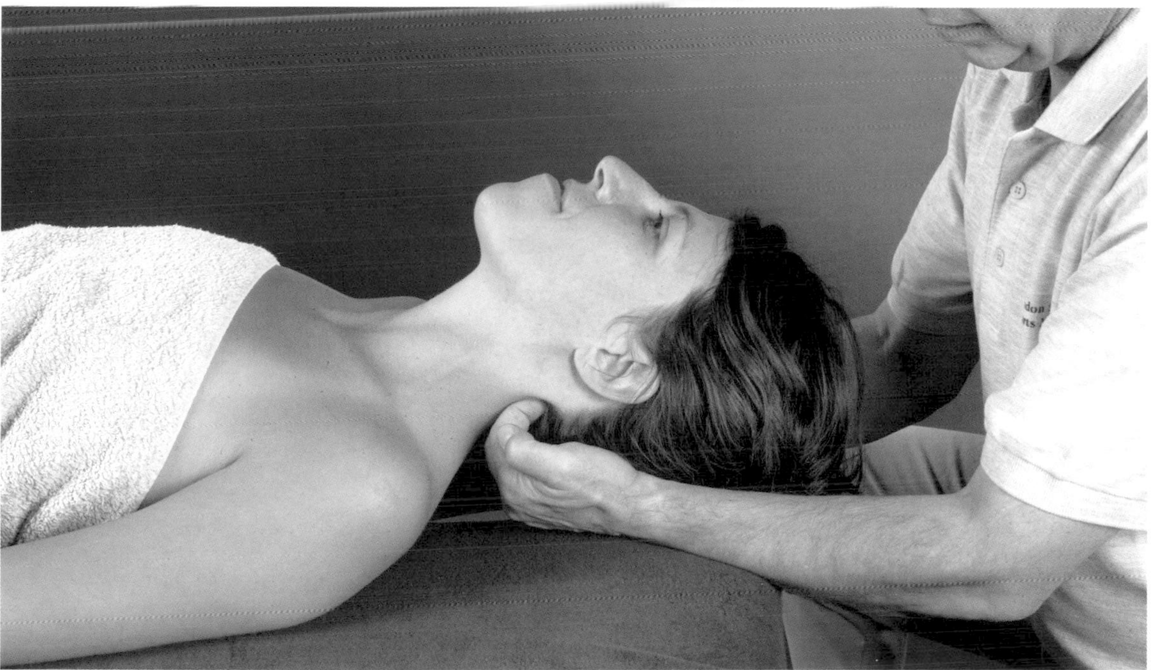

Photo 18. The therapist first pushes the cervical spine up to curl the head back and shorten all the posterior neck muscles. It is then easier to apply deep techniques to the muscles along the cervical spine and occipital ridge.

link from the body of one vertebra to the spinous process four to seven vertebrae above it. It does this from the sacrum all the way up to the cervical spine but is much more developed in the lumbar section where more strength is needed. It locks the vertebrae together and stabilises segments of spine. *(See fig. 46 & photo 19.)*

The **spinalis cervicis** muscles link between the upper C1–3 spinous processes and C6–7. They extend the cervical spine and become short and tight with excessive lordosis in people who hold their heads in a forward position.

The **semispinalis capitis** attaches from the transverse processes of C3 to T6 and inserts at

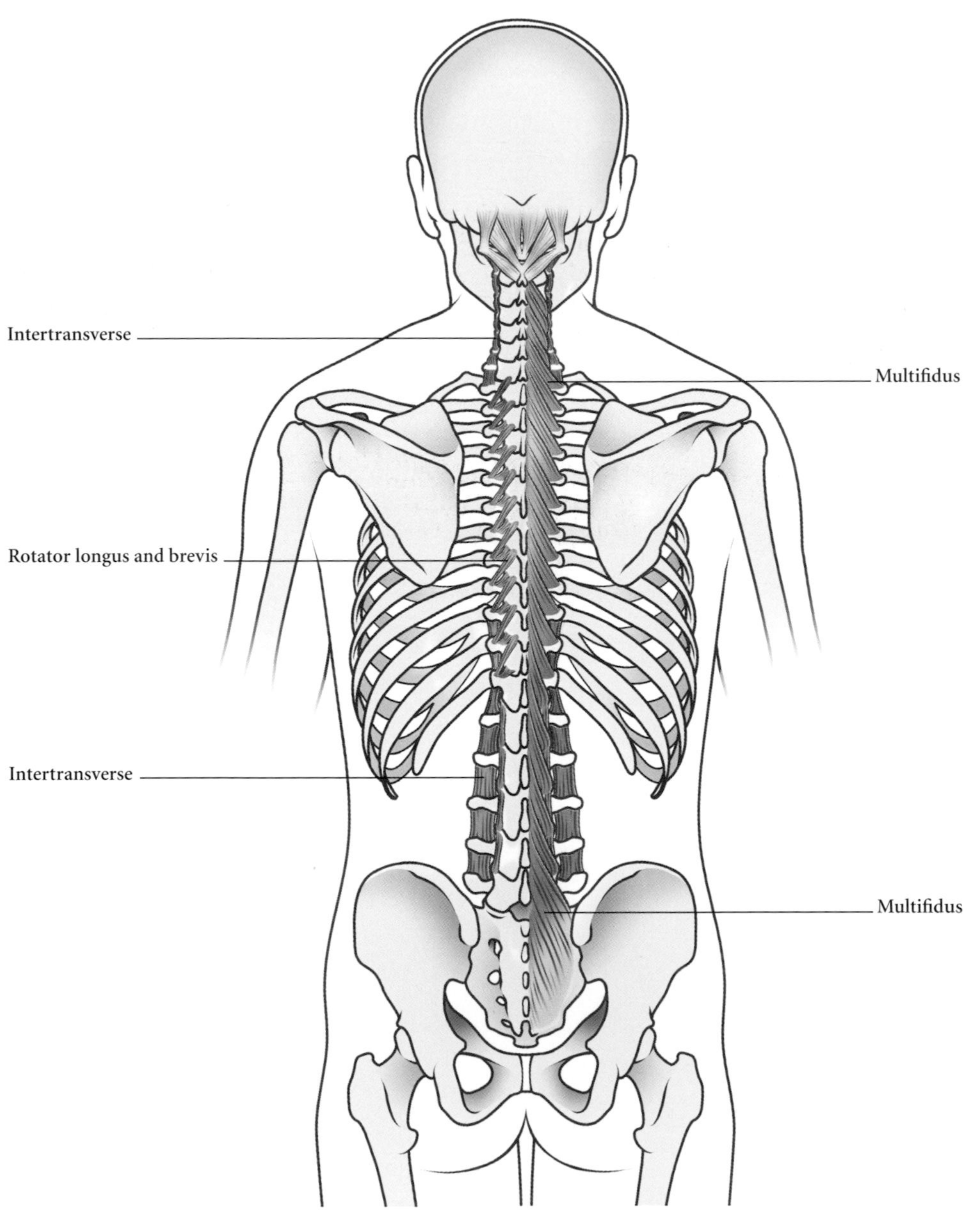

Fig. 46. Deepest spinal muscles

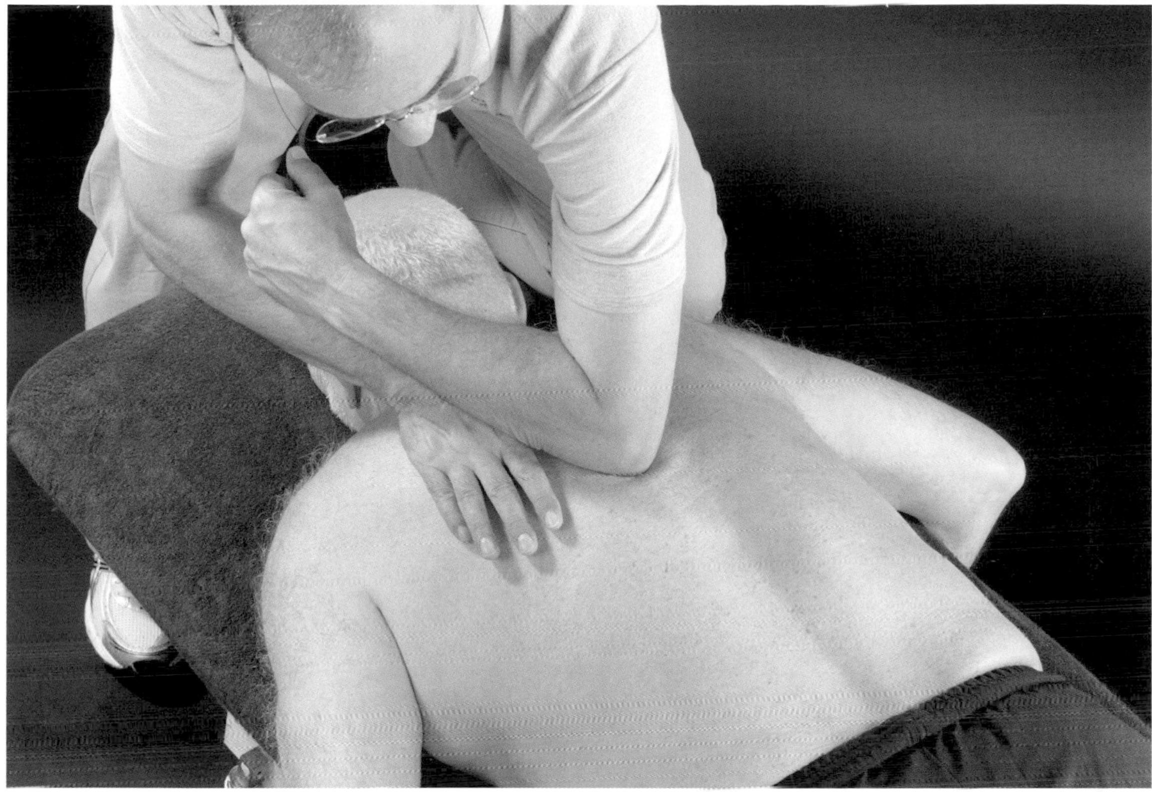

Photo 19. The deep spinal muscles can be treated with the elbow, but this must be done very slowly and carefully. Having the knee on the couch brings the therapist's body-weight forward over the client which makes this easier, and the other hand can be used to control the elbow.

the occipital ridge. It is a powerful neck extension. The semispinalis cervicis and thoracic attach from T1–10 and insert at the spinous processes C2–T4 and have more of a stabilising function, as they fix the upper thoracic and cervical spine in position.

The **spinalis thoracic** is a fairly large muscle which links between the upper 7 thoracic vertebrae and T11–L3. It extends the thoracic spine, but there is very limited range in this direction and its main role is to work statically to resist the gravitational force which encourages the torso to flex.

With increased thoracic curvature and protracted head positions, this muscle becomes stretched and the loading on it is greatly increased. This causes micro-trauma, and the muscle lengthens and becomes chronically tense. Although massage can effectively relieve the painful symptoms temporarily, they will quickly return in this postural situation.

The **splenius capitis** attaches from C7–T4 spinous processes, inserting at the occipital ridge by the mastoid process. The **cervicis** goes from T3–T6 and inserts at C1–2 transverse process. These extend, rotate and side-bend the neck and head.

The **longissimus** and **iliocostalis** are a complex network of muscles running laterally along the spine from the sacrum, connecting to

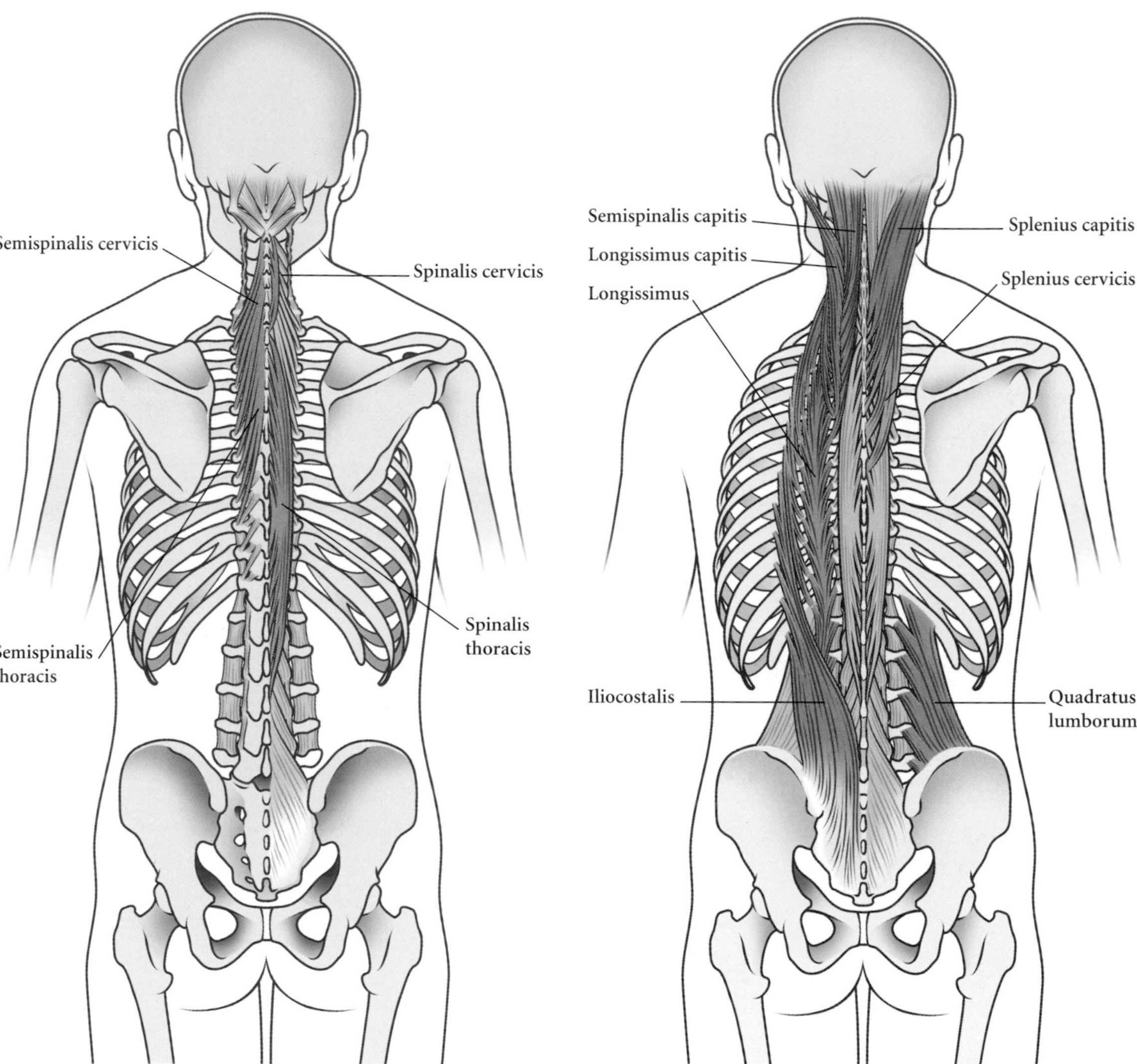

Fig. 47. Deep spinal muscles

Fig. 48. Spinal muscles

all the vertebrae and ribs with its final insertion at the mastoid process. They work actively to extend and side-bend the spine and help rotate the head. They also work statically to maintain spinal alignment (*see figs. 47 and 48*).

Collectively, all these muscles running along either side of the spine are called the **erector spinae** group, and they work together to create all extension and assist side-bending and rotation. Each muscle has its own unique function within the group, but this is often compromised through fascial restriction and so myofascial techniques aimed at releasing and separating them can be very effective. *(See photos 20–23.)*

The muscles along each side of the spine are interdependent with each other. Chronic tension on one side will restrict and inhibit the function of the muscles on the other side. Almost nobody has a perfectly straight vertical spine, with the erector spinae muscles evenly matched along both sides. Natural imbalances develop as the body adapts to a physical lifestyle. Movements predominate from one side of the body and so it is natural to find greater strength on one side of the spine in some sections. This may be counterbalanced by greater strength on the other side of the spine at the next level. These naturally developing imbalances can cause slight bends and twists along the spine.

The body can cope with a small degree of this asymmetry without it causing any problems. So when observing the spine and erector spinae muscles it would be wrong to consider trying to correct every apparent imbalance. It is good to work more deeply to release tighter areas and so help prevent potential problems developing, but deep remedial techniques should only be applied to areas that are likely to be contributing to a specific problem.

When the head is held in a forward position, the thoracic spine becomes fixed in an excessive kyphotic curve. The erector spinae muscles here have to work hard in a static and lengthened position to counterbalance the weight of the head extending in front of the body. Over time the muscles become tense and stiff. As well as causing chronic muscle pain, this thoracic restriction can also affect respiration. And the lack of thoracic mobility very commonly leads to overuse

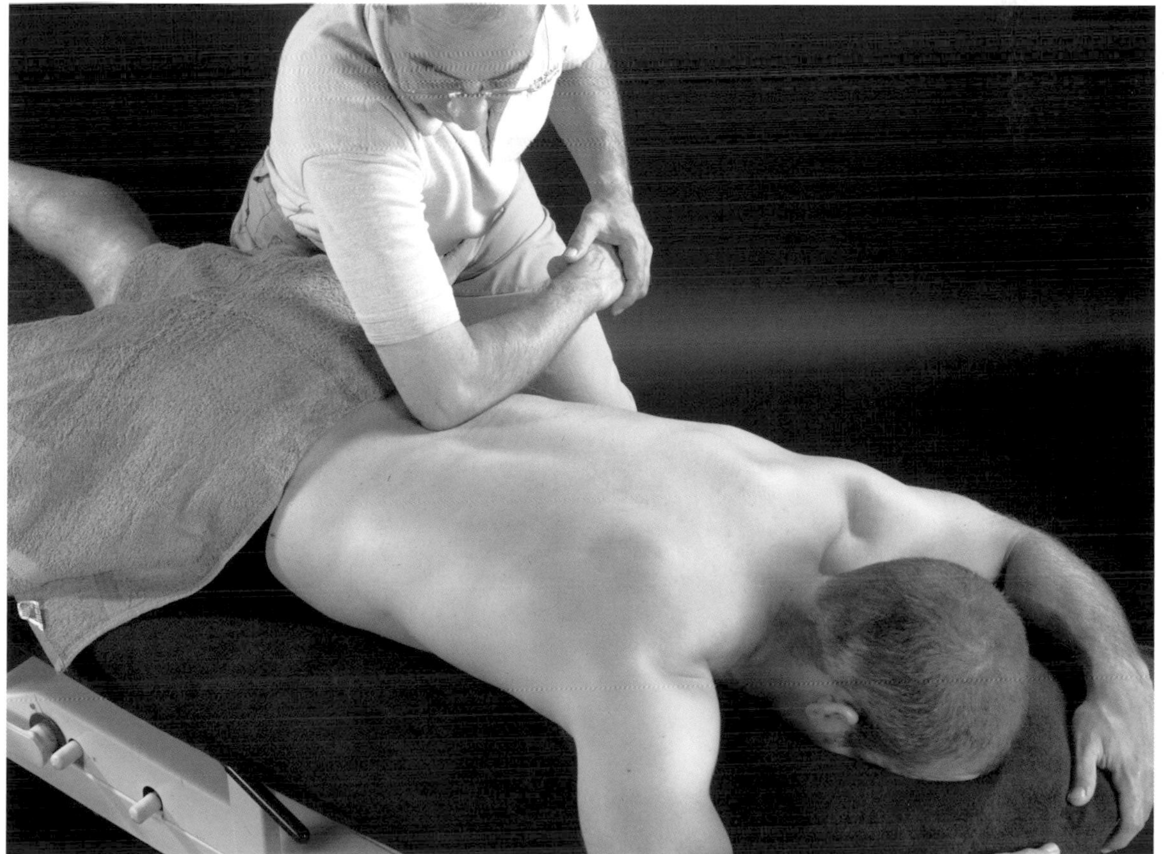

Photo 20. Treating the lower back muscles with the upper forearm and elbow.

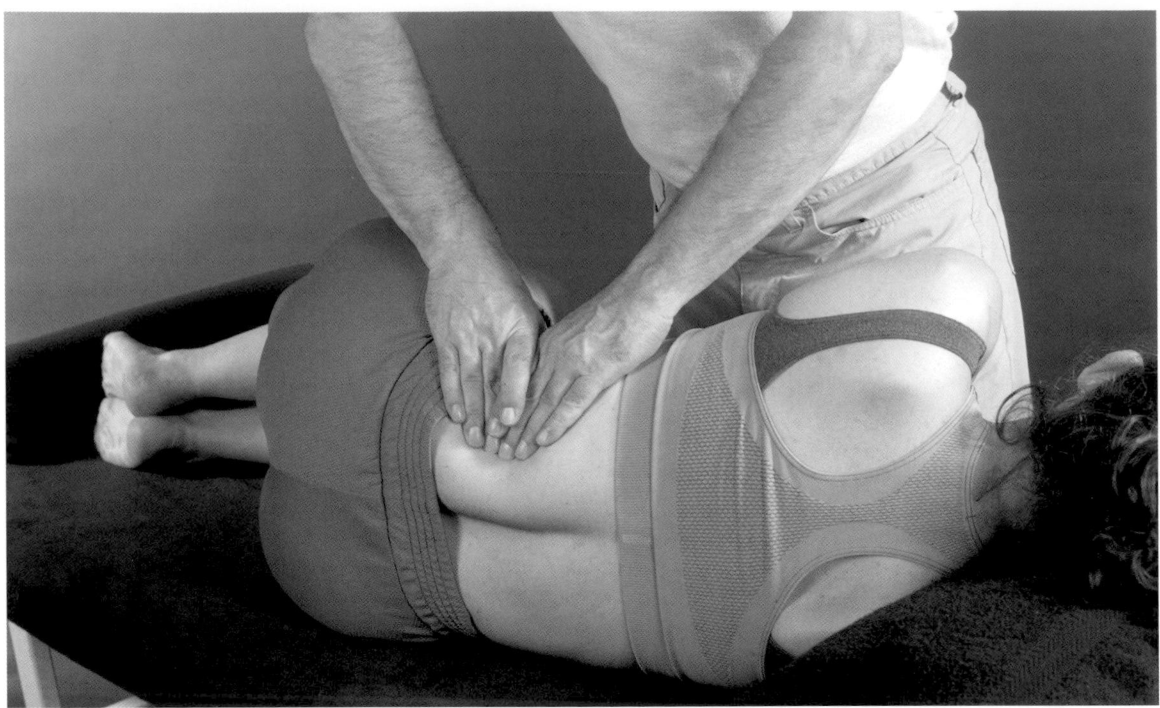

Photo 21. In the side-lying position, deep techniques can work behind the superficial muscles to reach the deep spinal muscles in the lower back.

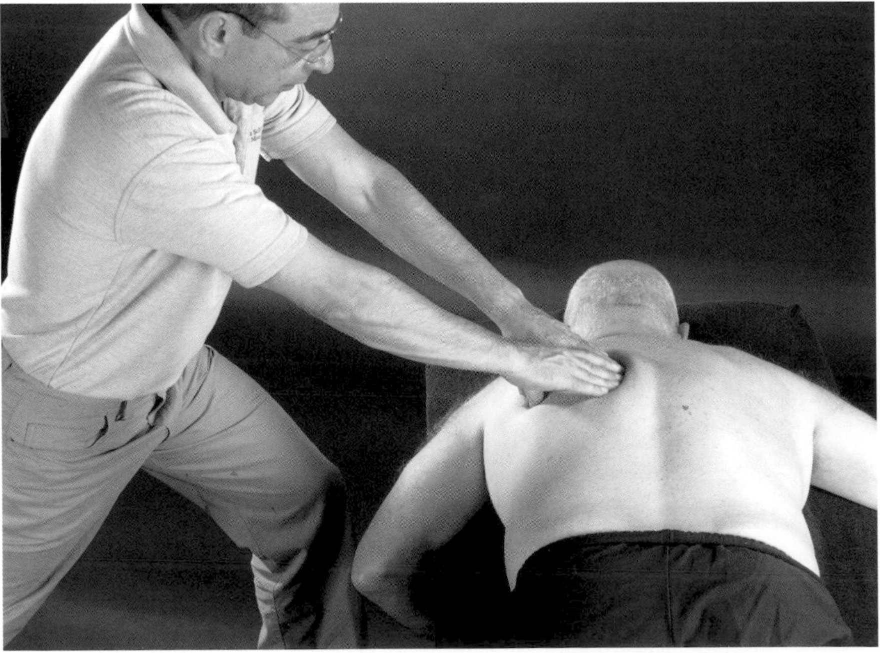

Photo 22. Deep friction applied to the lateral border of the rector spinae muscles.

problems in the neck, shoulders or lower back as these sections have to make up for the deficiency.

With increased lumbar lordosis, the erector spinae muscles here become chronically short and tight because they have to continually hold a strong short contraction to pull the spine back into its increased curve. Weak abdominal muscles mean they have to work even harder to support the torso, and excessive body-weight can add considerably to this. Chronic pain and sometimes spasm can occur here with an increased risk of acute strain when doing normal physical activities.

Deep in the lower back, the **quadratus lumborum** muscle attaches from the iliac crest diagonally up to insert into the bottom rib and transverse processes of the first four lumbar vertebrae. It holds down the ribcage during inhalation and also assists in side-bending the lumbar spine. When bending forward, the muscles work bilaterally to assist and stabilise trunk extension.

Where there is excessive lumbar lordosis, and/or long periods of sitting with the lumbar spine resting in this position the muscle will become short and tight. In this situation, chronic pain is common and acute injury becomes more likely in normal daily activity.

To reach the quadratus lumborum, the therapist has to get beneath the many lower back

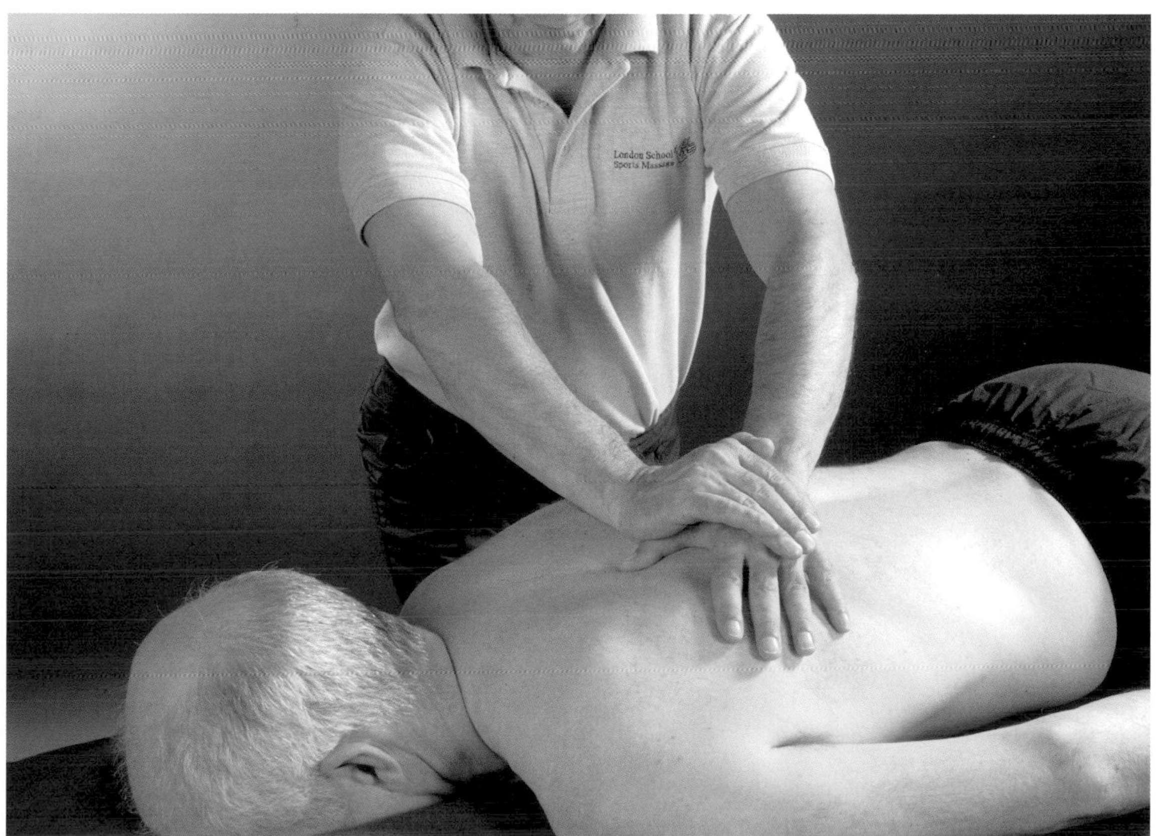

Photo 23. Protect thumb technique applied transversely across the erector spinae muscles.

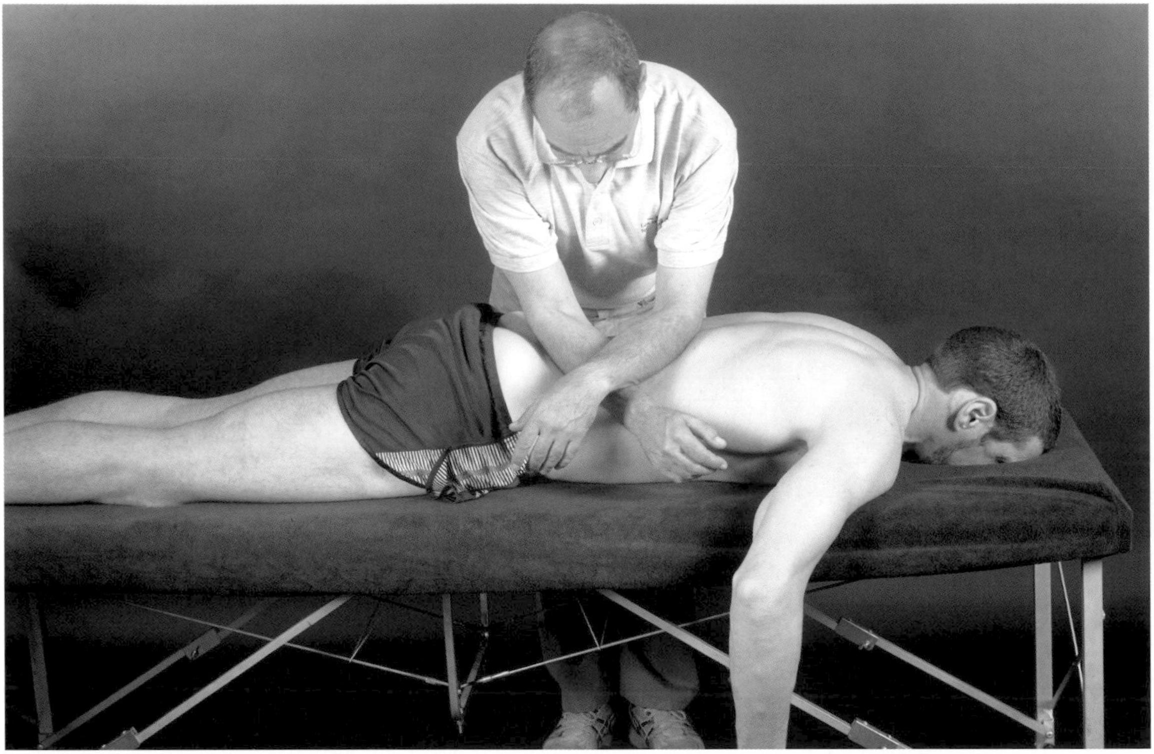

Photos 24 (above) and 25 (below). Using the forearms to apply stretching strokes along the back muscles.

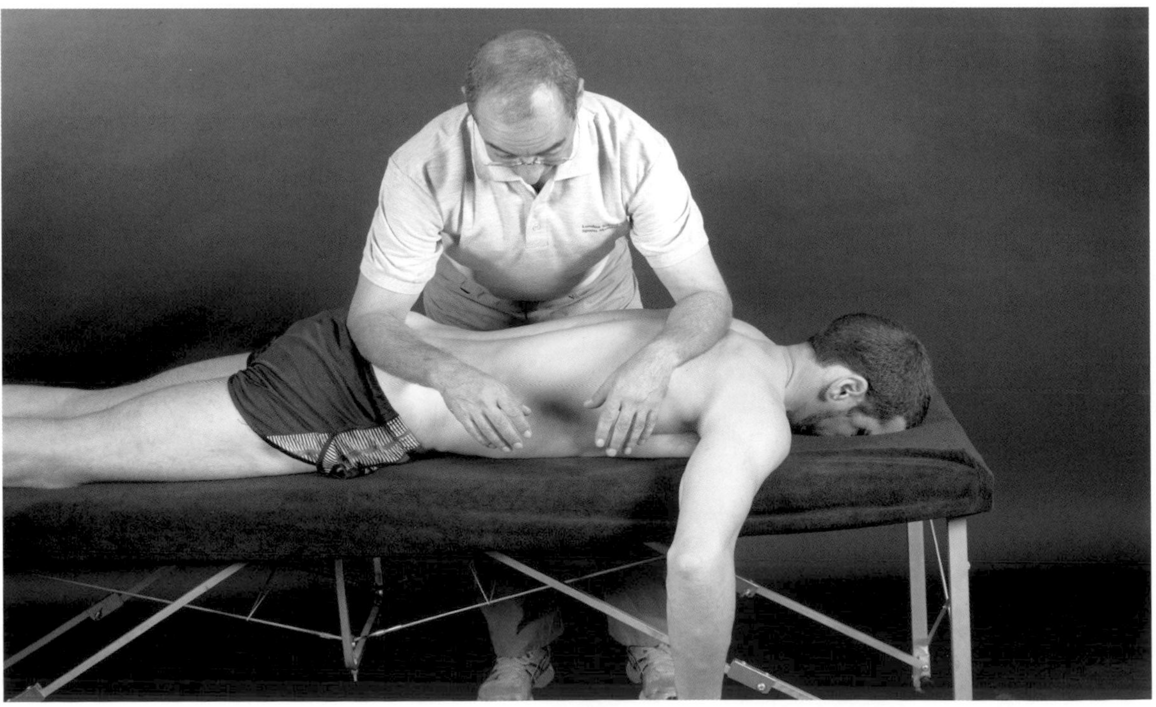

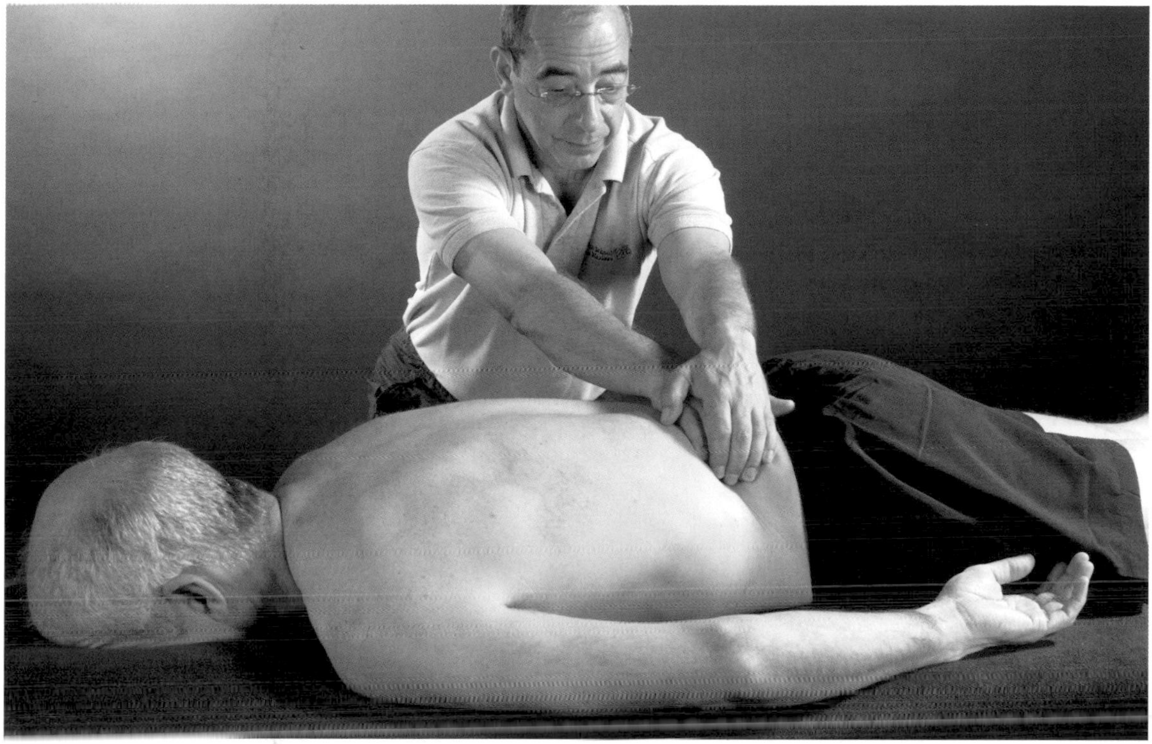

Photo 26. Applying a pull-back stroke to reach the quadratus lumborum. The therapist can lock onto the muscle and use their legs to rock their body back and forth to achieve a very deep friction into the muscle.

muscles which overlay it. This can be done by working in from the side with the clients in either prone or side-lying positions. *(See photos 26, 27 and 28.)*

The **rhomboid major** and **minor** muscles are found between the shoulder blades. They attach from the spinous processes of C6 to T4 and insert all the way along the medial border of the scapula. Their function is to hold the scapula down on the thoracic wall and move it medially towards the spine. It is an important stabiliser of the scapula and works reciprocally with its antagonist, the serratus anterior to do this. *(See fig. 49 overleaf.)*

In the protracted shoulder posture, the rhomboids are usually weak and overstretched and this can give the appearance of 'winged' scapula. Part of the weakness is due to reciprocal inhibition from opposing muscle tension across the front of the chest and this must be addressed first, otherwise the rhomboids cannot improve their tone. These muscles rarely need deep techniques to stretch them and usually require strengthening instead.

Between the neck and shoulder is the **levator scapula**, which attaches from the C1 to C4 transverse processes and inserts into the superior angle of the scapula. It lifts the scapula and also acts as a fixator, holding the scapula up when the arm is being weighed down. It becomes chronically tight in people who hunch up their shoulders or carry things on one shoulder or arm all the time.

With a forward head posture, the levator scapula and the other posterior neck muscles get considerably overworked. The levator scapula

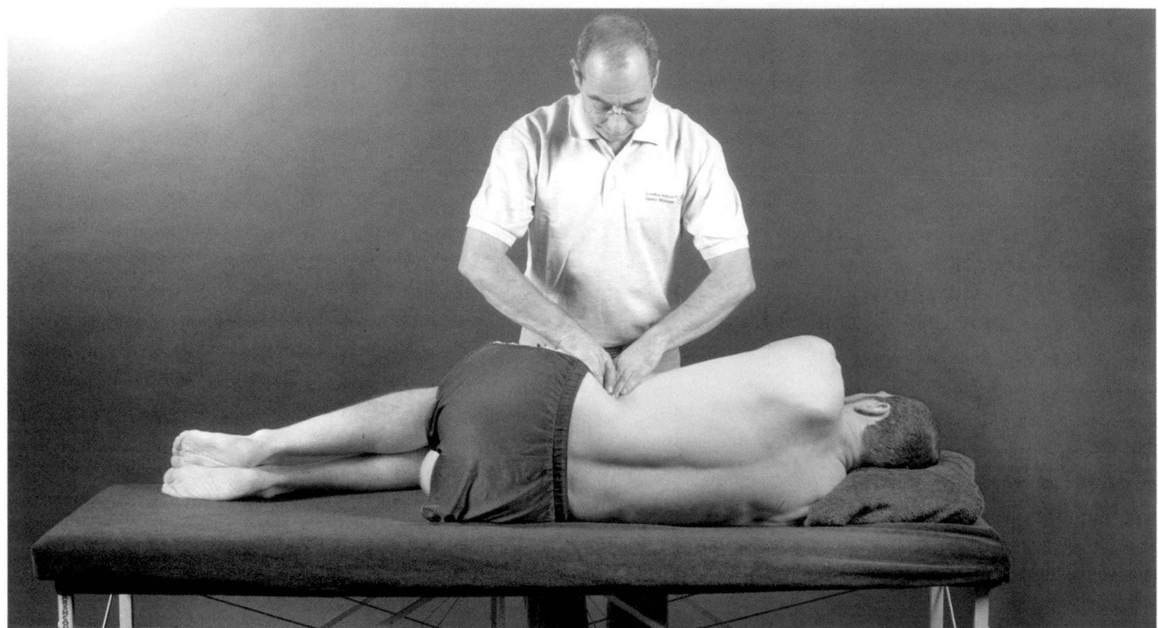

Photo 27. In a side-lying position, deep strokes can reach the quadratus lumborum beneath the overlying back muscles.

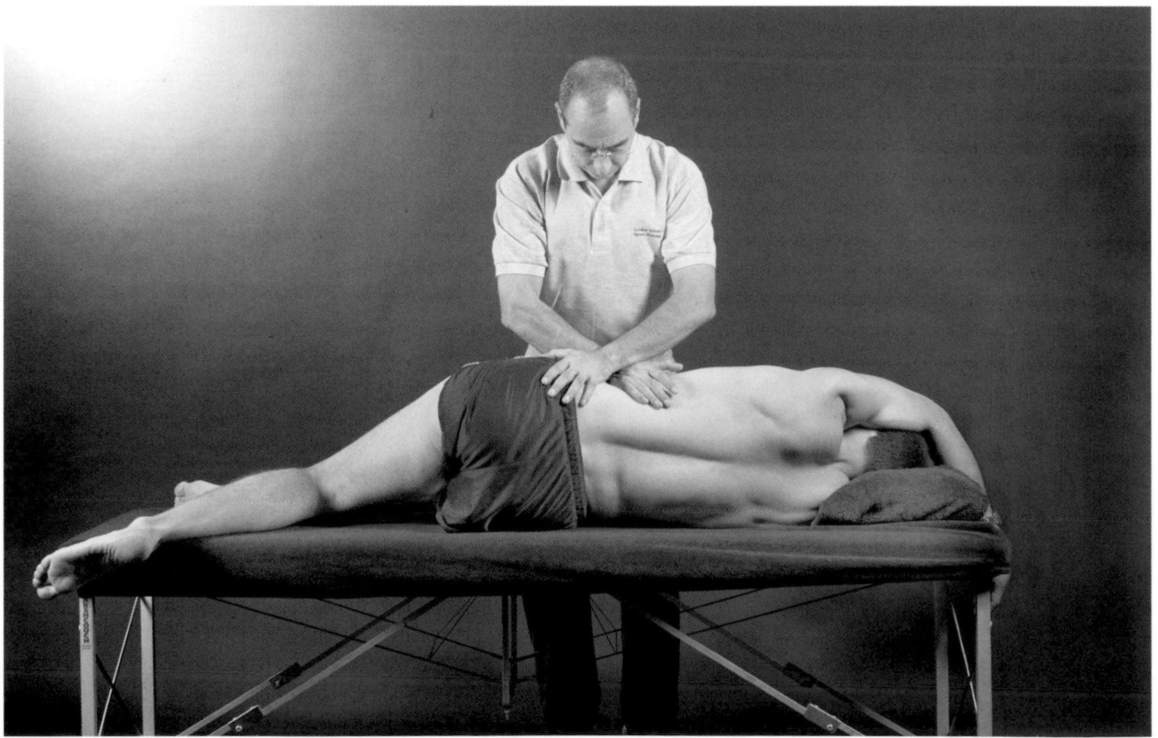

Photo 28. The quadratus lumborum can be stretched by applying strokes in opposite directions in the side-lying position. Note the position of the client's arm and leg, which adds to the stretching effect.

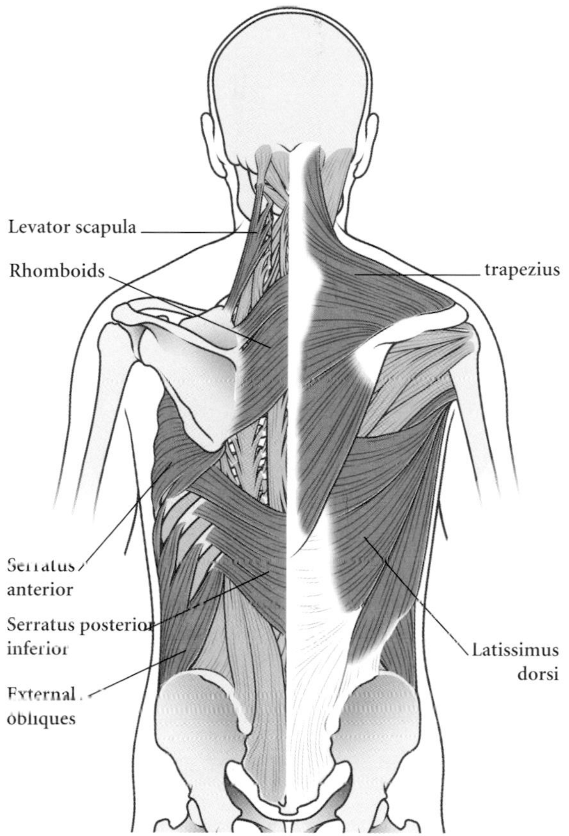

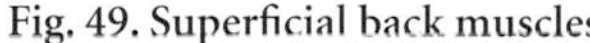
Fig. 49. Superficial back muscles

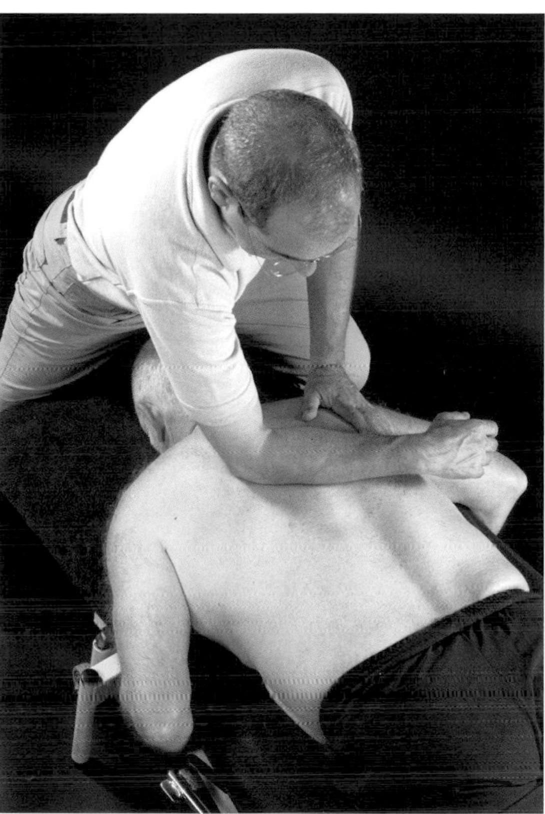
Photo 29. The forearm can be used to apply a deep stroke through the rhomboid and trapezius muscles. Note the therapist's knee on the couch brings their body-weight forward to make this much more effective.

has to support the extra weight of the extended head as well as side-bending the neck, because this becomes the only way to turn the head in this posture.

The extra load is increased even further when doing high-impact activities. When jumping down, the gravitational force on the protracted head is many times greater and these muscles can get acutely strained trying to resist this strong sudden force.

The levator scapula is often the first and most common muscle to suffer painful symptoms with the protracted head posture, and when a simple muscle injury appears to have occurred here it should always be considered in this wider postural context.

The **trapezius** is the large superficial muscle that covers must of the upper back and neck and can be considered in three sections. The upper part extends down from the occipital bone, inserts into the lateral third of the clavicle, and moves the neck and shoulders. The middle part has its origin from the C7 to T3 and it inserts into the acromion process and works with the rhomboids. The lower part extends up from the T3 to T12 to insert along the spine of the scapula and draws it downwards and in a medial direction.

With good posture, the trapezius should have a fairly static role fixing the position of the

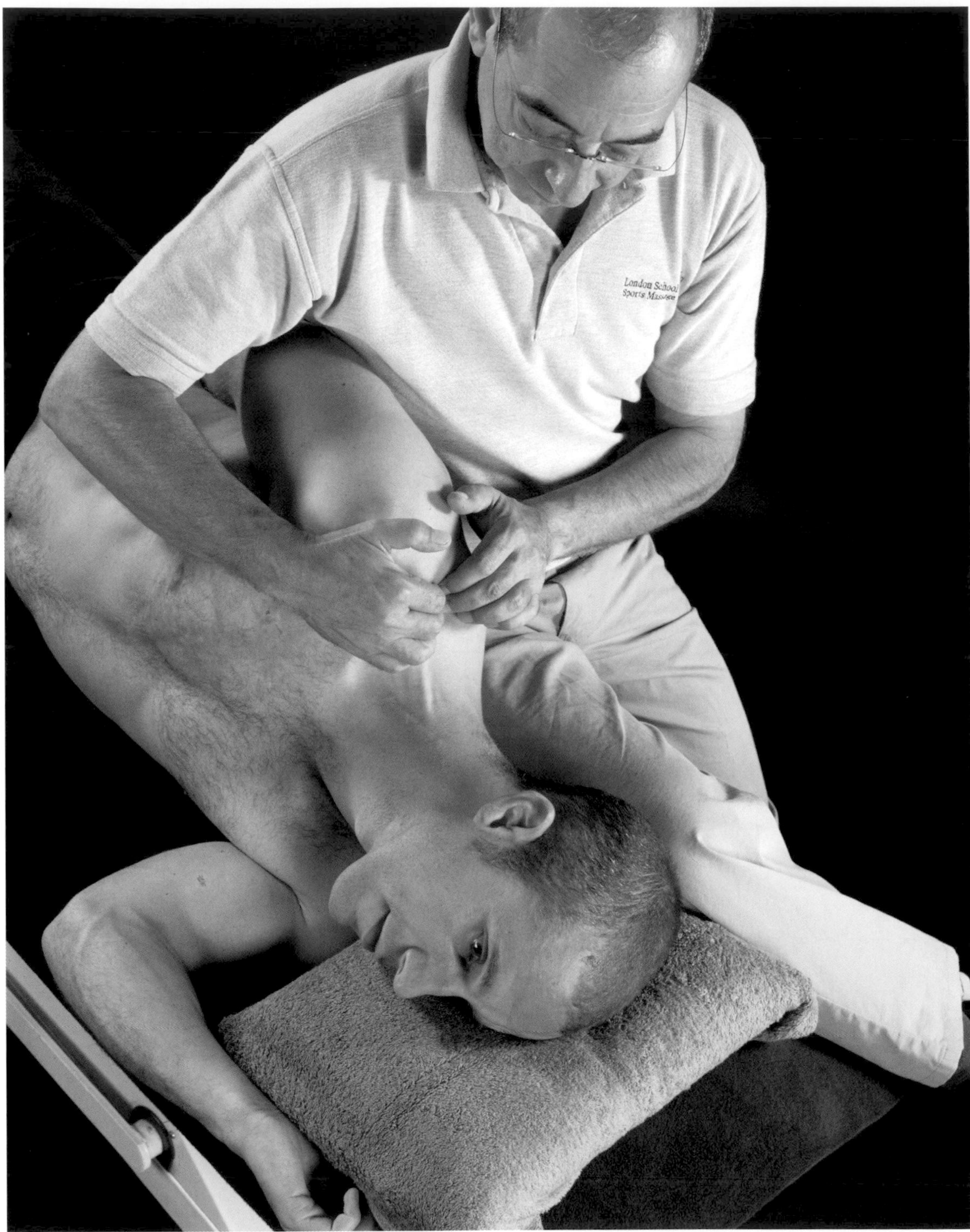

Photo 30. With the client side-lying and the therapist sitting on the couch behind them, the distal fibres of the trapezius can be effectively treated where they converge between the clavicle and scapula.

scapula. But it has to do far more than this when people have a protracted head, neck and shoulder posture. The upper part can suffer from overuse as it has to work much harder (with the levator scapula) to support the weight of the head and also to side-bend the neck when turning the head. The mid part suffers along with the rhomboid from being weakened and stretched. The lower part becomes stretched and weakened because it is reciprocally inhibited by hypertension in the opposing chest muscle.

When the muscle is correctly aligned, there is a large bulk of muscle fibres in the upper trapezius which are vertically aligned over the top of the shoulder. In this position, it can strongly support the downward force from a weighted arm. But in the protracted head posture, the muscle tilts forward and the thinner midsection of the muscle starts to become uppermost over the joint. With fewer fibres here, it is far less able to cope with this powerful function and overuse micro-trauma commonly builds up here.

The upper trapezius is often short and tight in people who hunch up their shoulders, which is particularly common when working behind computers or carrying shoulder bags. Micro-trauma commonly builds up towards the insertion between the clavicle and scapula. This is best treated with the client in a side-lying position where deep friction and stretching techniques can be applied very effectively. (*See photos 30, 31 and 32.*)

The **serratus posterior inferior** muscle runs from the lumbar spine out diagonally to the ribs

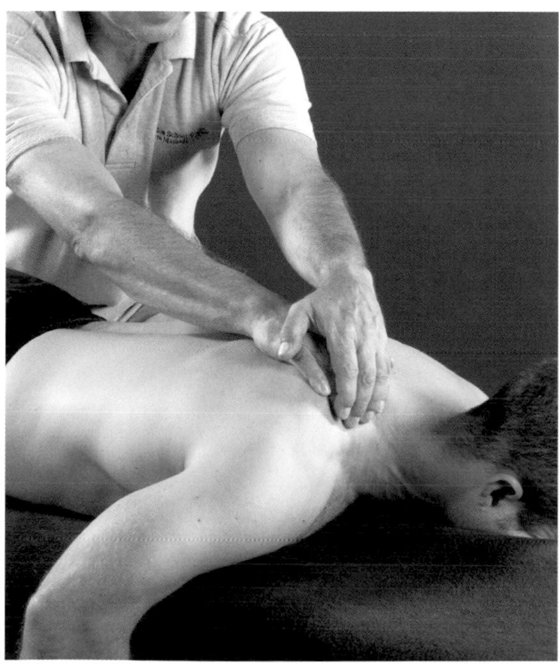

Photo 31. Using a pull-back stroke across the body to apply a deep stroke to the upper trapezius.

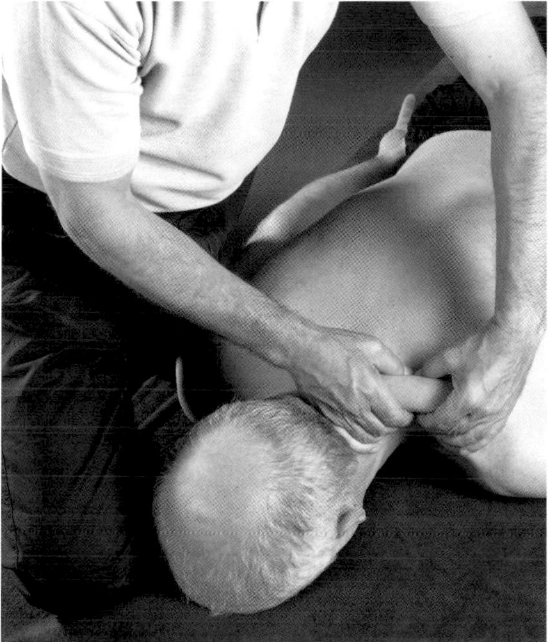

Photo 32. To efficiently treat the upper trapezius, the therapist should kneel as far across the couch as possible to get their body-weight over the shoulder they are treating. From this position, a variety of techniques can be applied.

and the corresponding **superior** muscle does a similar thing from the thoracic spine. These are incredibly thin muscles, and their function is to fix and move the ribs in respiration.

Hip and Legs

Posterior hip

The **gluteus maximus** is a very powerful muscle with a large attachment along the sacrum, sacrotuberous ligament, thoracolumbar fascia and iliac crest. Rather than inserting directly to a bone, however, it binds through strong fascia into the iliotibial band which connects it to gluteal tuberosity and down towards the knee. The muscle as a whole is the most powerful extensor and outward rotator of the hip, but the upper fibres also assist in abduction and the lower fibres in adduction. (*See fig. 50.*)

This muscle has to work powerfully in all walking and running activities, but it rarely gets injured. This is because when doing these activities the muscle contracts to extend the hip but then has a short rest and stretch during hip flexion. When standing, it has to maintain a mild static contraction to stabilise the hip joint in an upright alignment, but being such a strong muscle it can normally cope with this very well.

In the sway-back posture, the gluteus maximus is held passively in a shortened position. This causes a neural inhibition which weakens

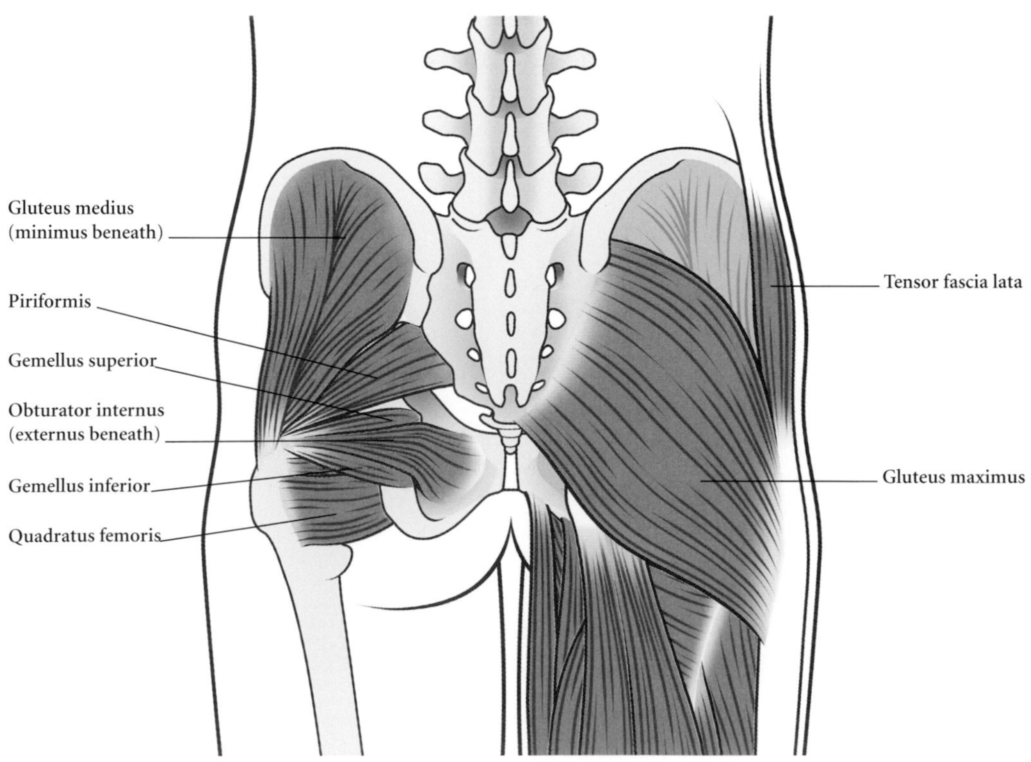

Fig. 50. Posterior hip muscles

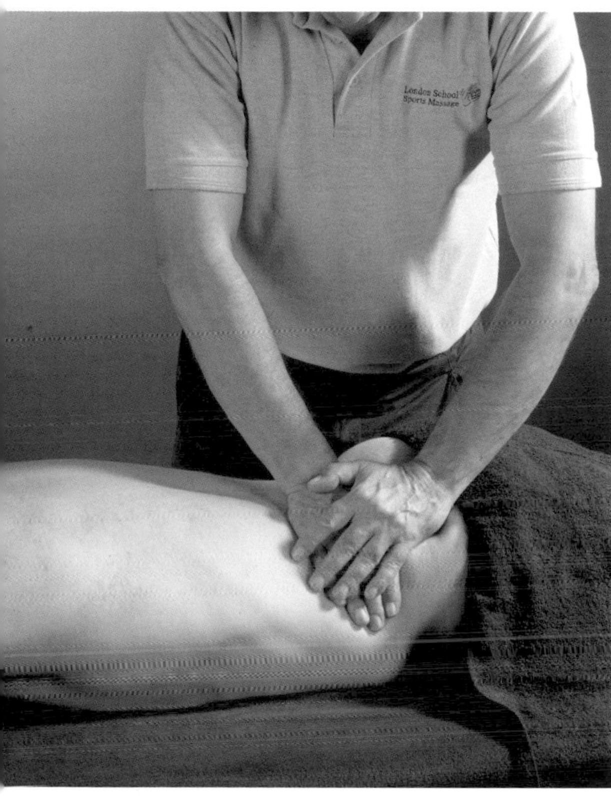

Photo 33. Using a protected thumb to apply deep strokes through the gluteus maximus.

the muscle and makes it function poorly when extending the hip. To make up for this deficiency, the hamstrings have to work harder and can suffer with overuse problems as a result. (*See 'Testing hamstring/gluteal balance', p. 110*)

The **gluteus medius** has its attachment along the upper posterior surface of the ilium, and the **gluteus minimus** is smaller and lies beneath it. They both attach to the great trochanter, and together their function is to abduct the hip. But the anterior fibres assist flexion and inward rotation and the posterior fibres assist extension and outward rotation. (*See photos 33 and 34.*)

They work mainly as stabilisers which control the hip joint through both flexion and extension when walking and running. Unlike the maximus which only works in one direction, the medius and minimus work during both extension and flexion phases and do not get a short recovery period in between. They also work in a fairly static way to stabilise the hip so there is less movement between the fibres, and fibrous adhesions are more likely to form in the muscle. This means that overuse micro-trauma and chronic tension are more likely in people who do a lot of running and walking activities, and it is these smaller muscles that usually require more attention than the much larger gluteus maximus.

The **piriformis** has a strong attachment on the anterior surface of the sacrum and crosses the back of the hip joint and inserts onto the great trochanter. As such, if it contracts and shortens, it creates outward rotation of the hip. But we rarely need to forcefully perform this action in normal activities, and instead its main function is to control and prevent too much inward rotation. To achieve this, it has to rapidly perform a series of intricate concentric, eccentric and isometric contractions as the hip goes through inward and outward rotations when walking and running.

In activities that involve a lot of running, this muscle has to perform its intricate task many thousands of times and with fatigue its efficient function can deteriorate and lead to injury. Biomechanical issues such as excessive pronation will cause the leg to inwardly rotate more during the weight-bearing phase of the running action. This means that the piriformis (along with other hip rotators) has to work harder to try to control this, and overuse injury can result.

In a small proportion of the population the sciatic nerve passes through the belly of the piriformis muscle. If this is the case, excessive tension or injury to the muscle could impinge on the nerve and cause neural symptoms running down the leg (**sciatica**).

When treating the piriformis, it is important to remember that its origin is on the anterior surface of the sacrum. To release excessive tension, it is necessary to reach the trigger points here where it is rich in Golgi tendon organs. This is difficult in the prone position unless applying deep techniques from the lateral side to get under the bone. It is usually easier to achieve this with the client in a side-lying position. *(See photos 35 and 36.)*

The piriformis often needs to be stretched as part of a treatment and as an outward rotator of the hip this would normally be done by inwardly rotating it. But when the hip is neutrally aligned its range of inward rotation is usually insufficient to achieve an effective stretch to it. However, when the hip is flexed beyond 60 degrees, the femur moves forward into a position which makes the piriformis inwardly rotate the joint instead of outwardly rotating it. By flexing the hip first, outward rotation then becomes a very effective way to stretch it. *(See 'Muscle Energy Technique', p. 191.)*

The **gemellus superior** and **gemellus inferior** are found below the piriformis with their origins at the ischial spine and tuberosity and insert into the great trochanter. They are quite small muscles, which assist outward rotation of the hip. The **obturator internus** is a bigger muscle with a large origin around the inner surface of the pubis and obturator membrane. It goes around the lip of the ilium then laterally out to the great trochanter. The **obturator externus** is the deepest muscle in this group and cannot be seen without removing all adjacent muscles.

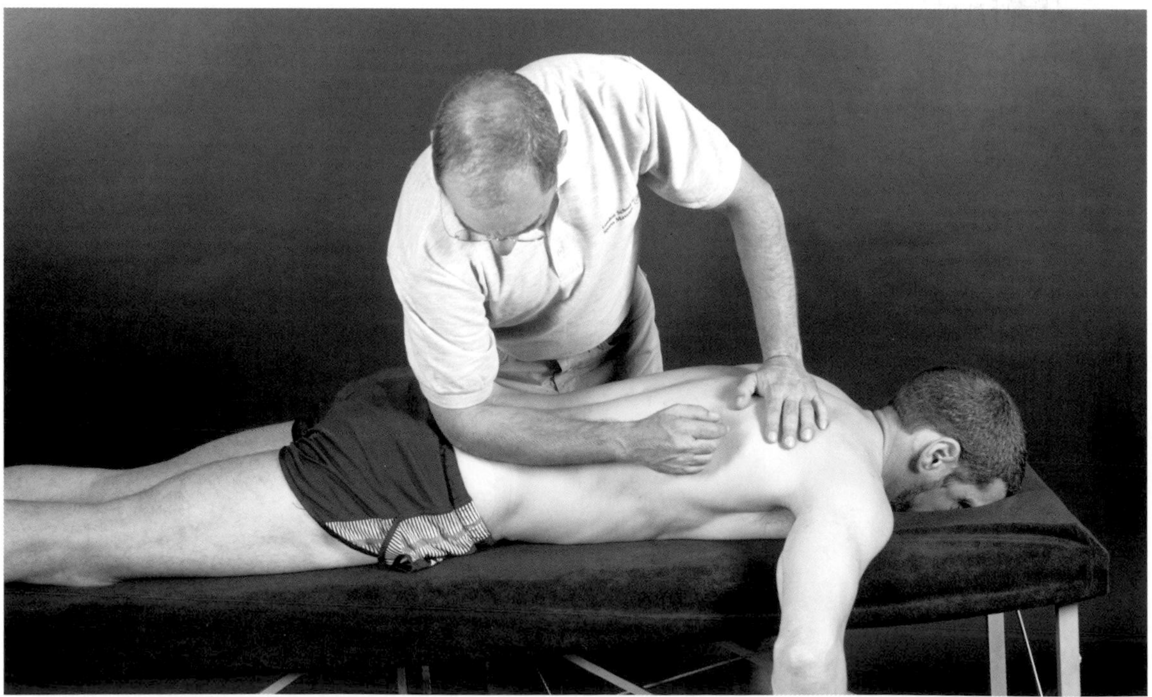

Photo 34. Very deep strokes can be applied with the forearm to all the gluteal muscles and along the piriformis. The therapist can rotate their arm at any point to use the elbow for deep friction. Note the way the therapist is leaning all the way across the couch to get their weight directly above the area being treated.

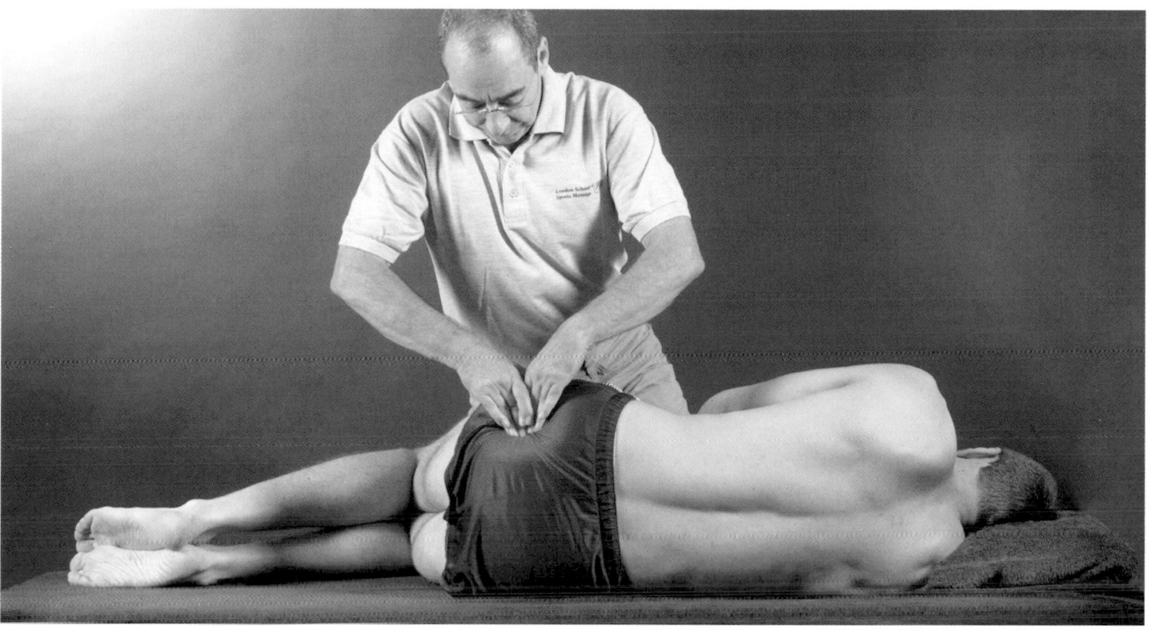

Photo 35. To reach the origin of the piriformis, it is necessary to apply deep pressure beneath the lateral border of the sacrum, and the side-lying position is a very good position to do this from.

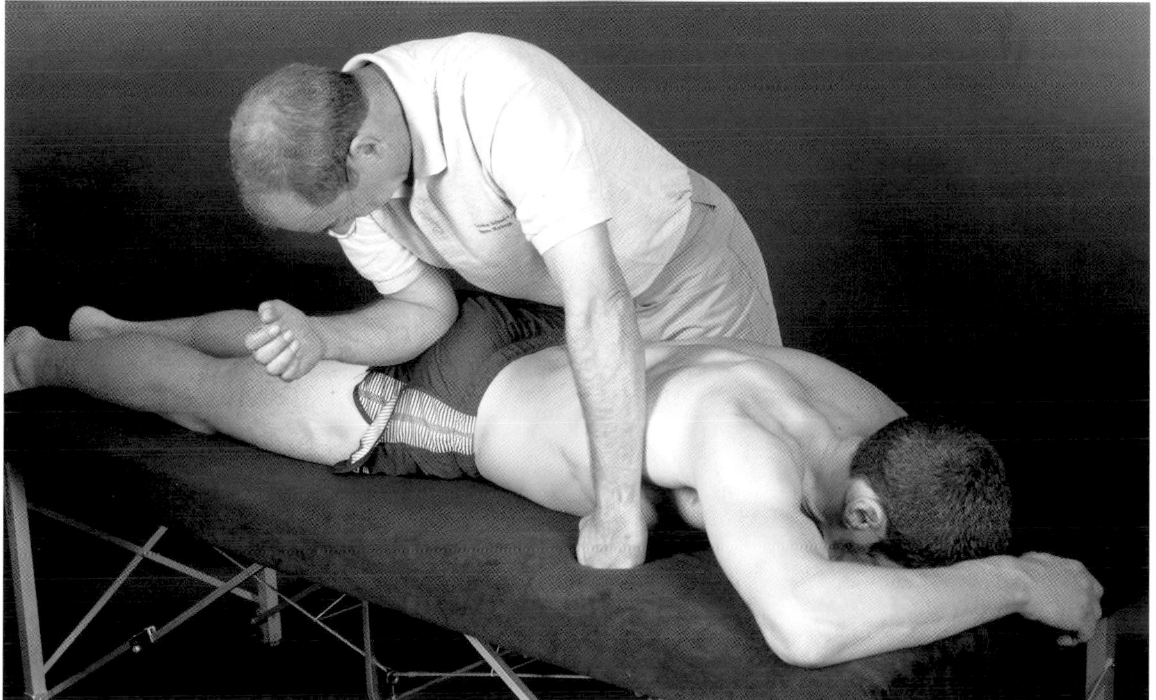

Photo 36. In the prone position, the piriformis can be reached with the elbow. Note the way the therapist leans fully over the couch so he can apply a great force in behind the bone.

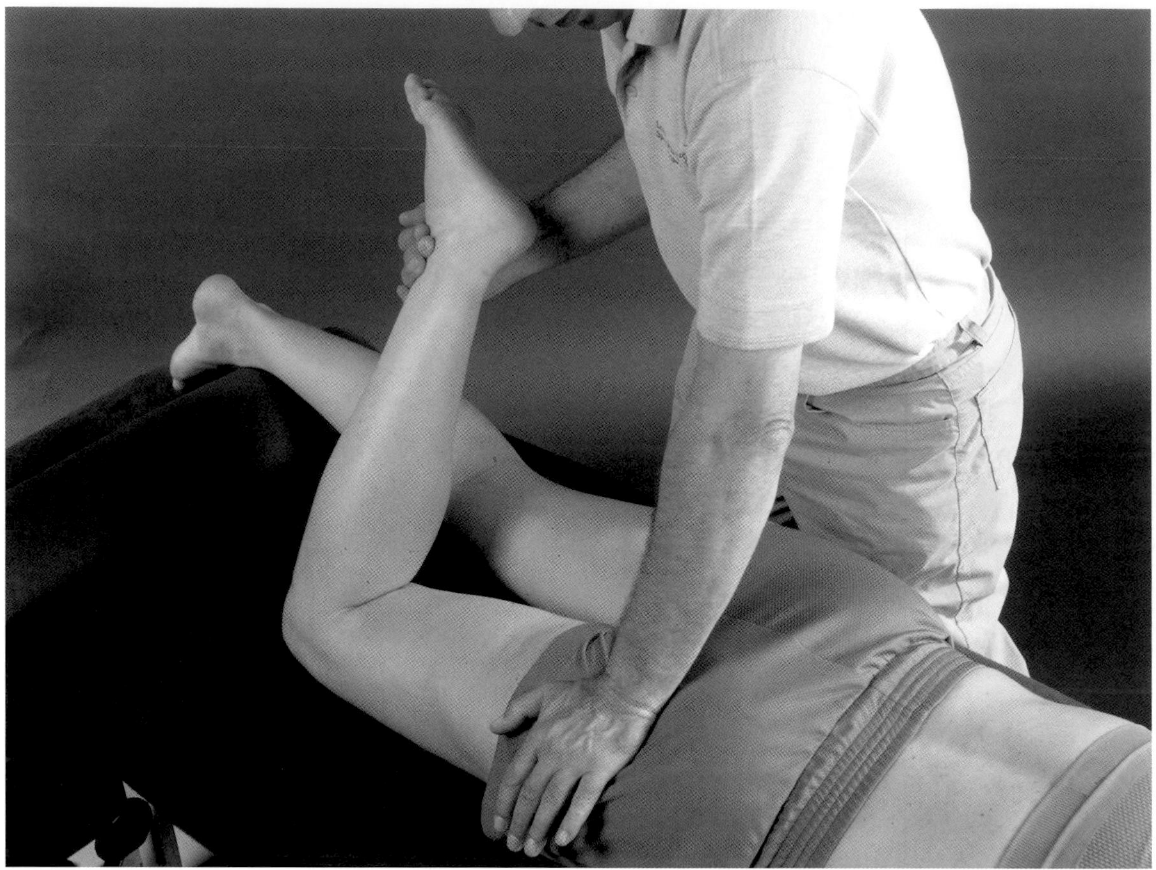

Photo 37. Treating the obturator, gemellus and quadratus femoris muscles using the heel of the hand. The strokes are being applied by rotating the hip to move the muscles in a form of Soft Tissue Release.

Its origin is on the outer surface of the pubis and obturator membrane, and it also attaches to the great trochanter. The obturators are more powerful outward hip rotator muscles than the gemelli. At the bottom of the muscle group is the short **quadratus femoris**, which goes from the ischial tuberosity and inserts below the great trochanter. This is a strong outward rotator and also adducts the hip. *(See fig. 50.)*

Because outward rotation of the hip is not an action we often need to do powerfully in normal activities, these are not particularly strong muscles and they work mostly to help stabilise the hip. Although acute injury may be rare, chronic overuse problems can develop in these muscles if they are put under greater stress trying to control other biomechanical issues such as over-pronation.

All these deep hip rotator muscles can be treated in the prone position in a similar way to the piriformis, and deep strokes need to be applied in from the lateral side to reach the attachments beneath the sacrum. The side-lying position is also good for this.

Posterior thigh

The **hamstring** group is made up of three muscles which are said to have their origin along the ischial tuberosity, but that is not quite correct.

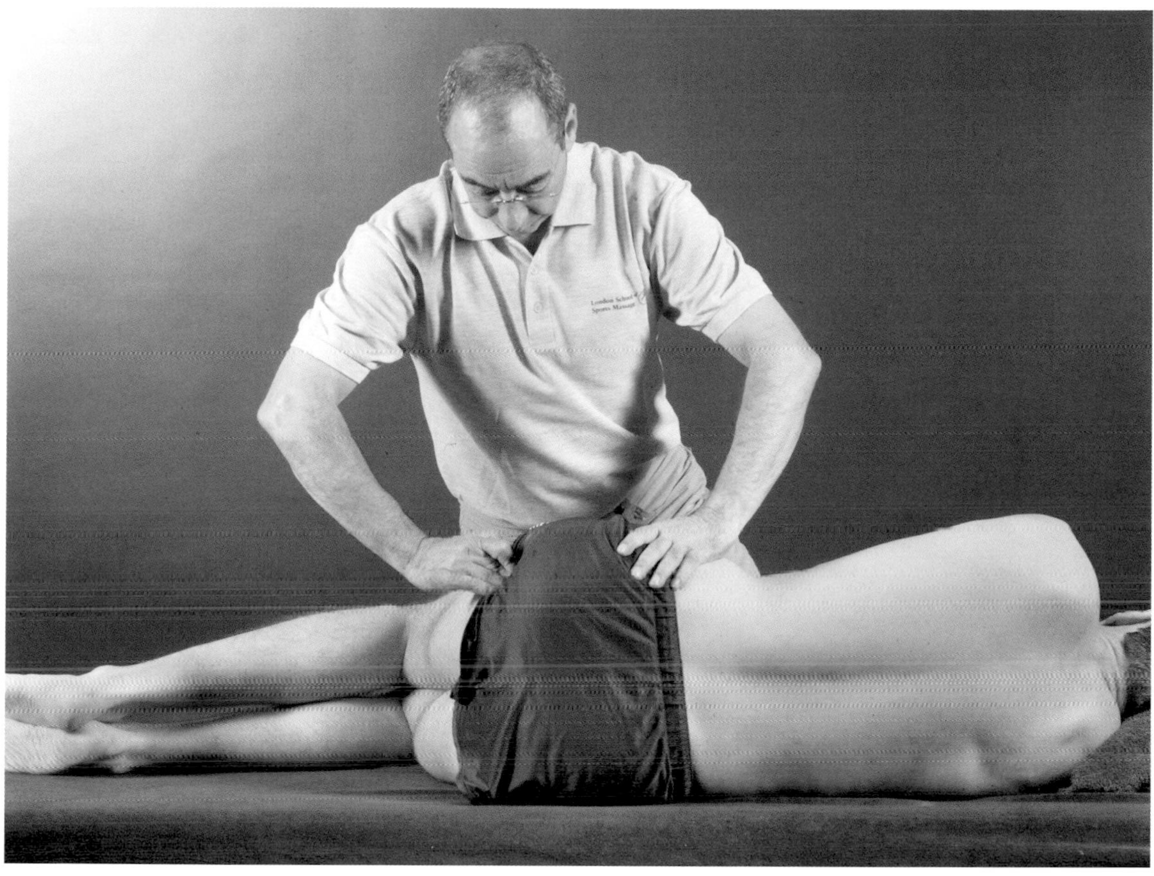

Photo 38. By fixing the ilium bone with one hand, the other can be used to apply deep friction along the hamstring's insertion with the ischium and also the sacrotuberous ligament which continues from it to the sacrum.

Although they attach there, a thick tendon-like structure (called the sacrotuberous ligament) continues on from the head of the muscles to insert into the sacrum and sacroiliac joint. This structure passes in between the gluteus maximus and the lateral hip muscles and, with good palpatory skill, it is possible to treat it all the way along it to the sacrum. *(See photos 38, 39, 40 and fig. 51.)*

The **biceps femoris** has two heads. As well as its common origin with the other hamstrings, it also has an attachment coming from the lateral lip of the femur. It runs down the lateral side of the thigh and inserts below the knee joint into the lateral tibial condyle and the head of the fibula. The **semitendinosus** runs down the medial side and forms a common attachment with the gracilis and sartorius muscles across an area of bone on the medial side of the tibial tuberosity called the *pes anserinus.* The **semimembranosus** runs alongside it and inserts into the medial tibial condyle, and through its fascia to the popliteus muscle and the joint capsule.

The hamstrings are commonly thought of as just being simple knee flexors, but their role is far more complex than that. Their attachment across the back of the hip joint makes them important hip extensors which assist the gluteus maximus. If the maximus is functioning poorly, the hamstrings have to make up for the deficiency and often suffer overuse problems if they become the primary hip extensors. (*See 'Testing hamstring/gluteal balance', p. 108.*)

As the hamstrings insert across the back of the knee joint, they are very powerful knee flexors. But the joint also needs to be able to rotate slightly when it is flexed and these muscles control this too. By pulling across the medial side of the joint, the semitendinosus and semimembranosus create inward rotation and, crossing the lateral side, the biceps femoris creates outward rotation. This movement is an essential biomechanical feature of the knee, and the two sides of the muscle group have to balance each other correctly to achieve the intricate control needed.

The hamstrings can suffer from poor strength-training methods. Gym equipment that requires the muscles to perform only a

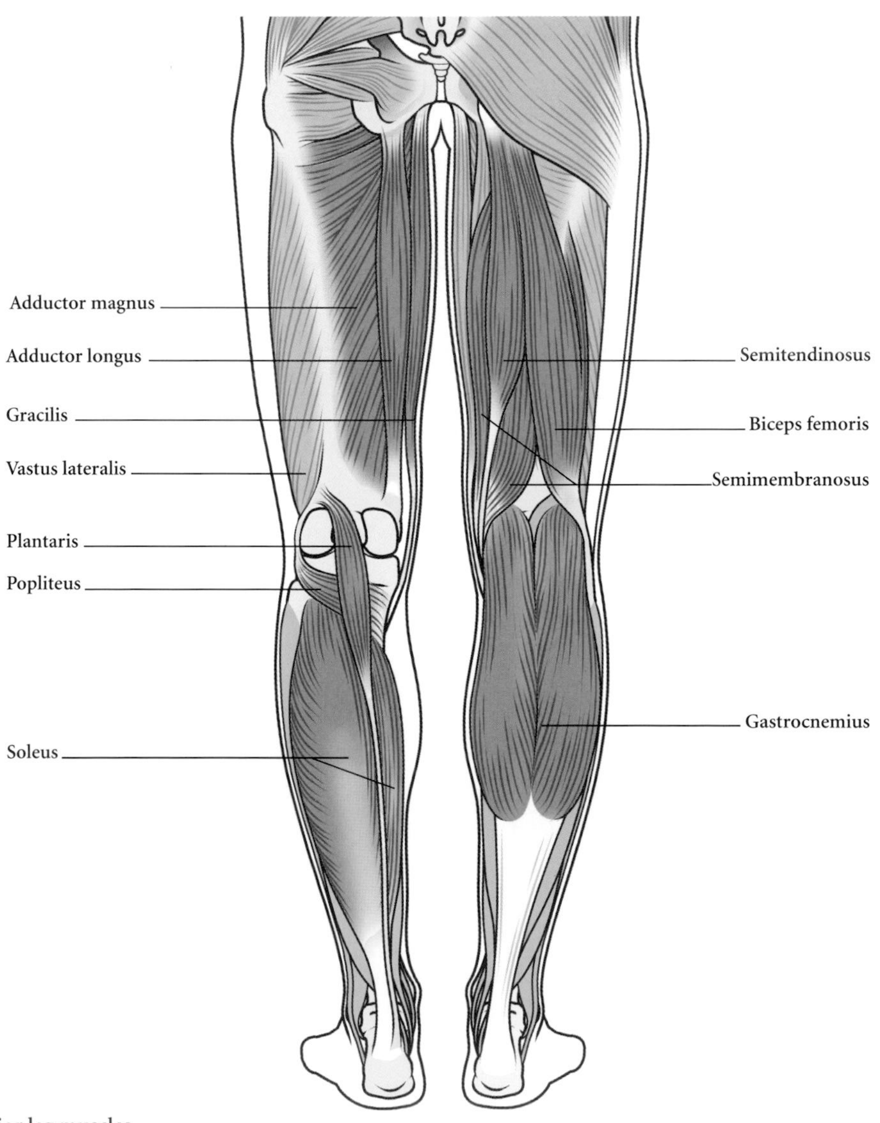

Fig. 51. Posterior leg muscles

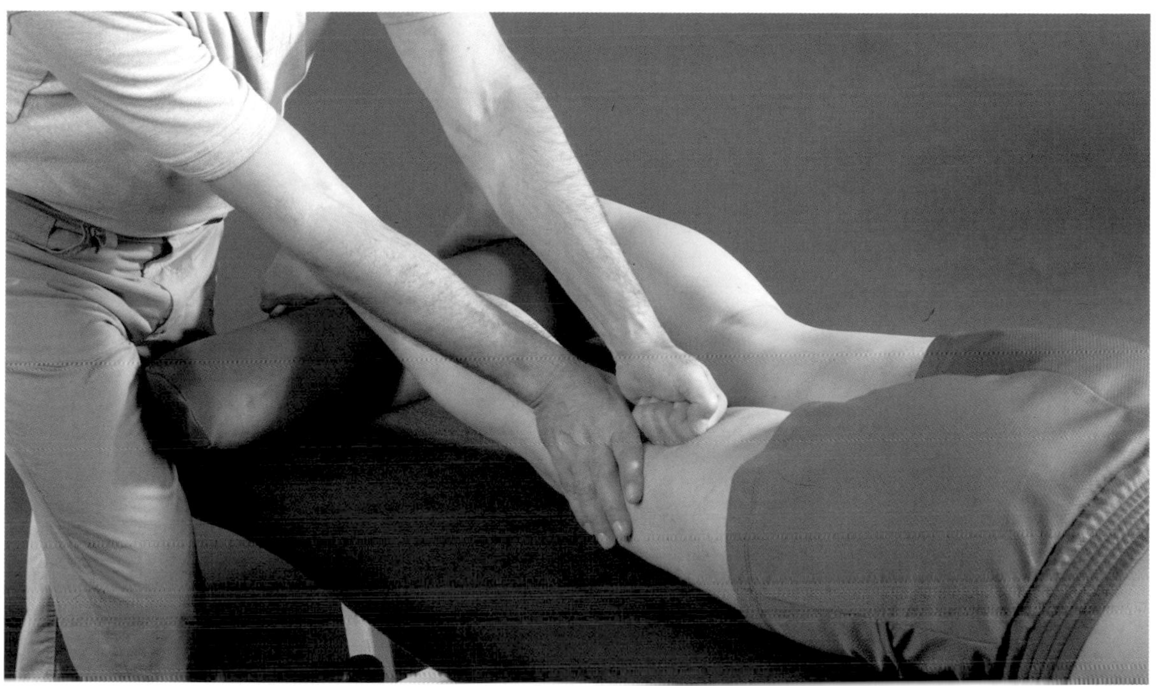

Photo 39. The hamstrings often require quite heavy massage strokes, and fist or elbows may need to be used.

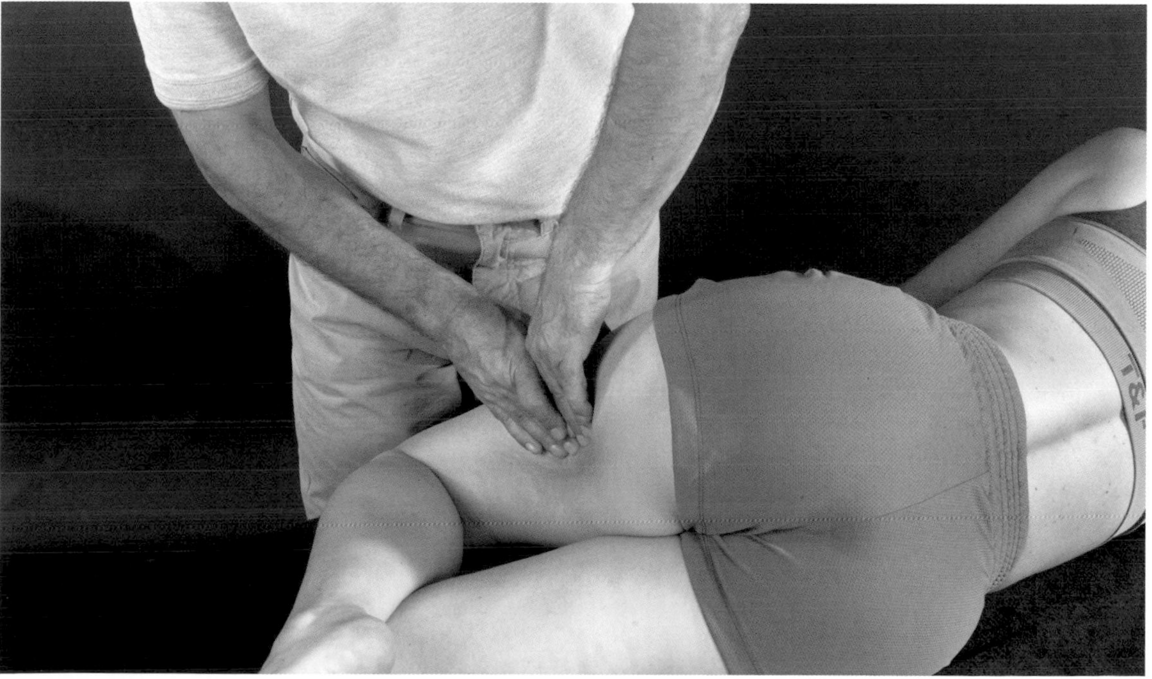

Photo 40. In a side-lying position, the bulk of the hamstring drops away, making it possible to reach the very deepest layers of tissue close to the bone.

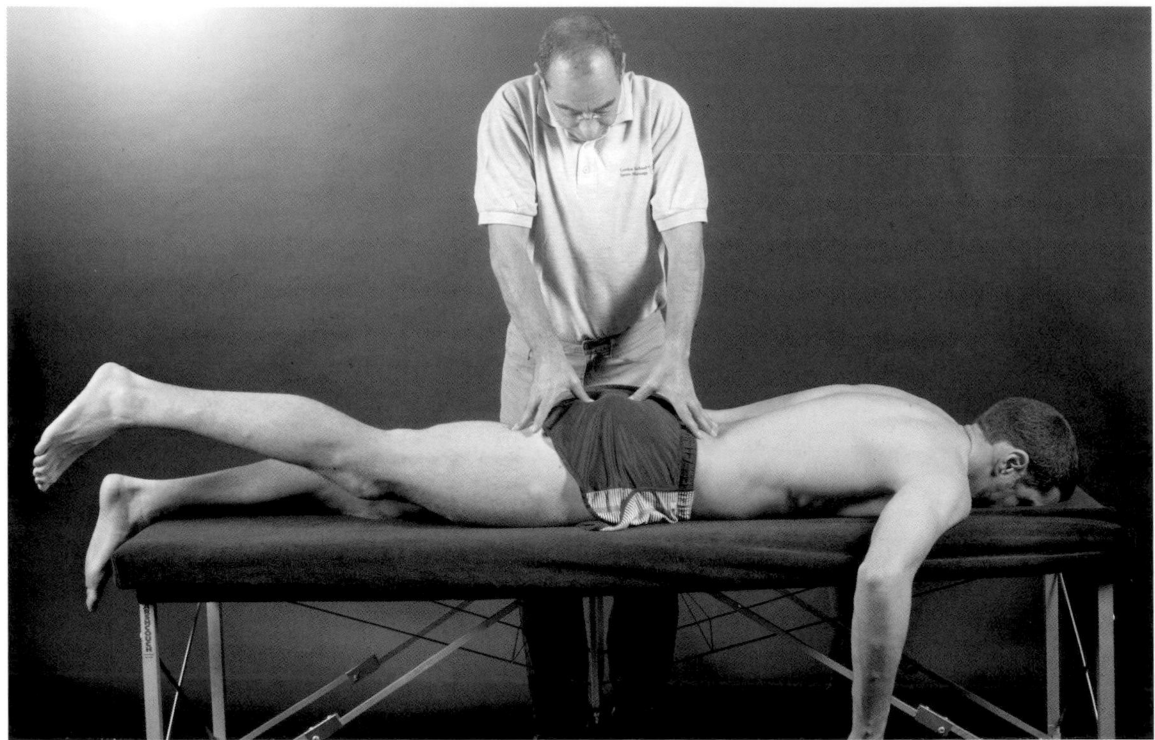

Photo 41. With the client lying prone and relaxed, the therapist's fingers and thumbs press deeply into the lower back and upper gluteus maximus with one hand, while the other presses into the lower gluteus maximus and the hamstrings. When the client extends the hip by raising the leg, the gluteus maximus should be felt contracting strongly as the primary muscle (as is shown here). This is often not the case, however, and instead the hamstrings contract strongly with the gluteus maximus contracting later, weakly or not at all.

short powerful concentric contraction through its inner range may possibly make them appear to be stronger. But this action is completely different to what the muscles have to do in normal everyday walking or running actions, and so it does little to help real function and in some cases can actually cause knee problems.

Testing hamstring/gluteal balance

The sway-back posture is possibly the most common tendency we see, and with this the gluteus maximus usually becomes weak and inhibited. This means that when performing normal hip extension movements (walking and running), the hamstrings have to take on the main role. In this situation, the hamstrings become tight and hypertonic and commonly suffer chronic overuse injury. It may also be the cause of lower back issues as well because this also has to make up for the gluteal deficiency.

- **To test for this:**

With the client lying prone and relaxed, with one hand the therapist presses their fingers very firmly into the lower erector spinae muscles and their thumb into the upper part of the gluteus maximus. The thumb of the other hand presses into the lower part of the gluteus maximus with the fingers pressing deep into the hamstrings.

The client first presses the front of their hip into the couch and then attempts to raise their straight leg up off the couch. In an ideal situation, there should be some contraction in the erector spinae muscles to stabilise the core an instant before the gluteus maximus contracts strongly to extend the hip with the hamstring muscles only assisting this. However, what often happens is the hamstrings contract instantly and strongly with little or no response from the gluteus maximus. This can be significantly different on either side of the body, and both should always be tested the same way. *(See photo 41.)*

- **To correct this:**

In the prone position, the therapist holds the knee in a comfortably flexed position which shortens the hamstrings and prevents them contracting. In this position, the client is asked to lift their knee off the couch. To do this, they can only use their gluteus maximus and initially may find this very hard to do. But after a few attempts the neuromuscular system learns to start functioning better. Repeating the straight leg raise test again usually shows a fairly instant improvement.

The client can feel the differences in muscle contraction quite clearly and the explanation is easy for them to understand. So although the results from the few brief exercises done in the clinic will not last long the client will be motivated to practice it themselves. To do this they should use some sort of strap so they can passively hold the knee in flexion, and then lift their knee off the floor. This can be developed further by doing it with the hip at different degrees of abduction and rotation so it activates the gluteus maximus in all its ranges.

Posterior lower leg

Deep in the popliteal space at the back of the knee is the small **popliteus** muscle which goes from the lateral femoral condyle and runs diagonally across to the posterior tibial surface. Crossing the back of the knee, it can flex the joint but being so small compared to the main knee flexors it only has a minor role in this action. When the knee flexes, however, it has an important role in creating and controlling its inward rotation. Although rarely injured, when this does occur it is usually associated with hyper-extended knee joints which can cause an overload and stretch on the muscle.

The **plantaris** is a long thin muscle which has its origin alongside the gastrocnemius at the lateral femoral condyle. It only has a short belly at the back of the knee and goes into a very long tendon, sweeping diagonally down between the gastrocnemius and soleus. It inserts with the Achilles tendon into the medial edge of the calcaneum bone. As its origin and insertion are the same as the gastrocnemius, it could be said to have the same function, but being so much smaller it can only have a very minor effect on this action. It is more likely to be significant in coordinating the rotational positions of the knee and ankle joints in walking and running actions. Not being involved in powerful weight-bearing activities it is seldom ever injured.

The largest muscle in the calf is the **gastrocnemius**. This has two large bellies which have their origins at the medial and lateral femoral condyles and merge with the soleus to form the Achilles tendon which inserts into the calcaneum. By crossing the back of the knee, it assists the hamstrings in flexing the knee, and crossing the back of the ankle this very strong muscle creates powerful plantarflexion. The two bellies can develop separately in response to the demands placed on them and it is quite normal to find different degrees of strength, tension, and even size, in the two parts.

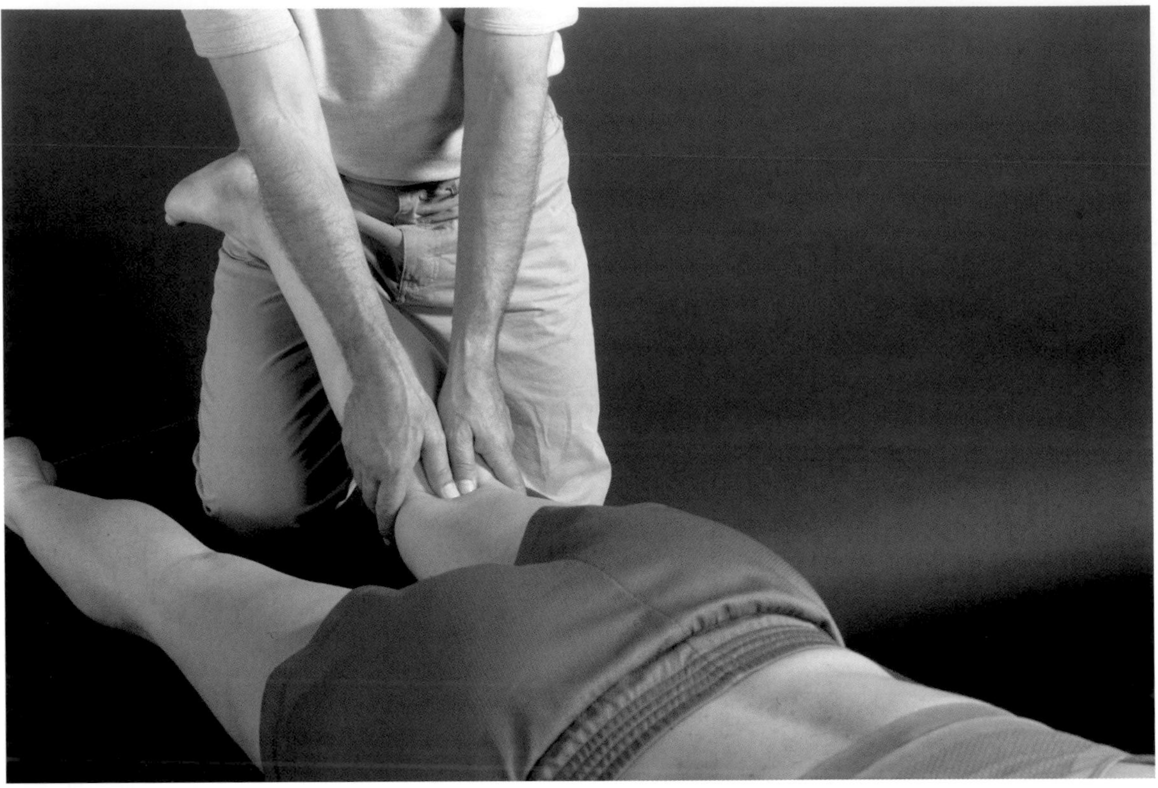

Photo 42. The client's lower leg is supported on the therapist's thigh to flex their knee. In this position, the popliteal space can be carefully palpated to find areas of soft tissue tension or damage which can then be treated with gentle friction.

When standing it maintains a mild contraction in conjunction with the dorsiflexors to maintain lower-leg alignment, which is not a problem for such a strong muscle. But with adverse postural tendencies the knees may be locked in full extension and have to support more of the body's weight to maintain balance. Chronic tension can develop in an effort to maintain this and, although it may not lead to painful symptoms, it can make the muscle more vulnerable to acute injury during physical activity.

The **soleus** lies beneath the gastrocnemius with its origin on the posterior surface of the fibula and tibia. It inserts through the Achilles tendon to the calcaneum and so it plantarflexes the ankle. In some postural situations, people may hold the knees in a slightly flexed position. This reduces tension in the gastrocnemius and so the soleus has to work harder to stabilise lower-leg alignments.

The gastrocnemius and soleus muscles merge into the **Achilles tendon** which attaches to the calcaneum at the heel. This strong tendon is subjected to great force and is difficult to rest if it gets inured. Although it is protected inside a lubricated paratenon sheath, it is vulnerable to rubbing, bending or twisting forces. Chronic stiffness is commonly felt first thing in the morning particularly in older clients who do a lot of sport. This is possibly due to poor circulation of lubricating fluid inside the sheath and light self-massage done regularly can be a remedy for this.

A **complete rupture** of the Achilles tendon

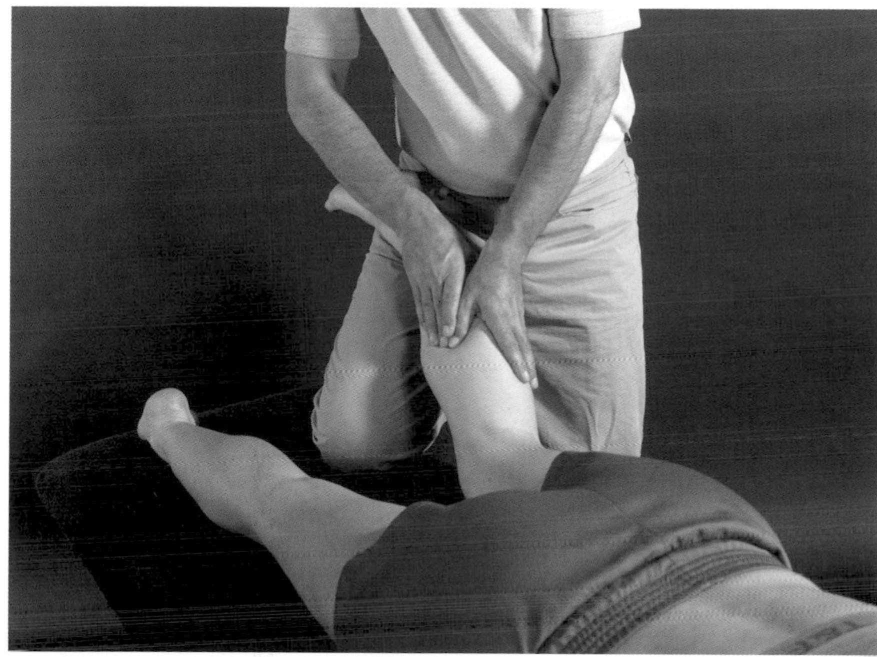

Photo 43. With the therapist kneeling on the couch and supporting the client's leg in a flexed-knee position, the gastrocnemius is shortened and relaxed, making it easier to work under it to reach and treat the soleus.

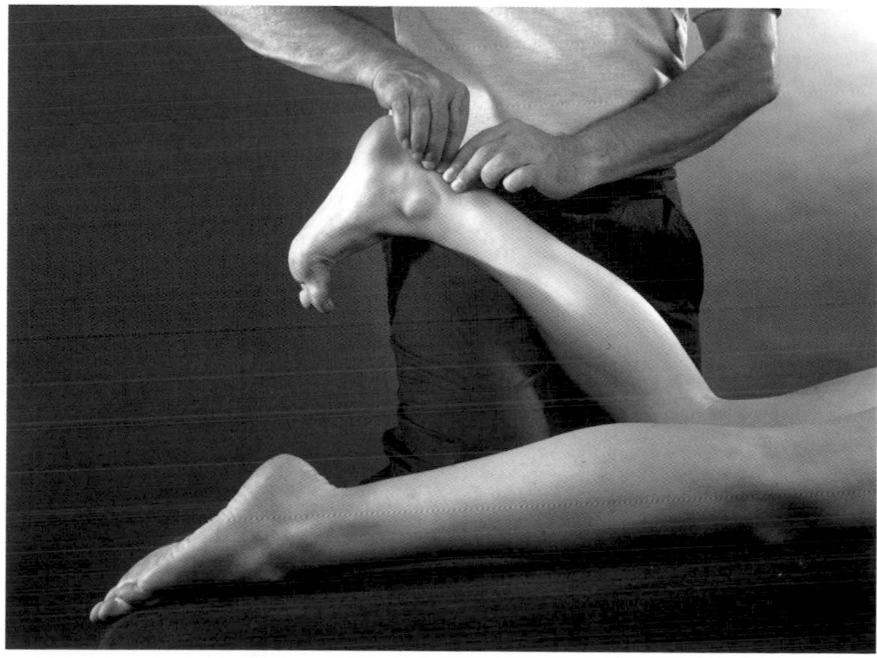

Photo 44. Supporting the lower leg on the therapist's thigh makes it easy and comfortable to treat the Achilles tendon.

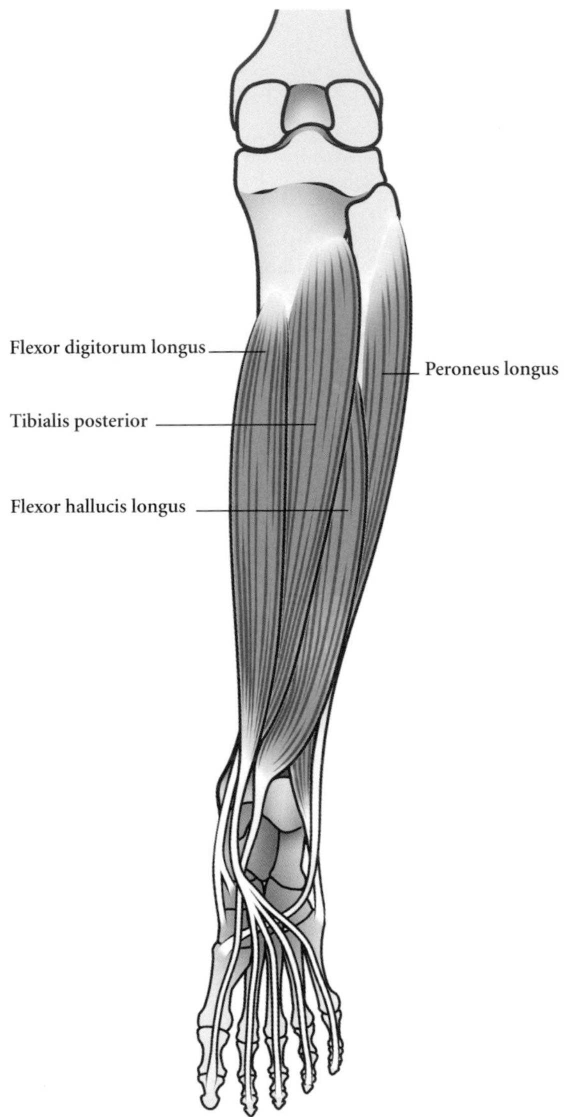

Fig. 52. Deep posterior compartment

can occur if there is a sudden powerful contraction of the muscles. This is more likely in older males who do a sport involving sudden running or jumping, especially if they are slightly overweight. Although they usually experience a loud snapping sound and sharp pain at the time, there may be little or no pain later. They will walk with a slight limp and any attempt to push up on their toes will be impossible. It is usually obvious that a complete rupture is likely from the client's description of the event, and the calf muscles will appear short and bunched up. To test this further, the client should lie prone with their foot hanging off the end of the couch. If the therapist squeezes the calf muscles, the foot will plantarflex slightly if the tendon is intact but will remain still if it has completely ruptured. This acute injury needs immediate medical attention as surgery may be the only effective remedy.

The **deep posterior compartment** of the lower leg is made up of three muscles which have long tendons that go round the medial malleolus to insert into the planter side of the bones in the ankle, foot and toes. These tendons run through a synovial sheath around the malleolus, which protects them from rubbing against the bone. Unlike the other muscles in the calf, these create movements in the foot rather than the ankle. Great strength is needed in the foot to control its function when weight-bearing and this requires big muscles. But large bulky muscles in the foot would prevent the intricate functional agility needed between all the small joints. So the body has evolved with the strength coming from large muscles contained in the lower leg which transmit their force through long tendons into the foot. (There is a similar situation with the lower arm, wrist and hand.) (*See fig. 52.*)

This muscle group has to function in two different situations. When not weight-bearing, they create foot and ankle movements against fairly minimal resistance, but in all weight-bearing actions they have to work strongly to control the biomechanics of the foot.

The central muscle of the group is the **tibialis posterior**, which has a large origin between the posterior surfaces of the tibia and fibula, and the interosseous membrane. The tendon passes under the malleolus and inserts through a broad fascia into the navicular and cuneiform bones. When the leg is not weight-bearing, it creates plantarflexion and supination (inversion) at the ankle joint. When standing, it lifts the inside of the joint to keep it correctly aligned and helps create the longitudinal arch of the foot.

On the medial side, the **flexor digitorum longus** has its attachment over the posterior surface of the tibia. In the sole of the foot, its thick single tendon divides into four thinner tendons which extend all the way through to insert into the distal phalanges at the end of the toes. It plantarflexes the foot and toes with slight supination when not weight-bearing. When weight-bearing, it is important in supporting the longitudinal arch through the sole of the foot and also lifts the transverse arch across the metatarsal/phalangeal joints.

On the lateral side of the group, the **flexor hallucis longus** has its origin along the lower posterior surface of the fibula and interosseous membrane. The belly of this muscle goes down further than the others and can be easily palpated behind the Achilles tendon. It has the longest and thickest tendon which runs all the way to the distal phalange at the end of the big toe. It produces plantarflexion of the big toe and when standing it supports the longitudinal arch.

Biomechanical problems in the foot will lead to overuse problems in these muscles as they have to work harder to try to control and stabilise the foot. A client may be suffering with calf pain but, if the gastrocnemius and soleus appear normal and only this deep compartment is tight and painful, then poor foot biomechanics is likely to be the cause of the problem.

Treatment to the foot as well as these muscles can reduce symptoms but assessment from a specialised podiatrist and properly prescribed orthotic insoles may be the most practical solution to these biomechanical issues.

The deep posterior compartment is contained within a strong fascial sheath, which restricts its ability to expand. If the muscles are in an overuse situation controlling the foot, over time these muscles will get stronger and need to expand. But, with the fascia preventing this, it can develop into a compartment syndrome, restricting blood flow to the foot.

These are difficult muscles to treat because they lie beneath the gastrocnemius and soleus and can only be reached from the medial and lateral sides. They can be treated through these big muscles, but the side-lying position usually gives better access to them. *(See photos 45 and 46.)*

Lateral hip

The **tensor fascia lata** (TFL) muscle is a very thin muscle found on the outside of the hip with its origin along the lateral part of the anterior iliac crest. Its posterior fibres run vertically over the lateral aspect of the hip, creating abduction, but the anterior fibres play a bigger role in hip flexion and inward rotation. The muscle as a whole helps stabilise the hip laterally and has to apply continual mild contraction to do this whenever standing, walking or running. *(See fig. 53 overleaf.)*

The muscle does not insert in the normal way through a tendon to a bone; instead, it binds strongly to the fascia along its outer surface, which extends down to become the iliotibial band. Through this, it connects with the lateral side of the knee. If the muscle becomes tight through overuse, rather than pain being caused in the muscle, the tension may continue down through the iliotibial band and cause lateral knee pain.

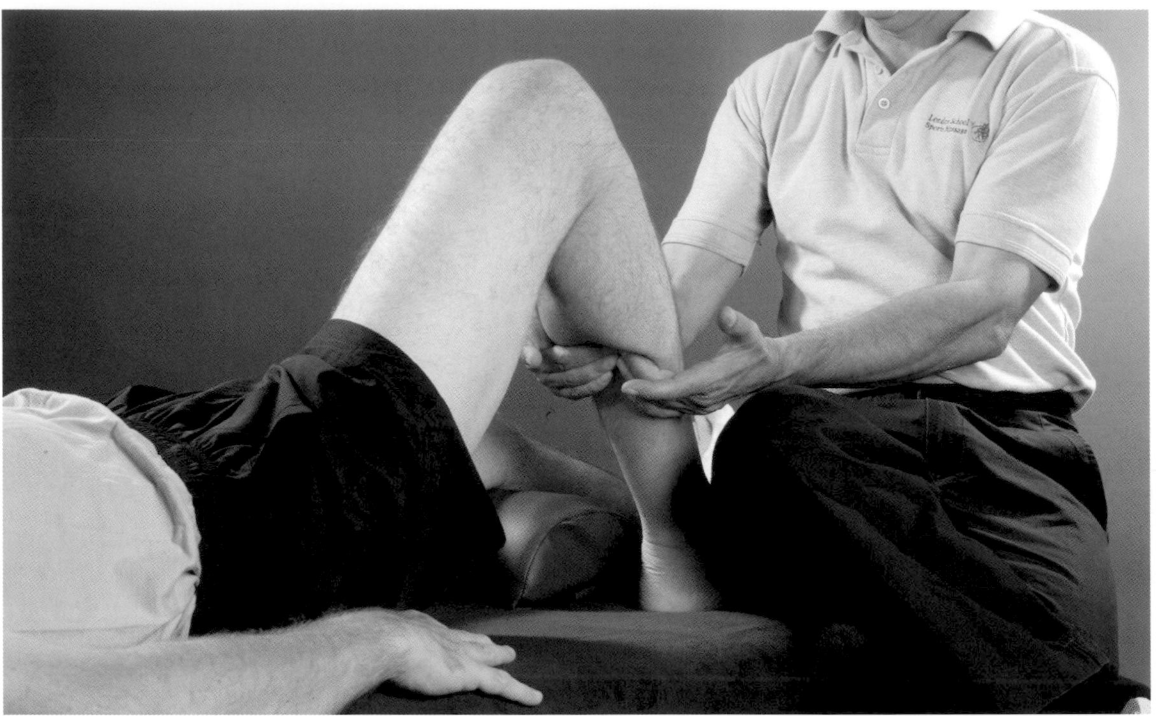

Photo 45. Sitting on the client's foot with their hip and knee flexed, the gastrocnemius and soleus muscles are shortened and relaxed. By pressing in between the two bellies of the gastrocnemius, it is possible to treat the deep posterior compartment. By leaning back, the therapist can apply a considerable force.

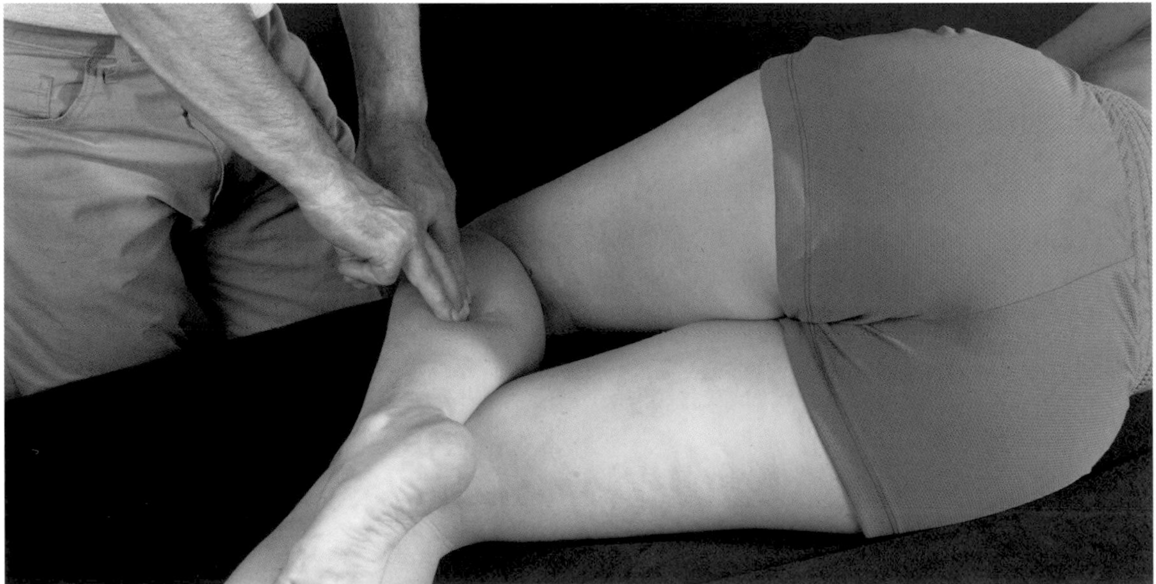

Photo 46. With the client side-lying and their ankle raised on their other leg (or a cushion), the gastrocnemius and soleus muscles drop away so it becomes possible to reach the lateral part of the deep posterior compartment.

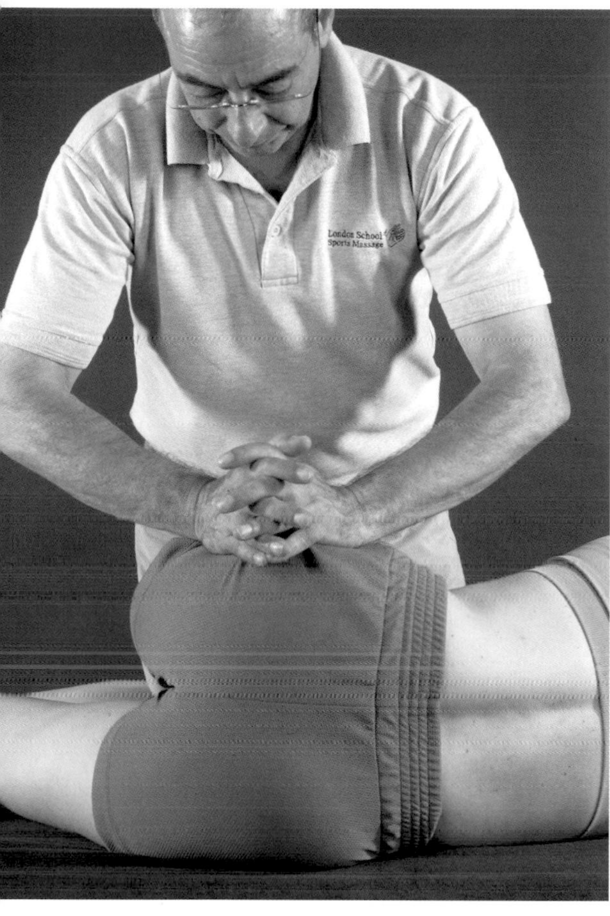

Photo 47. The client is side-lying with their knee and hip flexed (the therapist is blocking the client's knee against his thigh to fix the client's position). From this position, the therapist can lean down with their body-weight to apply deep squeezing movements with the hands to treat the tensor fascia lata and also the gluteus medius.

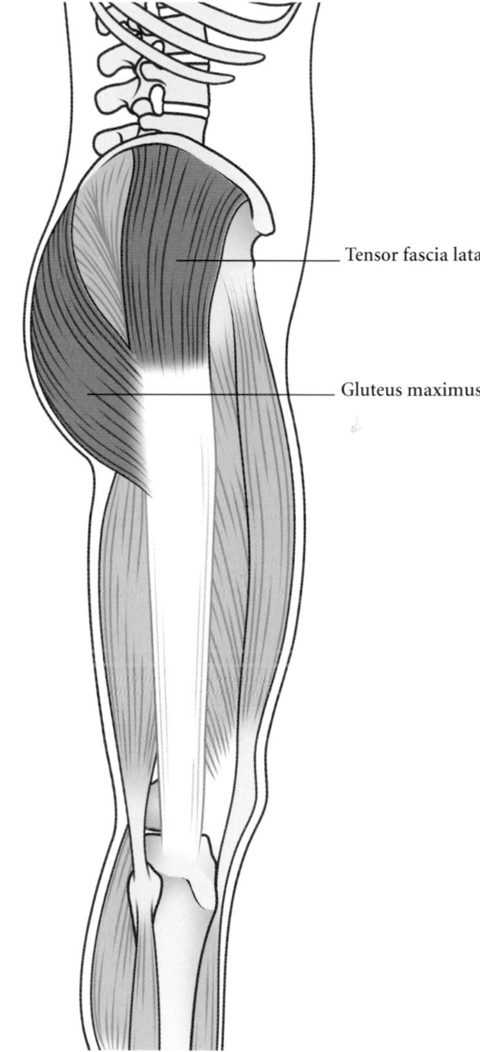

Fig. 53. Lateral hip muscles

Iliotibial (IT) band

The iliotibial band is not a separately identifiable structure but just a part of the deep fascial layer surrounding the whole body. It only appears on charts as a separate band because the rest of the fascia has been removed to just leave this part. But because it functions like a tendon for the TFL and gluteus maximus, the IT band needs to be shown in this way. The band can be clearly palpated because it has very strong and tightly packed parallel collagen fibres with much more elastic and mobile fascia on either side of it. As well as transmitting tension from the muscles above, the IT band can also become tight and restricted within the fascial layer through repetitive overuse. A tight IT band will pull on the lateral aspect of the knee and rub against the lateral epicondyle when running.

People often talk about tight Iliotibial Band Syndrome, but there is some confusion over this because muscle tension and fascial tension are not the same thing. Because it is made up of inelastic collagen fibres, it does not respond to muscular stretching and needs to be treated with myofascial techniques applied along and across the band. *(See 'Myofascial techniques', p. 225.) (See photo 48.)*

There has been a common practice of applying very deep strokes along the band to try to stretch it as if it were an elastic muscle. This only compresses the band hard against the bone, which causes considerable pain but has very little effect on releasing the fascial tension. The client may feel some looseness afterwards, but this will be due to the temporary neuromuscular effect on the muscles rather than any real tissue improvement to the iliotibial band.

Anterior thigh

The **adductor** group of muscles have their origin at the pubis and insert along the linea aspera along the femur and are very powerful hip adductors. Because they attach and pull on the posterior side of the bone, they create some outward rotation also. The **adductor minimus** inserts just below the great trochanter, the

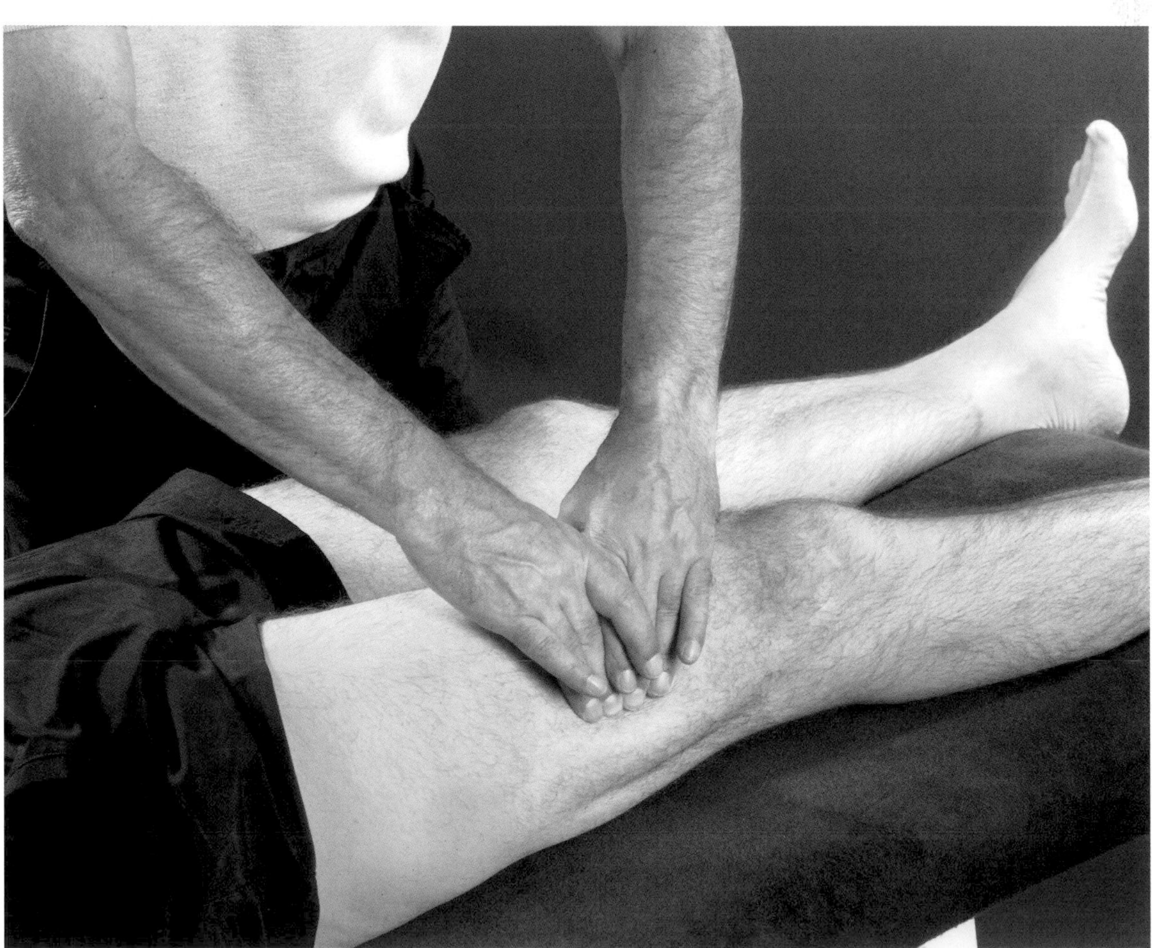

Photo 48. Transverse strokes can identify a tight iliotibial band, and fascial techniques should be used to release this.

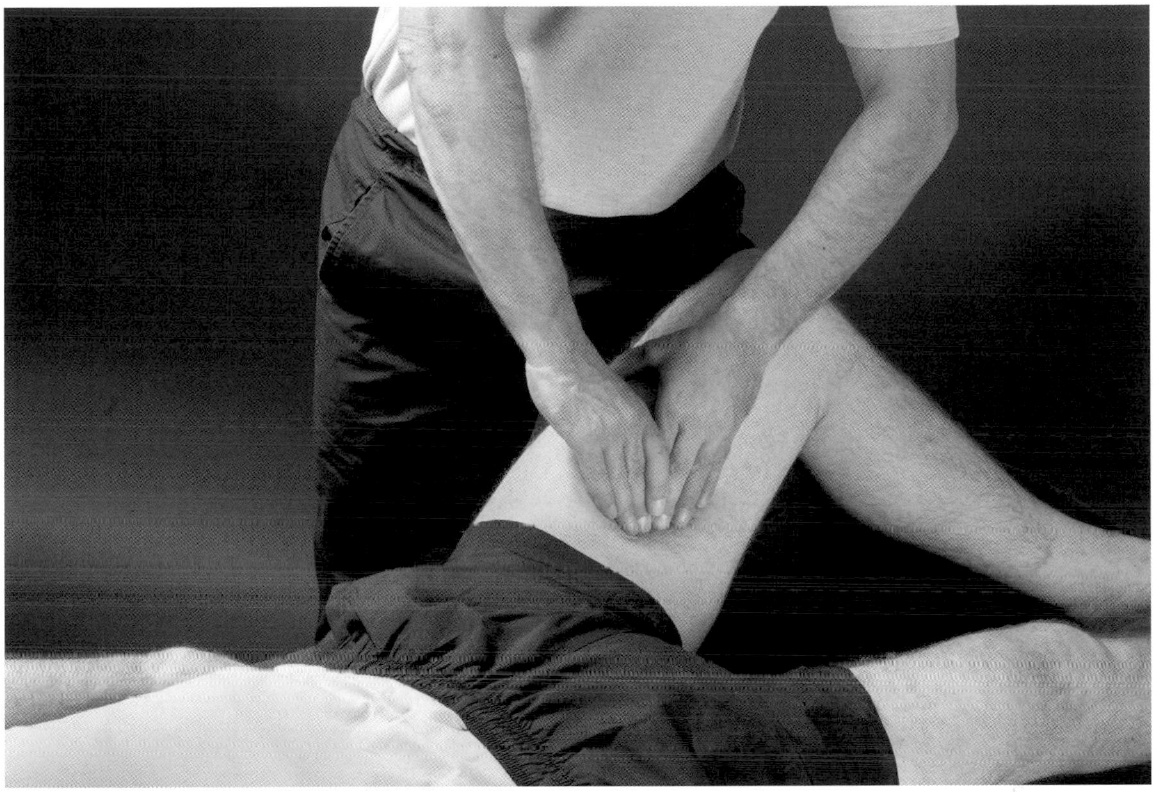

Photo 49. With the therapist kneeling on the couch, the client's leg can be supported on their thigh and deep strokes can be applied into the adductor muscles.

brevis along the upper third of the femur, and the **longus** along the middle third of the femur. The **pectineus** is found at the top of the inner thigh with its origin at the pubis and inserting just below the lesser trochanter. It is a strong adductor, inward rotator and flexor of the hip joint.

The **adductor magnus** is the strongest and largest of the adductor muscles and inserts all the way along the femur. Part of this muscle goes through a more prominent tendon which inserts into the adductor tubercle of the medial epicondyle, and this part assists inward hip rotation.

This describes the movements the adductors make with the femur when the pubis is the fixed origin. In the standing position, however, the femur is fixed through its connection to the ground, and it is the pelvis that will move when the muscles contract. The posterior fibres run from the back of the pelvis slightly anteriorly towards the femur, so when they shorten they pull the pelvis forward. This is a common situation with the sway-back posture, and the two are always linked. People with a sway-back will have tight adductors and people with tight adductors will often develop a sway-back.

The **gracilis** is a long muscle with its origin by the pubis symphysis and goes down past the knee joint to insert through the pes anserinus at the tibia. It can assist in flexing the knee, but when the knee is extended it adducts the hip.

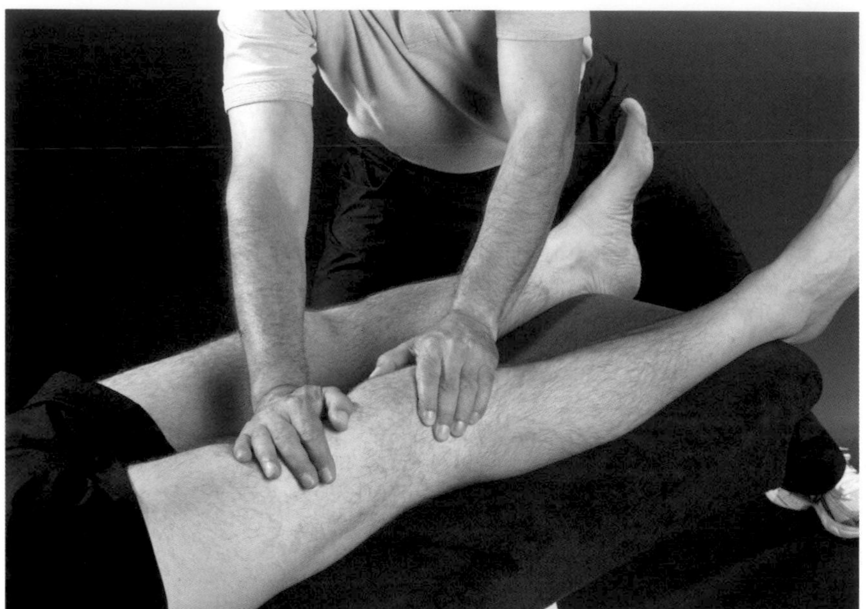

Photo 50. Leaning across the couch, the therapist can efficiently apply deep strokes along the adductor muscles. The therapist is using the other hand to fix the position of the leg, and this can also be used to pull the leg medially and greatly increase the power of the stroke. A similar approach can be used on the medial hamstrings with the client lying prone.

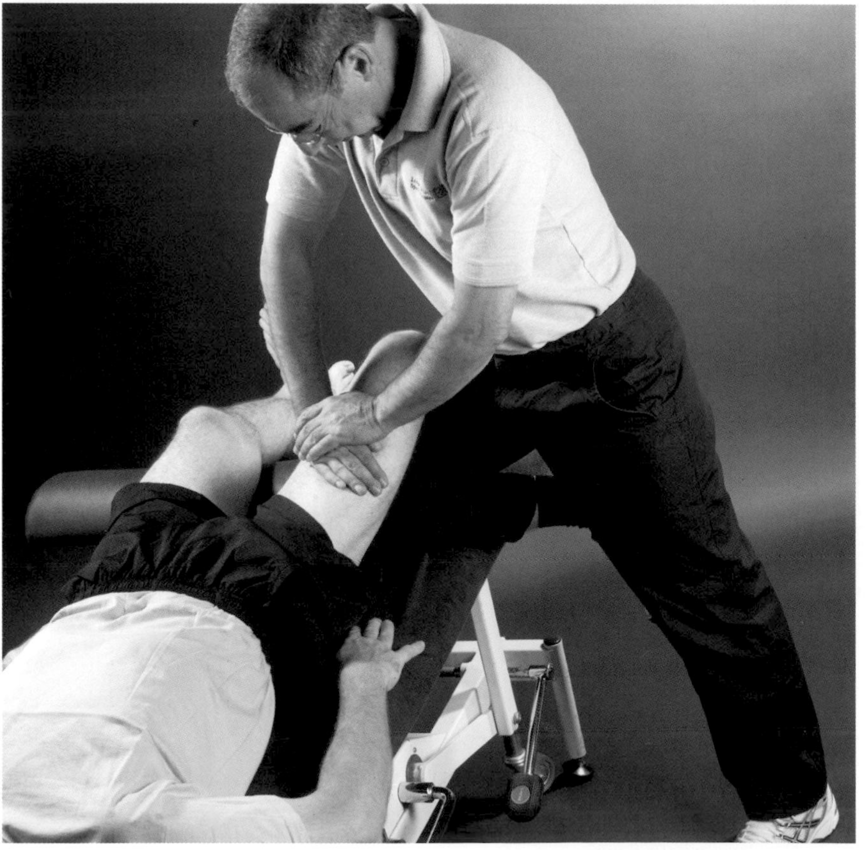

Photo 51. Kneeling on the couch and supporting the client's leg is very strong and efficient way of treating the abductor muscle.

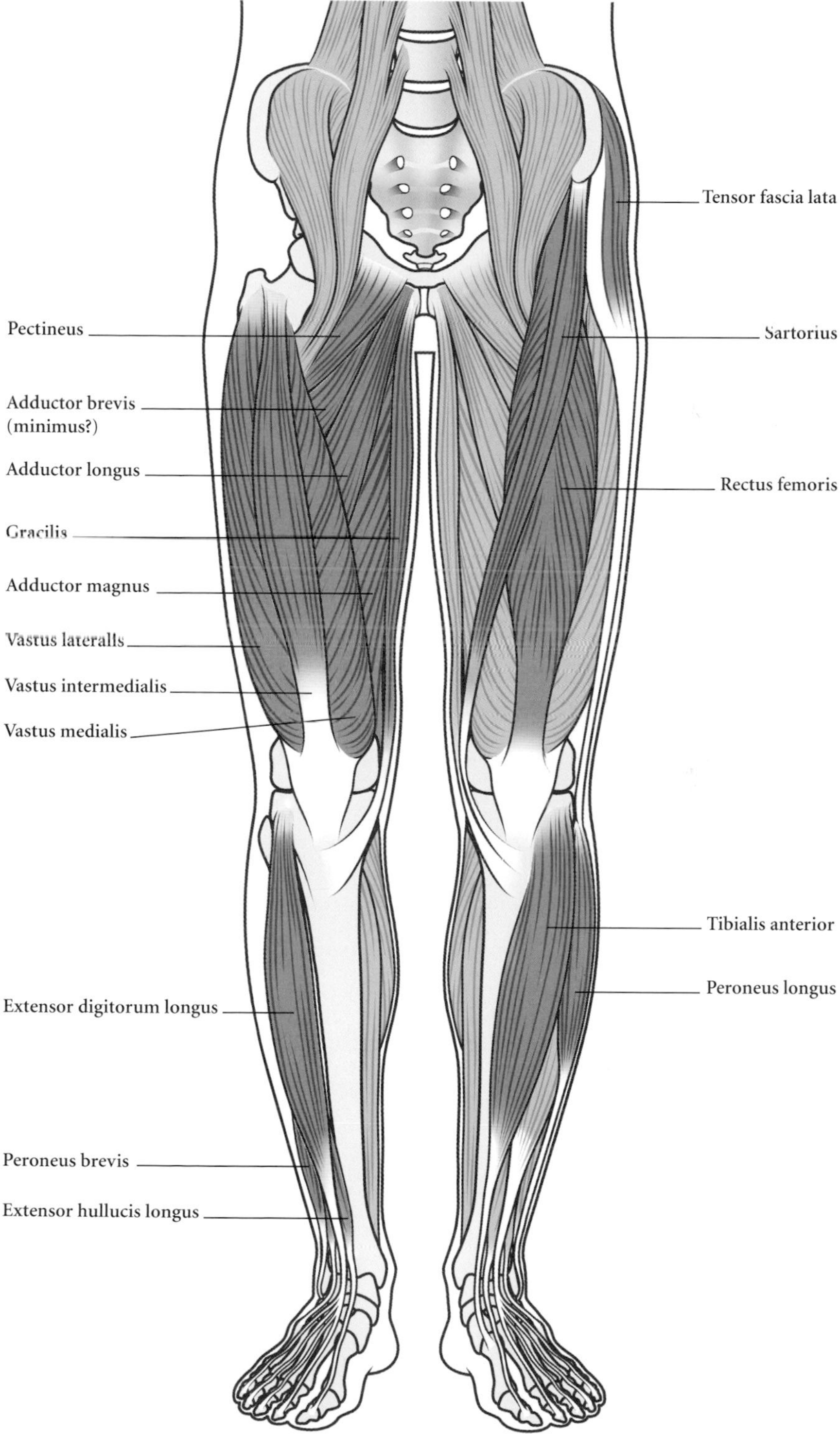

Fig. 54. Anterior thigh muscles

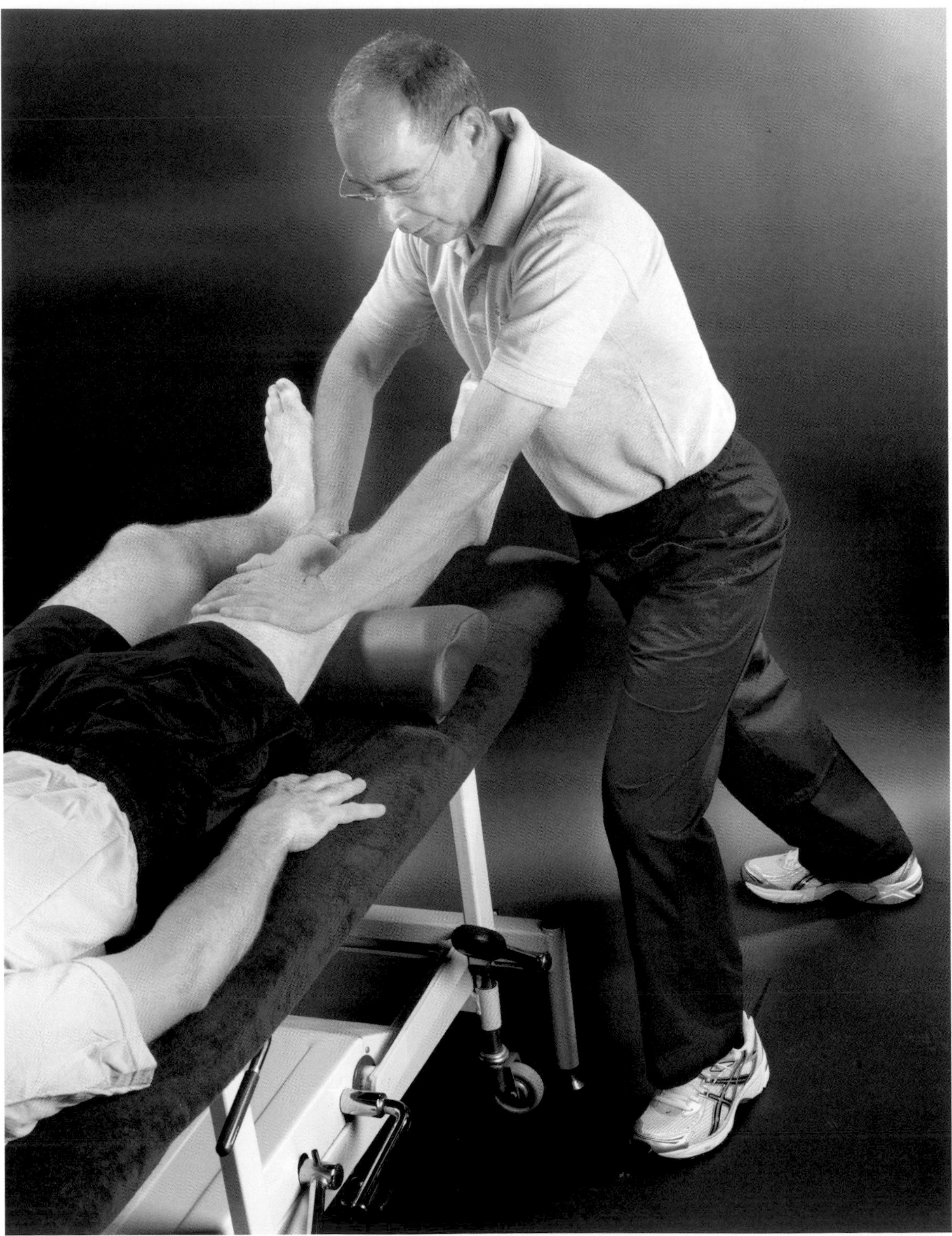

Photo 52. The quadriceps often require heavy massage strokes and good postural alignment and technique are essential.

The four muscles which make up the **quadriceps** group all cross over the front of the knee joint and are very powerful extensors. They converge into a single tendon, which contains the patella and continues on to a very strong attachment at the tibial tuberosity.

The **rectus femoris** is significantly different to other quadriceps and needs to be considered separately. It is the largest of the group and is the only one that crosses two joints. With its origin at the superior inferior iliac spine, it is a very powerful hip flexor as well as a knee extensor. This also gives it an important postural function as it holds the hip and knee joints in correct alignments. Because it functions differently from the other quadriceps, it is subjected to different stresses and needs to be treated separately.

With a sway-back posture, the rectus femoris is under a constant mild overload which causes it to increase tension. It is also often found to be quite tight in athletes due to overtraining and poor stretching. The hip needs to be in extension when the knee is flexed to stretch this muscle. If not, only the three vastus muscles get stretched. If the muscle is tight, it can cause the patella to press down and rub against underlying structures as the knee flexes. Pain and inflammation may appear at the knee joint without there being any apparent symptoms in the muscle.

The **vastus medialis, intermedialis** and **lateralis** all have their origin along the upper shaft of the femur and they run down the medial, central and lateral aspects of the thigh, merging together at the patella. This means the muscles' fibres pull across the joint from a range of angles which together control the tracking of the patella as it glides between the condyles when the knee moves.

At the distal end of the vastus medialis, the fibre alignment changes and they run towards the patella from a very oblique angle. This holds the patella in its medial plain and prevents any lateral displacement. Any tissue damage or weakness in this part of the muscle can significantly affect patella tracking and cause joint problems.

The vastus lateralis is commonly found to be stronger and more developed, especially in athletes, and hypertonicity here can inhibit and cause the opposite weakening effect on the medialis which opposes it across the knee. This can allow the patella to be pulled laterally as the knee flexes, causing it to rub against the lateral femoral condyle and lead to inflammation there.

Adolescents who do a lot of strong exercise involving knee extension can develop inflammation at the quadriceps insertion with the tibial tuberosity. This is because the excessive force on this point affects the growth plate and the bony prominence overdevelops, remaining permanently enlarged (**Osgood-Schlatter** condition).

The **sartorius** is a very long thin superficial muscle with its origin at the anterior superior iliac crest. It sweeps down and medially over the quadriceps, around the medial aspect of the knee and inserts into the medial tibia at the pes anserinus. The actions that would take place when this muscle shortens are hip flexion with outward rotation and knee flexion. But there are much bigger stronger muscles to perform these actions, and so the sartorius almost never gets overused or injured. The shape of the muscle is quite unusual. When a muscle contracts and shortens, it is naturally pulled into a straight line, but the sartorius does not take the shortest straight line between its attachment points. This muscle would seem to be more of a control muscle that coordinates the positions of the hip and knee (similar to the plantaris muscle in the lower leg). *(See fig. 54.)*

Anterior lower leg

The largest muscle running down the front of of the lower leg is the **tibialis anterior** which has a large attachment over the lateral surface of the tibia and interosseous membrane. It has a thick tendon which passes under a strong retinaculum in the fascia at the ankle before it attaches across the joint between the medial cuneiform and first metatarsal. It dorsiflexes the ankle and slightly inverts it. If the muscle suffers overuse, it can develop a compartment syndrome where the tight fascial sheath around the muscle prevents the muscles expanding.

The **extensor digitorum longus** attaches along the anterior surface of the fibula and passes under the retinaculum before dividing into four long tendons which insert into the distal ends of the toes. Beneath this, the **extensor hallucis** and **digitorum longus** attach from the medial surface of the fibula and have a long tendon which inserts into the distal end of the toes. These work similarly to the tibialis anterior but also dorsiflex the toes.

When standing, these three muscles work reciprocally with the calf muscles to control and balance the alignment of the lower leg at the ankle, but this can be influenced by certain

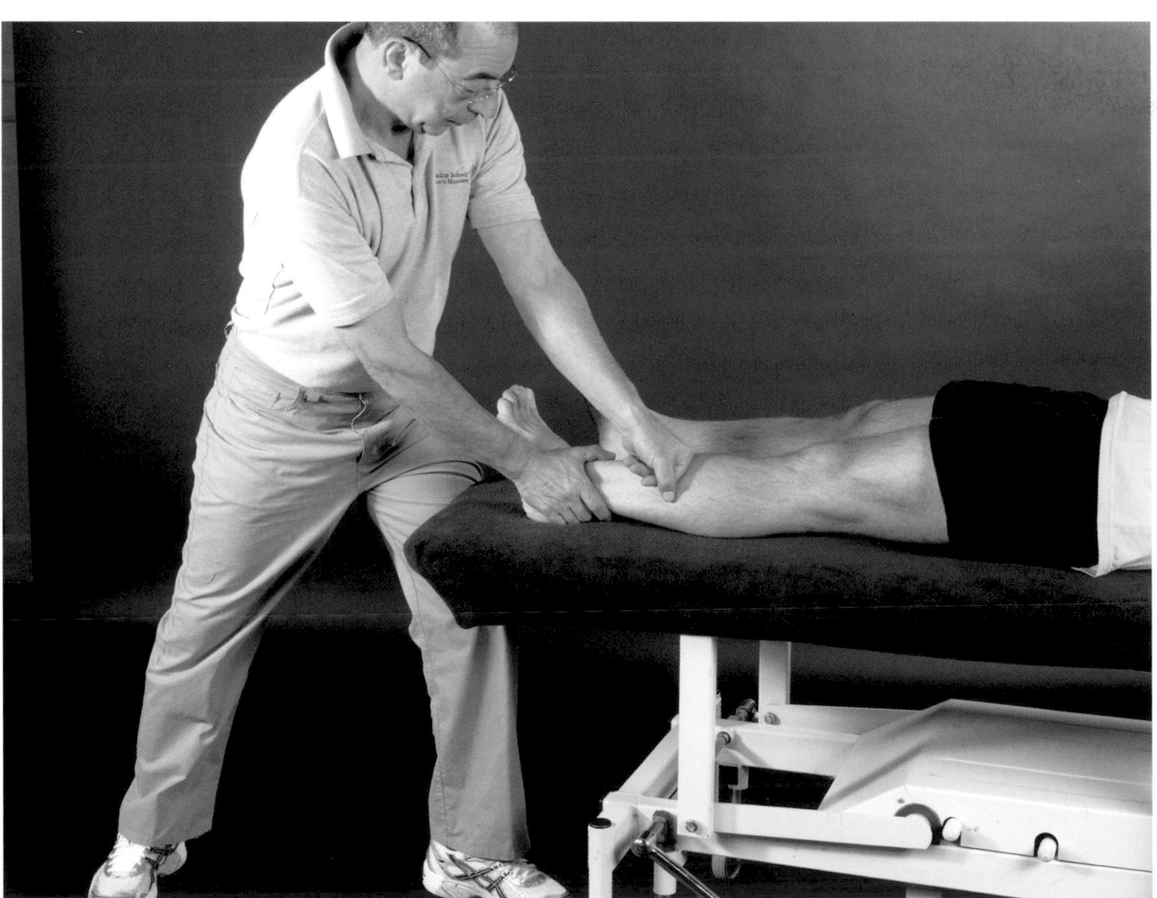

Photo 53. Applying a longitudinal stroke along the tibialis anterior.

postural tendencies. In the sway-back posture, more weight is supported by the calf muscles which can lead to weakness and poor function in these anterior muscles. In other postures, the knees may be held in a slightly flexed position which means the ankle has to slightly dorsiflex to balance it. These muscles then have to maintain a shortened contraction to do this and chronic tension can result from this.

Pain felt along the medial border of the tibia, usually in people who do a lot of hard running activities, is commonly referred to as **shin splints**. This occurs when fibrous adhesions form between the soft tissues and the bone. This restricts the movement of the fibres, which leads to further damage. Providing it is a chronic condition with no acute inflammation, deep transverse friction techniques are painful but very effective in relieving this. *(See photo 54.)*

Lateral lower leg

The **peroneus longus** attaches along the lateral side of the upper fibula and forms into a strong tendon which curls round the lateral malleolus and across the plantar aspect of the foot to insert into the fifth metatarsal. The **peroneus brevis** attaches along the lower fibula, and its tendon goes through a common sheath with

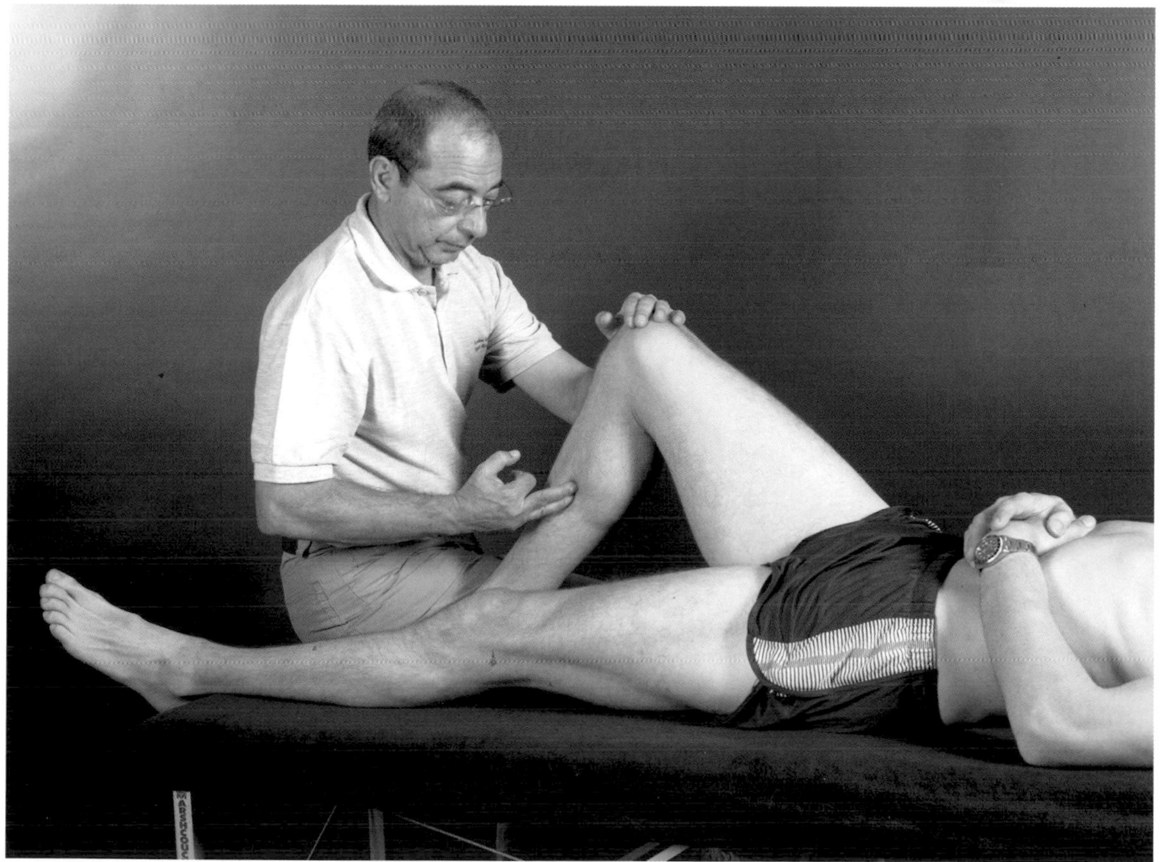

Photo 54. Sitting on the client's foot and supporting their leg with one hand, the fingers of the other hand can be curled round the inner border of the tibia to apply friction to break down scar tissue associated with 'shin splints'.

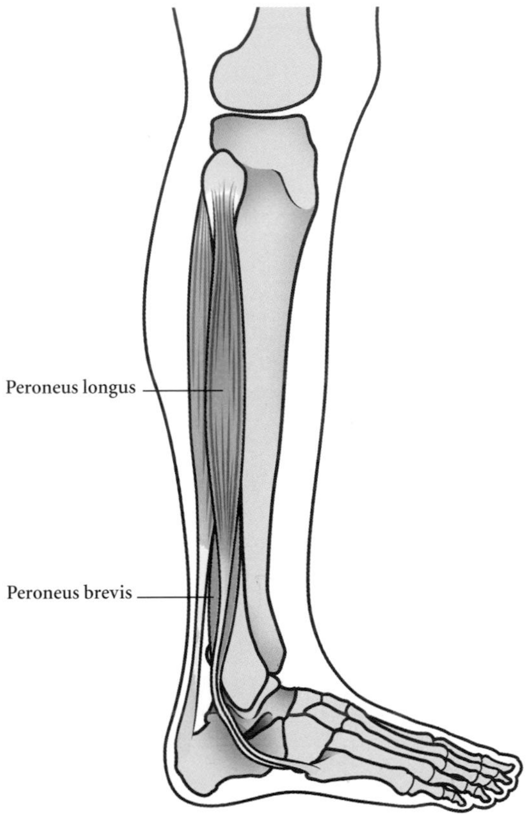

Fig. 55. Lateral lower leg muscles

the longus, around the malleolus and insert into the fifth metatarsal. They plantaflex and evert the ankle. When weight-bearing, they stabilise the ankle joint on the lateral side. *(See fig. 55.)*

Being very superficial, they merge with the strong fascial band running down the outside of the leg in a continuation of the iliotibial band. This gives the peroneal muscles considerable strength and tension, which can make them feel painful when deep massage techniques are applied, but this may not be the sign of any injury. Excessive tension can occur here if the muscles have to overwork to control ankle instability and are best treated with fascial techniques.

Dorsal foot

The **extensor digitorum brevis** muscles have their origins along the upper surface of the calcaneum, have fairly short muscle bellies with long tendons extending to the second phalange of the second to the fourth toes. In the case of a dropped transverse arch, this muscle becomes short and the tendons appear prominently across the arch on top of the toes. The **extensor hallucis brevis** is medial to the brevis and extends the big toe, and together they all dorsiflex the toes.

Plantar foot

All the muscles in the sole of the foot are covered by the planter aponeurosis which is made up of thick fascial bands which run longitudinally and transversely across the whole area. This provides a lot of the tension to the sole of the foot and adds strength to the muscles. If the longitudinal arch drops or flattens, this fascia gets stretched and the muscles have to work harder in an effort to make up for this weakness.

The main muscles on the medial side of the sole, the **adductor halluces**, extend from the calcaneum, and the shorter flexor, **hallucis brevis**, from the medial cuneiform. Both insert into the base of the proximal phalanx of the big toe. They plantarflex the foot and big toe and help raise the longitudinal arch. Excessive pronation puts much greater loading on the inside of the foot and these muscles have to overwork to try to support the arch. Micro-trauma tends to build up gradually without causing pain until it reaches a critical level when the muscle can no longer flex the toe.

The main muscle along the centre of the sole is the **flexor digitorum brevis**, which runs from the calcaneum into long tendons which insert into the middle phalanx of the second to fourth toes. This muscle flexes the toes and lifts the transverse arch between the metatarsal/phalangeal joints. If this arch drops, the muscle will be weak and its ability to plantarflex becomes limited.

On the lateral side of the foot, the main muscle is the **abductor digit minimi**, going from the calcaneum to the first phalanx of the fifth toe. It also helps support the arch and plantarflexes the little toe.

There is also a network of very small deep muscles attaching from the tarsal bones to the distal end of the metatarsals. These plantarflex and move the forefoot.

We often see poor toe alignment with some toes crossing over the top of other toes and pressing down on them during walking and running actions. This means the plantarflexor muscles of the toe underneath do not have to work as the toe on top is doing the job instead. These planter muscles weaken and also lengthen which allows the transverse arch of the foot to drop.

The Shoulder and Arm

Shoulder

Deep in the shoulder are the **rotator cuff** group of muscles (supraspinatus, infraspinatus, teres minor and subscapularis), which all stabilise the joint by contracting horizontally across it from the scapula out to the humerus. This holds the head of the humerus correctly in the glenoid cavity. The glenohumeral joint is not bound together by strong ligaments but instead it relies on the function of these muscles to keep the humeral head stable in the socket. Each muscle within the group also has a separate movement function which it performs at the same time as maintaining the joint's stability. *(See figs. 56 and 57.)*

With protracted shoulders, the alignment of the girdle and joint tilt forward and this dramatically alters the function of all the rotator cuff muscles. When a client has shoulder pain without there being an apparent physical activity that caused it, poor shoulder girdle

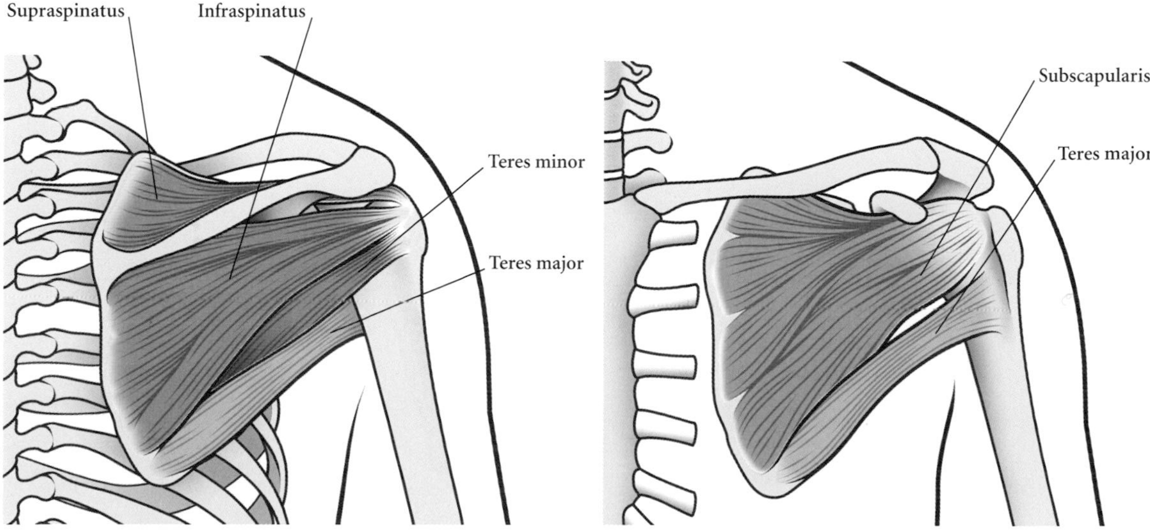

Fig. 56. Posterior rotator cuff muscles

Fig. 57. Anterior rotator cuff muscles

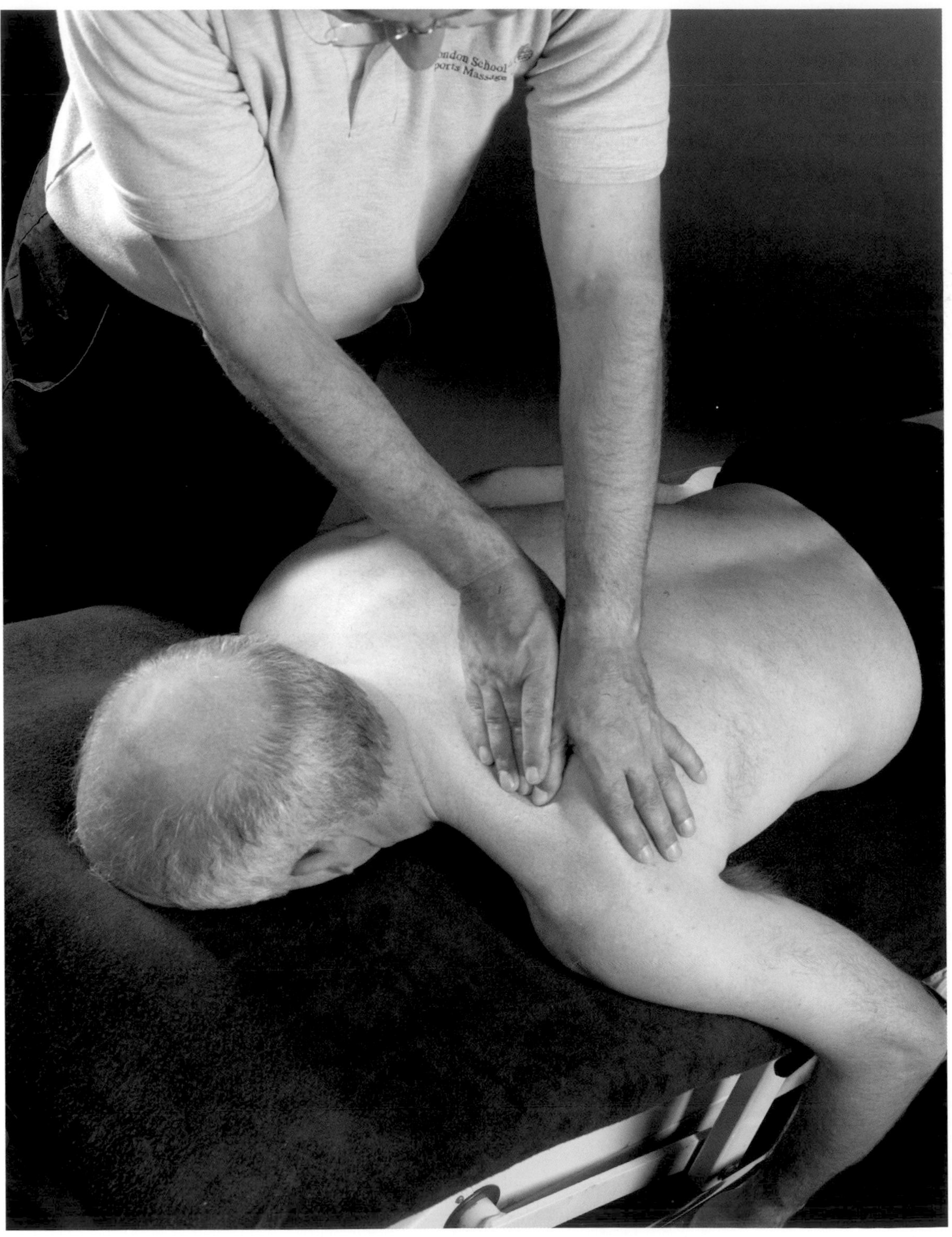

Photo 55. Deep stroking and friction along the supraspinatus using a protected thumb.

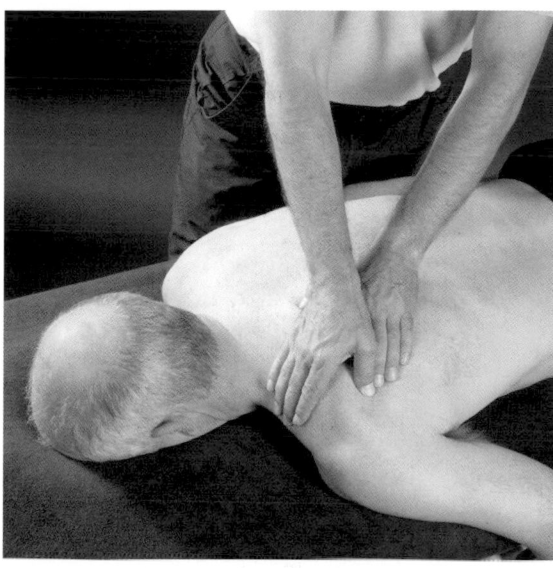

Photo 56. Deep stroking and friction along the infraspinatus and teres minor.

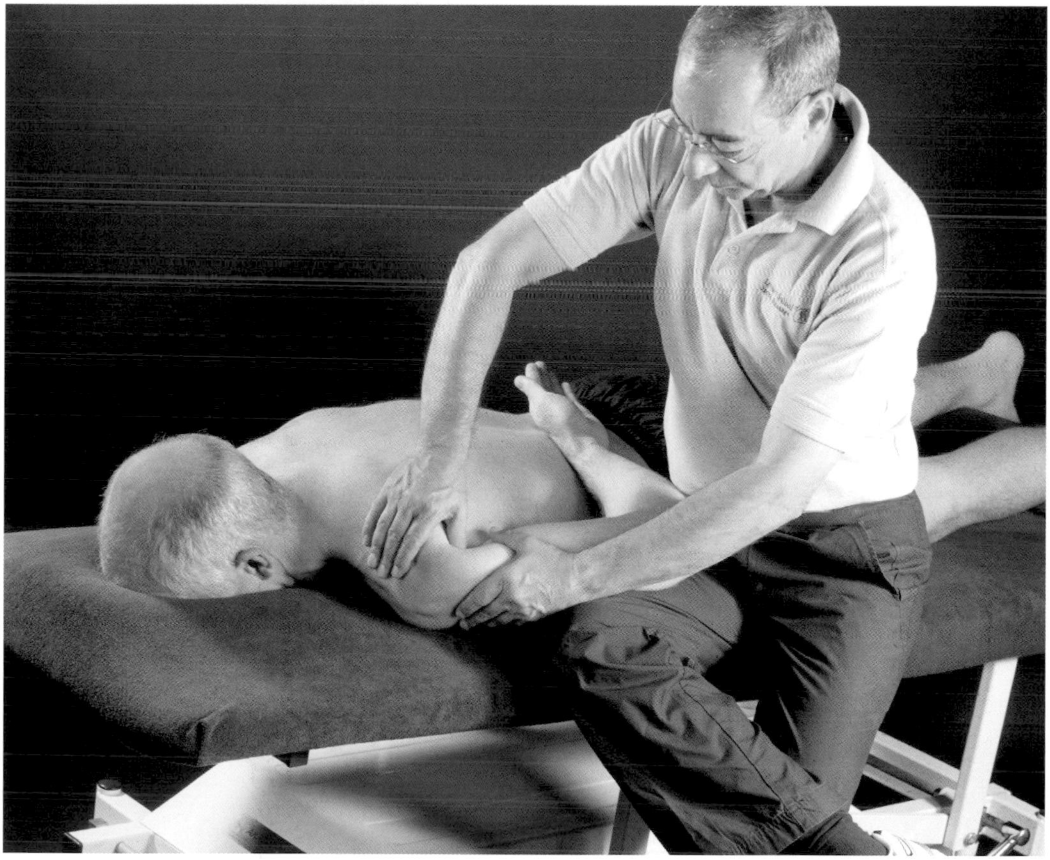

Photo 57. With the therapist sitting on the couch and supporting the client's arm on their thigh, deep friction can be applied with the thumbs to the rotator cuff insertions to the humerus beneath the deltoid.

alignment is the most likely underlying issue that needs to be addressed. Even when there is a link to particular physical activity, it is still likely that poor alignment has compromised the efficiency of the muscles and is at the centre of the problem. *(See photos 55, 56 and 57.)*

The **supraspinatus** is above the spine of the scapula and runs from the posterior surface of the superior angle. It passes under the acromion process, crosses over the top of the joint and inserts into the greater tubercle of the humerus. This is a small muscle with limited strength and its role is to initiate the first few degrees of shoulder abduction before the larger deltoid muscle is able to take over the role. *(See fig. 58.)*

With protracted shoulders, the muscle does not align properly over the top of the joint and its ability to abduct it is compromised. The muscle has to pass through a very narrow space beneath the acromion process, and this can close if the joint is misaligned. This compresses against the muscle, which restricts its movement and can lead to inflammation. Any swelling and thickening of the tissues in this confined space adds to the problem and can lead to an impingement syndrome.

The **infraspinatus** is a wider muscle which covers most of the posterior surface below the spine of the scapula. It crosses the back of the joint to attach to the greater tubercle and so it outwardly rotates it.

With protracted shoulders, the scapula is tilted forward and this moves the infraspinatus

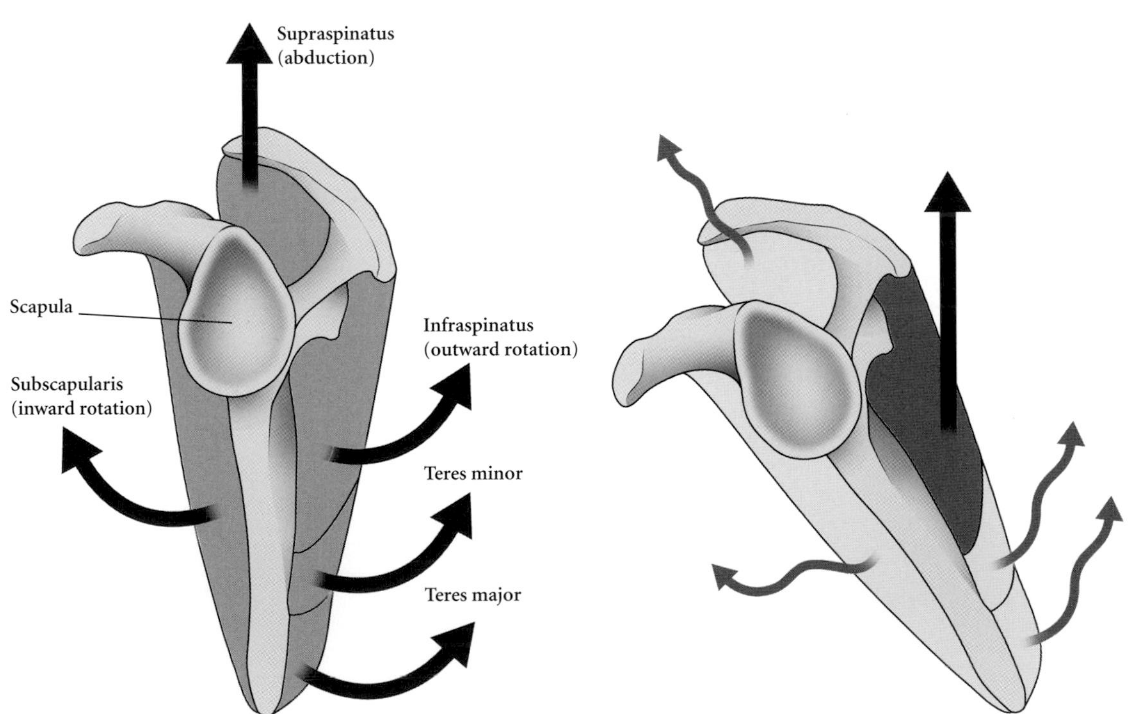

Fig. 58. Cross-section of scapula and rotator cuff muscles

over towards the top of the joint. In this position it becomes more of a shoulder abductor than an outward rotator, and this requires much more strength because it has to lift the long lever of the arm against gravity. This causes it to suffer overuse problems and micro-trauma gradually builds up, particularly towards its insertion at the joint. Deep friction can effectively break down the scar tissue but it will build up again if the shoulder alignment issue is not corrected.

Below this, the **teres minor** runs from the medial border of the scapula to insert just below the infraspinatus on the humerus and it also outwardly rotates the shoulder. But with protracted shoulders this muscle also becomes involved in extension, assisting the deltoid, and can suffer overuse in this situation.

The **teres major** goes from the inferior angle of the scapula and joins with the latissimus dorsi to pass anteriorly around the front of the joint to insert into the humerus. It is not one of the rotator cuff muscles because it does not run horizontally and hold the head of the humerus into the socket. Instead it crosses the joint at an angle, which makes it adduct and extend the joint as well as inwardly rotating it.

On the anterior surface of the scapula, deep between it and the ribcage, is the **subscapularis** muscle which extends across the front of the joint to insert into the lesser tubercle. This muscle inwardly rotates the shoulder joint.

With protracted and inwardly rotated shoulders, the subscapularis is underused and becomes weak and short but is rarely the source

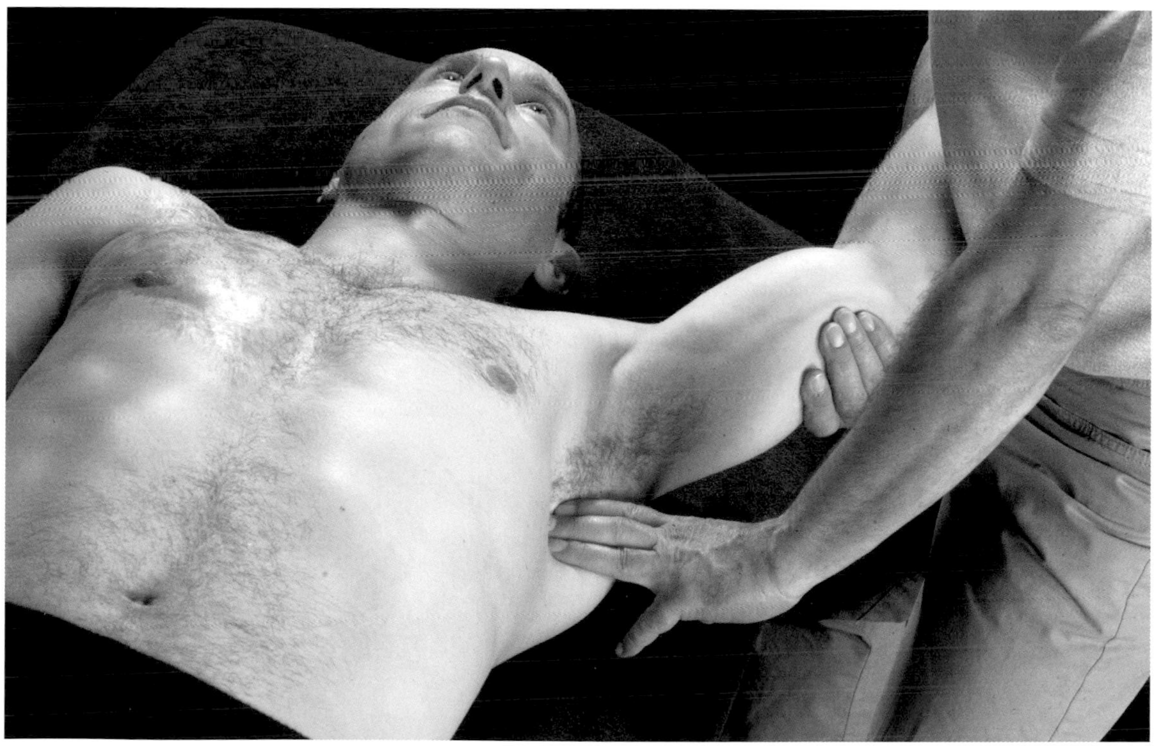

Photo 58. Supporting the client's arm in abduction, the scapula is drawn laterally from the torso. By abducting and flexing the shoulder the therapist presses down on the anterior surface of the scapula and then applies deep strokes and friction medially along the subscapularis.

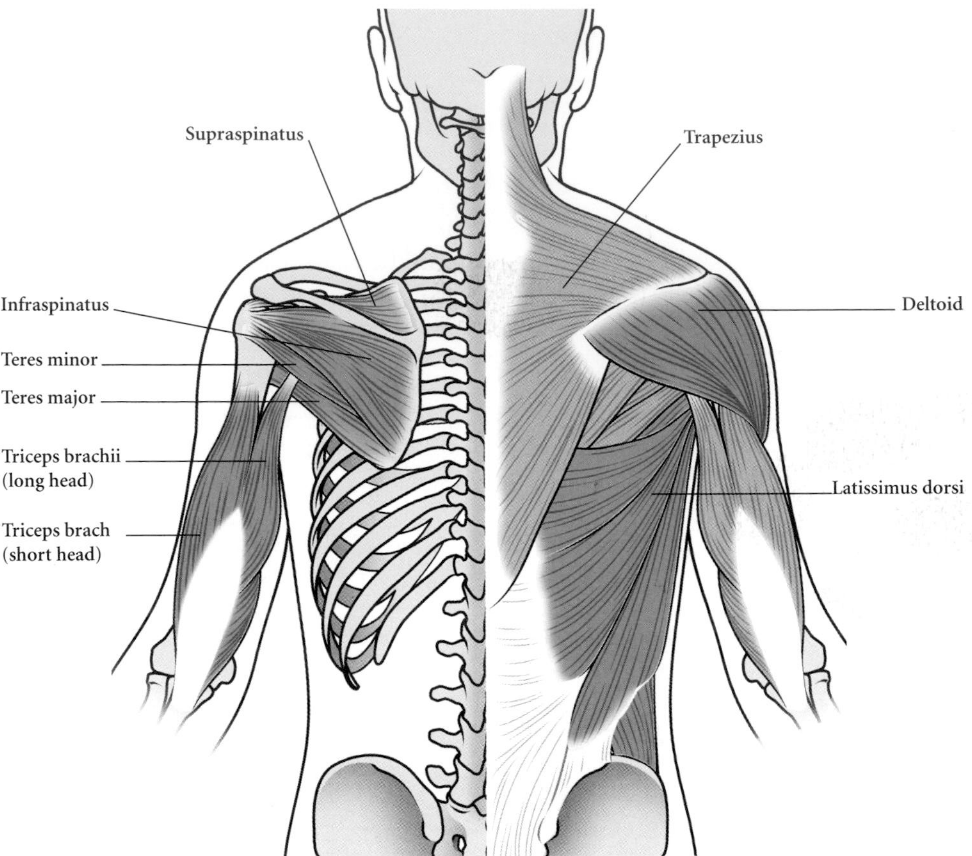

Fig. 59. Posterior shoulder muscles

of any pain. The subscapularis is a difficult and painful muscle to treat but should always be considered when dealing with any shoulder condition or protracted head and shoulder posture. *(See photo 58.)*

The **latissimus dorsi** is the superficial muscle at the side of the upper back. It emerges from the very thick strong thoracolumbar fascia which comes from the ilium, sacrum, lumbar and thoracic spine. This very broad muscle forms into a thick tendon as it extends towards the shoulder joint. This passes round the inside of the humerus to insert into the bicipital groove along the front of the bone. The most powerful action of the muscle is adduction of the shoulder, but it is also a strong extensor and inward rotator of the joint.

The **deltoid** is a large muscle around the outside of the shoulder joint and can be divided into three sections. The anterior part attaches along the lateral third of the clavicle, the midsection at the acromion process and the posterior part along the spine of the scapula. All these parts converge to insert into the deltoid tuberosity halfway down the humerus. The muscle as a whole is the most powerful abductor of the shoulder. The anterior part flexes and inwardly rotates the joint, and the posterior part assists extension and outward rotation.

Protracted shoulder posture changes the alignment of the deltoid with the posterior

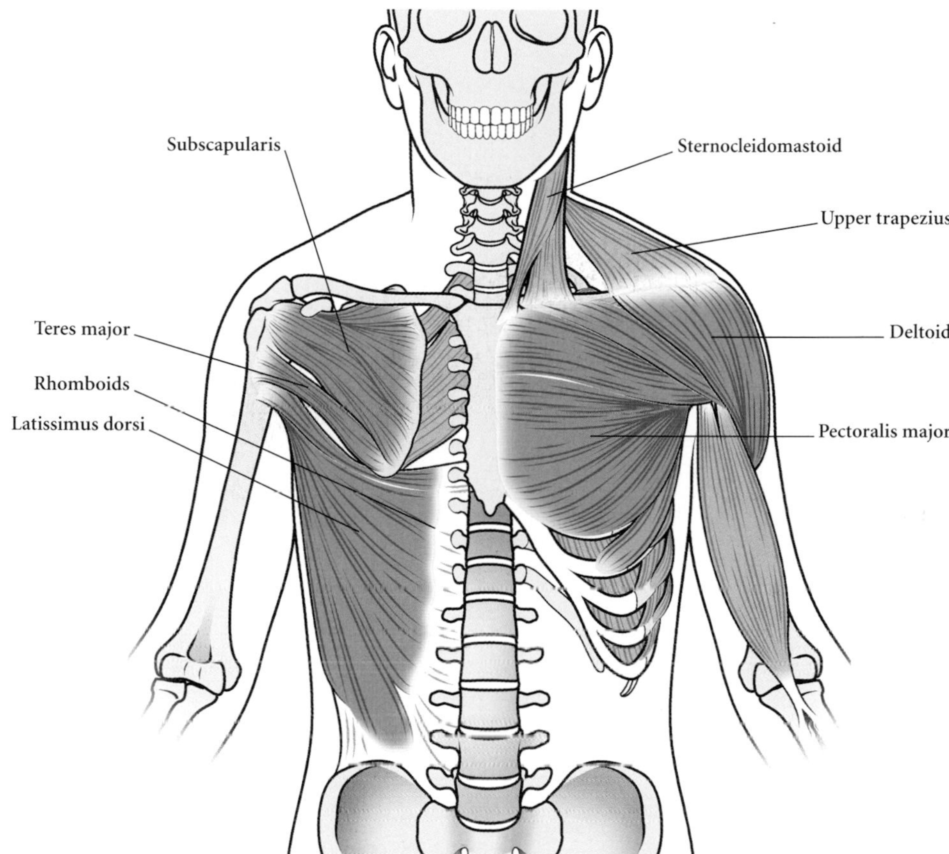

Fig. 60. Anterior (view) shoulder muscles

fibres taking on a greater role in shoulder adduction and the anterior fibres becoming short and tight as the joint hangs in a slightly flexed position. *(See figs. 59 and 60.)*

Upper arm

The **coracobrachialis** has its origin at the coracoid process and extends down the arm to insert halfway along the medial border of the humerus. Its action is to assist flexion and inward rotation at the shoulder joint, but it also works statically to hold the head of the humerus up into the acromion process, which is crucial to the joint's stability.

With protracted shoulders, the scapula is tilted forward and the humerus hangs down and away from the socket. The coracobrachialis has to overwork constantly to lift the humerus and keep the joint correctly aligned. Although it is rarely the obvious source of pain, it is commonly found to be tight and often causes pain to be felt inside the joint. This muscle should always be assessed when treating people with shoulder alignment issues. It can be found by palpating the tissues on either side of the short head of the biceps tendon. *(See fig. 61.)*

The **biceps brachii** is the large muscle on the anterior side of the upper arm. Its long head originates from the supraglenoid tubercle on the scapula, and its tendon passes laterally over the head of the humerus. The short head has it origin very close by at the coracoid process

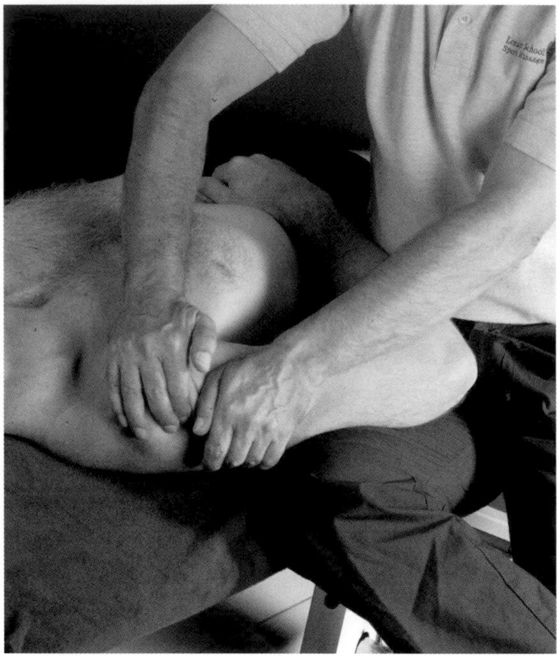

Photo 59. Sitting on the couch with the client's arm resting on the therapist's thigh creates an ideal position to treat the deltoid and coracobrachialis as well as the pectorals and upper arm muscles.

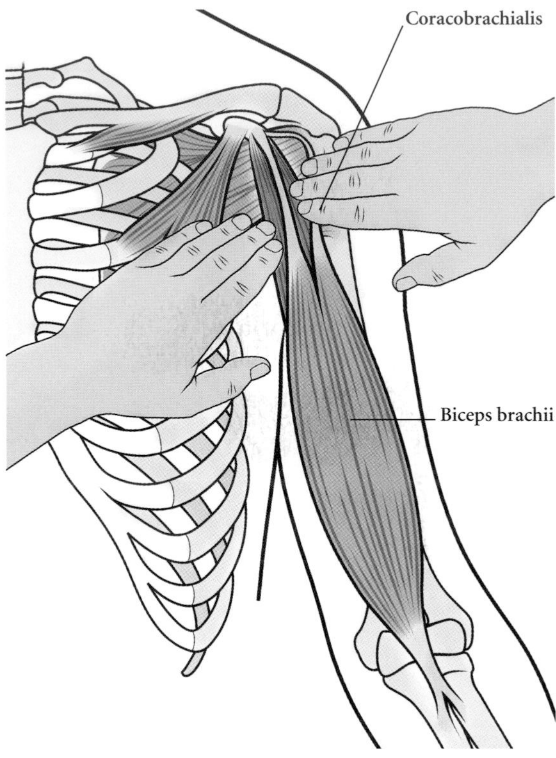

Fig. 61. Locating the coracobrachialis

and passes down the front of the joint. The two heads merge into a large muscle which has two insertions at the elbow. A main tendon attaches to radial tuberosity and a shorter, broader tendon merges into the fascia around the muscles on the ulna side of the forearm.

The biceps is commonly thought of as a simple flexor of the elbow, but the muscle has a more complex function. It is a very powerful supinator of the forearm and can only flex the elbow when the joint is in this supinated position. As the tendons cross the front of the shoulder joint at the top they also assist flexion here.

The muscle can develop great strength through exercise and heavy manual work, but without good stretching it can become short and tight. This can prevent the elbow from fully extending and leads to overuse injury which in extreme cases can include a complete rupture of a tendon.

In people who have protracted shoulders, the long head of the biceps tendon does not pass normally through the bicipital groove at the top of the humerus. Instead it rubs hard against the bone, particularly with shoulder movements that involve flexion and inward rotation. This inflames and thickens the tendon which restricts its movement even more. It can then become acutely inflamed and very painful when any shoulder flexion is attempted. Complete rest is the only way to effectively stop the inflammation, but this is hard to achieve with this joint so recovery is often slow. The dysfunction soon affects the deltoid and rotator cuff muscles, and by the time the tendon has recovered these have often become secondary sites of pain and

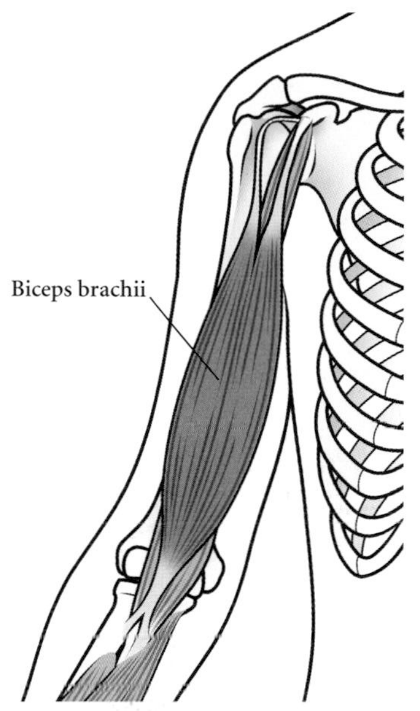

Fig. 62. Anterior upper arm (superficial)

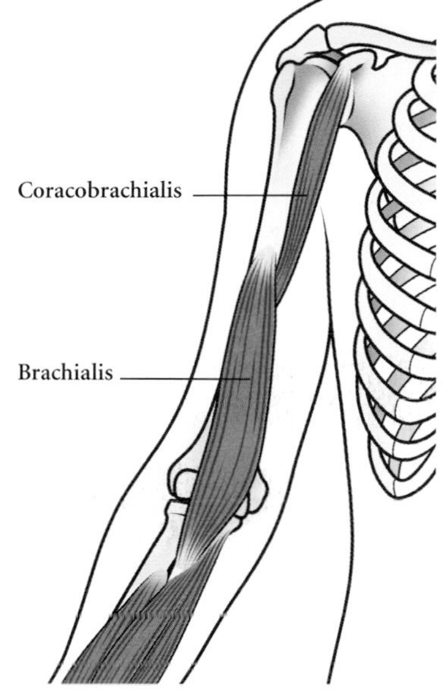

Fig. 63. Anterior upper arm (deep)

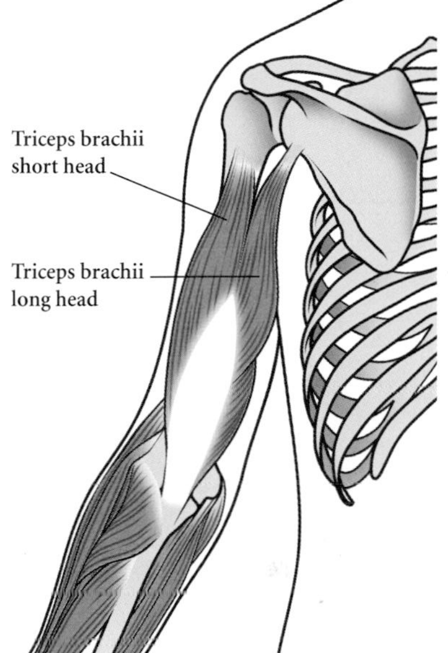

Fig. 64. Posterior upper arm

restriction. Although the tendon should not be treated with manual techniques when inflamed, treating the associated muscles to prevent these secondary problems is important.

Beneath the biceps lies the **brachialis** muscle. This has a large origin covering the lower anterior surface of the humerus, and it crosses the elbow to insert into the ulna tuberosity and the joint capsule. It is also a powerful flexor of the elbow, working in conjunction with the biceps.

The triceps brachii runs down the posterior side of the upper arm. Its two shorter heads have large origins on the lower posterior surface of the humerus. But the long head has its origin at the infraglenoid tubercle of the scapula, making it a two-joint muscle. All three merge into a flat common tendon which inserts into the olecranon process of the ulna. The main action is to extend the elbow but the long head crossing the back of the shoulder joint assists in extension and adduction of the shoulder joint. *(See figs. 62, 63 and 64.)*

The triceps is a smaller muscle than the biceps because elbow extension in the normal upright position is assisted by gravity and requires little or no muscle contraction. But many occupations (such as massage) and some sports do require powerful elbow extension and this muscle can develop considerable strength when used this way. The long head which extends the shoulder gets fairly constant use when swinging the arms in normal daily activities. It is usually this part of the muscle that can suffer with overuse problems. It is not possible to get a good stretch on the muscles by flexing the elbow only; it is necessary to fully flex the shoulder joint first to effectively get a stretch all the way through the long head.

Forearm

The muscles of the forearm are primarily involved in the movements of the wrist, hand and fingers. Great strength is needed in the hands to be able to grip and hold on to things,

Forearm, Palmer-side

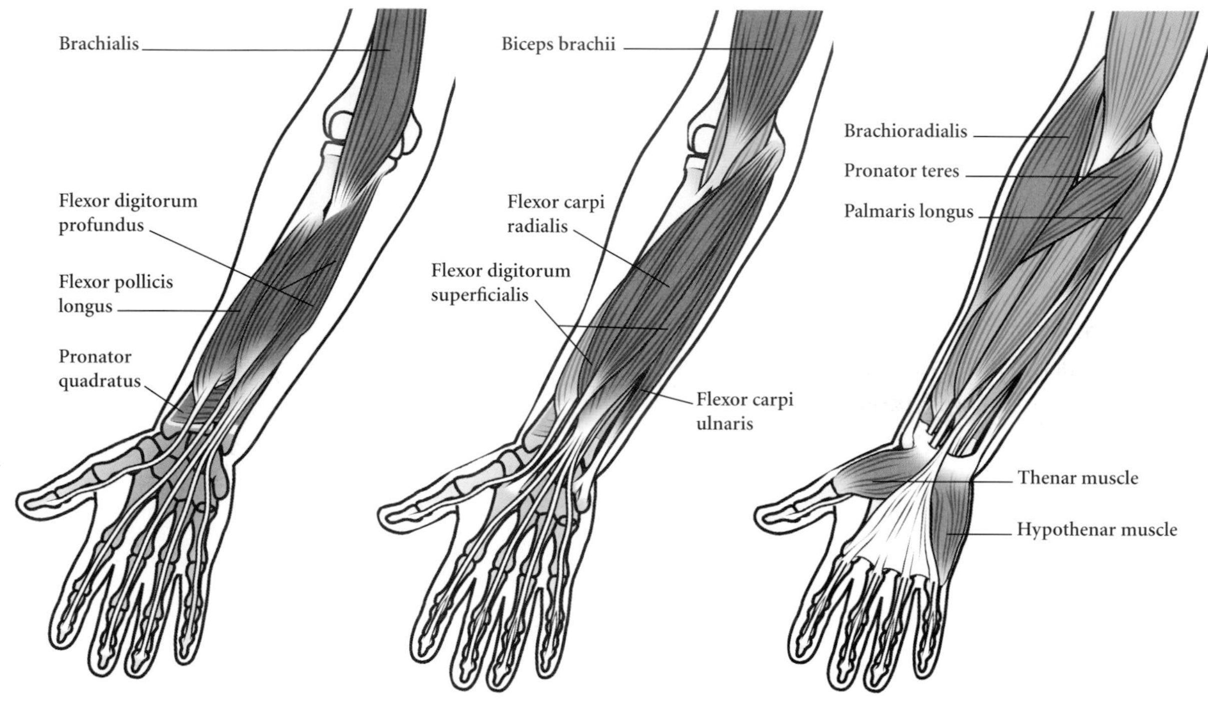

Fig. 65. Deep

Fig. 66. Intermediate

Fig. 67. Superficial

and this requires large muscles. But if there were big muscles in the hand it would be too bulky to allow the dexterity needed for intricate finger movements. So instead there are powerful muscles in the forearm which transmit their strength into the fingers through long tendons. These tendons are kept in place at the wrist by a retaining ligament and thick fascial sheath, which form the carpal tunnel on the palmer side.

Whilst considerable strength is needed on the palmer side to flex the wrist and fingers, the extensor muscles on the other side do not have a powerful role in normal activities so are much smaller. But this does not ideally suit modern computer keyboards which require the extensor muscles to do most of the work. They have to isometrically contract to hold the hands above the keyboard, then gravity is the main force used to strike the keys with the extensor muscles still working to control this. These muscles can be put under a greater repetitive stress than they are able to cope with and chronic tension builds up. Fascial release techniques are usually the best way to release the painful restriction this causes. *(See photos 60 and 61 overleaf.)*

On the palmer side of the forearm, there is a group of muscles with their origins at the medial epicondyle of the humerus. They all cross the elbow and are involved in flexion and pronation of that joint. The **palmaris longus** is a fairly short muscle with a very long tendon which inserts into the fascia in the palm, so it acts in all palmer hand movements. The **flexor carpi radialis** is a larger muscle which inserts through a strong tendon to the proximal end of the second metacarpal and it palmer-flexes the wrist. The **pronator teres** crosses the forearm to insert halfway down the ulna and this pronates it. The **flexor digitorum superficialis** runs along the side of the ulna to insert into the pisiform bone in the wrist, where it flexes and creates ulna-adduction.

On a deeper level, the **flexor digitorum profundus** has its origin on the palmer surface of the ulna, with four long tendons extending to the phalanges at the end of the second to fifth fingers, and they flex the hand and fingers. The **flexor pollicis longus** attaches from the palmer surface of the radius and interosseous membrane to the distal phalange at the end of the thumb, and it powerfully flexes it.

Deep across the lower forearm, the **pronator quadratus** runs from the palmer surface of the ulna to the palmer surface of the radius and pronates the lower arm.

On the radial side of the forearm, the largest muscle is the **brachioradialis**. With its origin at the lower lateral humerus, it has a long thick tendon extending to its insertion at the distal end of the radius. Only crossing the elbow, it does not affect the wrist or hand. It pulls the lower arm into a midway position between pronation and supination, and in this alignment it then becomes an elbow flexor. *(See figs, 65, 66 and 67.)*

The **anconeus** is a small muscle that runs from the lateral epicondyle of the humerus and inserts at the olecranon process and proximal part of the ulna. It connects through its fascia with the triceps brachii and assists in extending the elbow and also stabilises it during pronation and supination. The extensor **carpi radialis brevis** and **longus** have their origins at the lower lateral humerus and insert into the base of the third (brevis) and second (longus) metacarpals. They are weak flexors of the elbow but more significant as a wrist extensors.

On the dorsal side of the arm there are three superficial muscles which emerge from a common fascia attached to the lateral epicondyle of the humerus. The **extensor digitorum** and **digiti minimi** have long tendons running beneath a retaining ligament at the wrist and extending to the distal phalanges of the fingers. These extend the wrist and fingers. The **extensor carpi ulnaris** inserts into the fifth metacarpal and does not move the finger as the name suggests. It is a strong ulna adductor of the wrist.

Deep in the upper dorsal forearm, the **supinator** is a short flat muscle which has its origin at the lateral epicondyle of the humerus and supinator crest of the ulna. It inserts into the radius and supinates the forearm. Below this, a group of deep muscles emerge from the lower surfaces of the radius, ulna and interosseous membrane. The **abductor pollicis longus** is a short muscle with a very long tendon which extends through the wrist to insert into the base of the first metacarpal. Its main function is to abduct the thumb, but also flexes and abducts the hand. The **extensor pollicis longus** and **brevis** extend through long tendons to the phalanges of the thumb and extend and abduct it. *(See figs. 68 and 69 overleaf.)*

Hand

On the palmer side of the hand, the main group of small **thenar** muscles run from the carpal tunnel and carpal bones to the sesamoid bones at the distal end of the first metacarpal and powerfully flex and adduct the thumb. The **adductor pollicis** links between the first and third metacarpal and adducts the thumb. The **hypothenar** muscles also attach from the carpal bones and insert at the end of the fifth metacarpal, flexing the

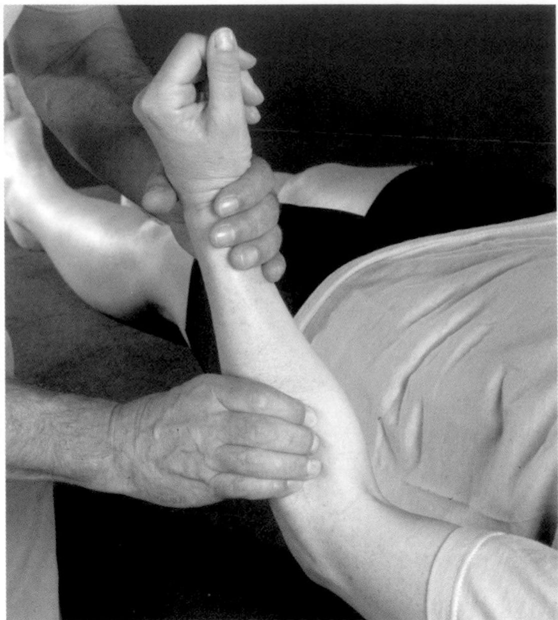

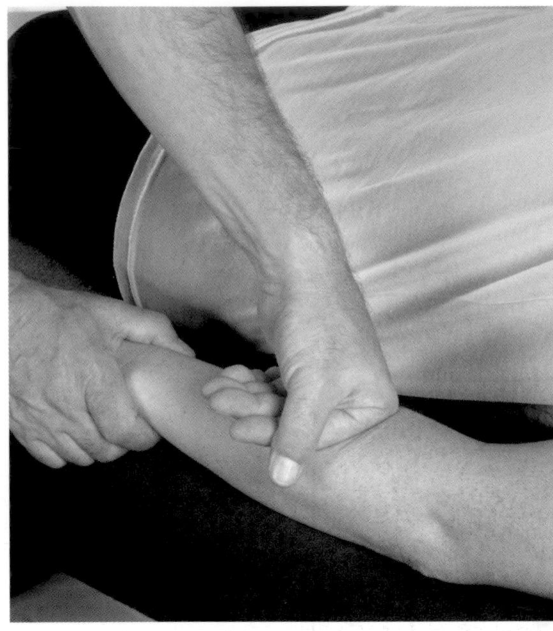

Photos 60 and 61. Friction and stroking techniques applied to the forearm muscles.

Forearm, Dorsal-side

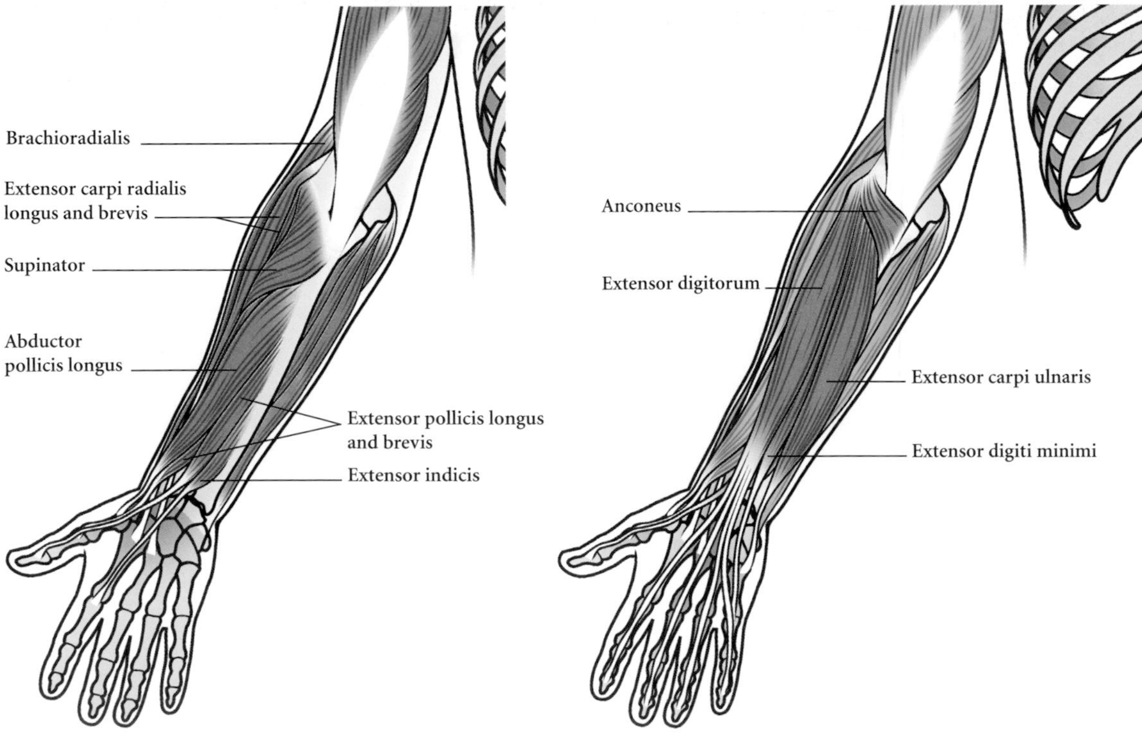

Fig. 68. Deep

Fig. 69. Superficial

5 The Peripheral Joints

Remedial massage is effective in treating the soft tissues, primarily muscles, tendons and ligaments, but joint injuries can involve damage to the bones and inner structures. Although it might be better if all joint injuries were seen first by an orthopaedic specialist and then referred to a therapist for soft tissue work when required, this is not realistic. A great many joint problems are quite minor and can be effectively treated with soft tissue techniques and would unnecessarily overload the limited supply of specialists.

But the client cannot be expected to self-diagnose the nature and severity of their own injuries and so some may go to the massage therapist first, even though they have a more serious condition. It is therefore essential to correctly assess a joint to find out if it is a minor soft tissue problem or not.

Newly qualified therapists who may lack experience should not be afraid to deal with joint injuries. Providing there are no signs of inflammation, massage should always be safe to perform. All the soft tissues around the joint should be thoroughly treated within a comfortable range. If the client's injury is only minor, this should produce an excellent result. But if there is an underlying structural issue, they will probably find that the joint may feel looser but the same painful symptoms remain or very soon return.

Even though a joint injury may appear to be a minor soft tissue problem, the client should be referred on for further investigation if it fails to respond to treatment. Similarly, if a problem keeps recurring for no apparent reason, the client should also be referred.

Joint injuries often occur because of a particular physical activity which is done to excess, with poor posture or technique. If these factors are not corrected, then the problem will inevitably return. There is a danger that regular massage treatment may remove the painful symptoms and because of this the client continues doing the activity with the same bad overuse habits. This can allow a minor injury to develop into a more serious structural problem.

Common Joint Conditions

Joint sprains

The sprain is an acute trauma which occurs when a joint is forced beyond its normal range of movement. The inelastic ligaments which act to prevent this get torn apart and, because they are also often an integral part of the joint's synovial capsule, this gets damaged too. The ligaments have a limited blood supply so bleeding from this may not be that great, but it does cause bruising and some discolouration under the skin. It is, however, usually the leakage of synovial fluid which causes most of the extreme swelling around the joint.

The ligaments act as a line of defence for the bones, and if the tear is considerable then there is a greater risk that there may also be some bone damage. For this reason, all joint sprains should ideally be seen on an X-ray first to check for this.

- **Treatment:**

Normal acute procedures (Appendix 2; rest, ice, compression and elevation) should be applied in the initial stage. It is very important that the joint is fixed in a neutral position so the ligaments repair at the correct length. If they set in a shortened position they will restrict joint movement and be easily re-torn. If the joint is fixed with the ligament in a lengthened position, so the torn ends are held slightly apart, then scar tissue will form across the gap. This results in the ligament being too long and loose, which makes the bone structures much more vulnerable to damage if the accident occurs again.

The muscles are often not injured at the time of the incident, but they may lose strength and tone during the early recovery stage through lack of use. This can be prevented to some extent by fixing the joint firmly within its pain-free range and have the client perform isometric muscle contractions in all directions. This maintains a degree of muscle function without adversely affecting the repairing ligaments.

The strength of a ligament depends on the correct alignment of the collagen fibres. If it repairs with them poorly aligned and tangled with scar tissue, it can easily tear again if tension is put through it. To prevent this, light friction whilst also making joint movements as part of the post-acute treatment can help the repairing fibres realign correctly.

Joint dislocations

Joints can be dislocated in severe traumatic incidents which force the articulating bones apart. This causes a massive amount of damage to the synovial capsule, ligaments, bones and other inner-joint structures. The shoulder joint is the most common to get dislocated, because the arm is a long powerful lever and the joint itself is not bound together by thick strong ligaments which can resist this. The main thumb joint is also quite commonly injured this way in traumatic situations. People with hypermobility issues often have slack or elastic ligaments which cannot control the limits of joint range, so they are also much more prone to dislocations.

Dislocations must be assessed by an orthopaedic specialist first, because structural issues must be correctly dealt with as a priority before any soft tissue treatment begins. A considerable amount of soft tissue treatment is normally required in the post-acute stage.

Inflammatory Joint Conditions

Osteoarthritis (OA)

This is caused by the wearing away of the articular cartilage which protects the bone surfaces inside the joint. It only affects those particular joints which have been subjected to the excessive wear and is more common in weight-bearing joints like the knees and hips, especially in older people who are overweight.

Poor joint alignment is a common contributing factor, since this creates uneven pressure and wear on the joint surfaces. Previous acute joint trauma can also be a causative factor because this may result in scar tissue forming inside the joint that can become an irritant which over time wears away the articular cartilage.

As the cartilage gets worn away in small patches, the debris builds up around it and the bone surfaces become pitted and rough making joint movement even more painful and difficult. Without the protective cartilage, the bones start to rub together, becoming inflamed, and swelling occurs from inside the synovial capsule. When this happens, the joint becomes severely restricted and this affects the associated muscles. The combined deterioration in both joint and muscle function makes this a very degenerative situation.

Rheumatoid arthritis (RA)

There are many variant forms of RA, some of which affect just one or two joints, others involving many or even all the joints of the body. The most common type we see affects older people and usually only involves the weight-bearing joints in the lower leg and the hands. Some rarer forms do affect younger people and can be very debilitating.

The inflammatory joint symptoms appear to be the same as with OA, but the underlying pathology is very different. With RA, the body's immune system treats the synovial membrane as if it is a foreign body and tries to destroy it. This causes the capsule to become inflamed, which leads to considerable pain and swelling in the joint.

- **Soft tissue treatment for OA and RA:**

These arthritic conditions usually go through periods of inflammation in between periods of remission, with a general deterioration over the longer term. When a joint shows signs of inflammation (swelling, heat, redness), soft tissue treatment is contraindicated at the joint itself, but it can be very beneficial when it is not acute. The joint often remains stiff and swollen after a period of inflammation, and gentle friction in and around the joint can break down this scar tissue, loosen the surrounding fascia and disperse the congestive fluid. It may be advisable to recommend (or apply) ice treatment afterwards as a precautionary measure to prevent inflammation if accidentally over-treated. It is also important to treat the associated muscles and keep them in good condition. Exercise to improve muscle and joint function during non-acute phases is very important.

Bursitis

Bursae are small fat pads which are found within and around joints and act as cushions to prevent friction between the moving structures. Excessive and/or repetitive pressure or rubbing against these can cause them to become inflamed and cause pain and swelling. Poor technique when performing repetitive movement in sports or occupations can often lead to this type of joint problem. It is an overuse condition that may also be aggravated by poor joint alignment or extreme muscle/tendon tension which increases the pressure on underlying bursae.

As this problem is caused by pressure and friction, it does not respond too well to deep soft tissue techniques which do the same thing. Resting the joint is the primary way to allowing the inflammation to subside, but unless the specific overuse factors causing the problem can be identified and corrected the problem is likely to recur.

Assessing and Treating Peripheral Joints

When assessing a joint injury, it is vital to observe what is happening throughout the body as well as the joint in question. Clients may unknowingly be moving other parts of the body to compensate for a dysfunction in a particular joint. For example, instead of abducting their shoulder joint fully, they may elevate the shoulder girdle to achieve the same overall result. A painful overuse problem in one joint may be caused by underuse from a restriction in another area, so it is important to look at the whole body.

When testing a joint's function, all movements should be performed slowly and smoothly, and the therapist needs to observe the quality of the movement throughout the range. If a client only seems able to perform a movement quickly this is usually a sure sign that the muscles are not functioning well. Any shaking or hesitation may suggest that there is a neuromuscular issue involved.

Postural Assessment

The client's posture should be assessed with particular regard to how this may affect the alignment of the injured joint. Even though the injury may appear to have been caused by a particular activity, joint misalignment through poor posture may be the underlying cause of the problem.

Particular attention should be paid to the spinal alignment in the neck with arm joint injuries, and the lumbar section with leg joint injuries. Postural tendencies here, usually excessive lordosis, may cause nerve compression which can lead to painful symptoms appearing anywhere along the limb.

Active Movements

The client actively takes the joint through all its anatomical ranges of movement and describes where they feel any pain or resistance as they move. This should always be the first test as it shows the therapist their safe and comfortable range before making any manual movements with it.

Resistive Movements (Optional)

Active movements may not test the joint enough to produce any clear result so, to increase the force, the therapist can apply a resistance throughout the range. A muscular overuse issue will cause greater pain when more force is applied.

Passive

The non-contractile joint structures need to be assessed and tested passively so no muscular activity is involved. The client remains relaxed, and the therapist moves the joint through all its ranges of movement. It is important to make sure that only the joint being tested is moving and the rest of the body is fixed, still and relaxed. As well as moving the joint and controlling the client's body position, the therapist should also try to have one hand palpating the joint that is being assessed to feel what is happening there. *(See photo 62.)*

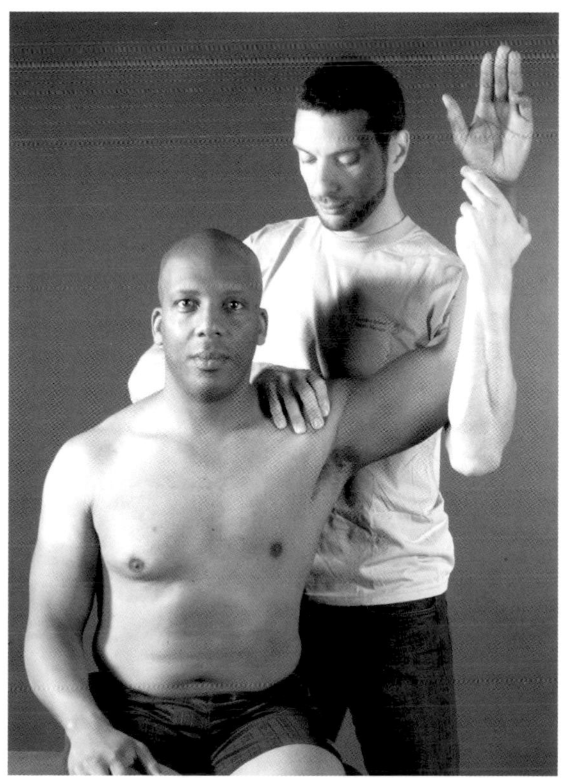

Photo 62. The therapist is using one hand to feel the joint and control the shoulder girdle alignment. With the other arm and hand, he supports the whole arm and takes the glenohumeral joint to the end of its range, and a mild overpressure is applied to test the joint.

Passive Over-pressure

To further test the ligaments, the therapist needs to assess the joint's end-feel by applying a slight over-pressure at the end of the range. In a normal healthy joint, the ligaments are capable of resisting a very strong force without causing any pain. So the therapist should start cautiously with mild pressure but then build up to a reasonable force at the end-of-range to test how it feels. *(See photo 63.)*

Interpreting the Results

If the client feels pain when doing active and resistive movements (when their muscles are doing the work) but no pain when it is passively moved, this clearly suggests it must be a muscle/tendon problem. But pain with both active and passive movements will indicate a problem in the joint structure (ligaments, capsule and/or inner joint structures).

The end-feel

- Resistance and pain which gradually increases towards the end of the range with a soft springy end-feel usually indicates a muscle/tendon issue.
- A sharper resistance and increased pain felt only in the last few degrees of overpressure, with a short and slightly soft end-feel usually indicates some ligament/capsule damage.
- A sudden hard end-stop with an abrupt sharp onset of pain suggests a bone or joint structure issue. It could also be caused by scar tissue in the soft tissues around the joint being compressed.

It is important to know the anatomy of the joint and be aware of what the end-feel should be. For example, the knee joint should fully extend with a fairly firm, hard end-feel as the bones lock together. But if the joint is being restricted by a problem in the hamstrings (muscle, tendon or attachment points), there will be less extension and a softer, more elastic end-feel.

Individual characteristics also have to be taken into account. A flexible client may have a hard bony end-feel at the front of the ankle joint when it is fully dorsiflexed, because this is as far as the bones will allow the joint to go. In this case, no attempt should be made to try to increase this. But a less flexible client will reach the end of range with a spongier muscle/tendon restriction coming from the calf/Achilles area. If this is not excessive and is the same with both legs, it is probably normal for that client and less likely to be the cause of any problem.

Comparison test

When assessment shows a positive sign by causing pain or restriction, the same test must be carried out on the other side of the body to compare. Not only can this further validate the findings, but the comparative difference can also be used as a test at the end of the treatment and on future visits to monitor progress. Clients may also be able to carry this out themselves as a home exercise, which is particularly useful with athletes who can use it judge how they progress with their rehabilitation and training.

Palpation with friction

Therapists should thoroughly palpate all the tissues around the joint and its associated muscles to identify any areas that feel irregular and/or cause pain. This needs to be done slowly and methodically with small, focused, friction-like movement, using different pressures to explore every tissue layer and bone surface. The

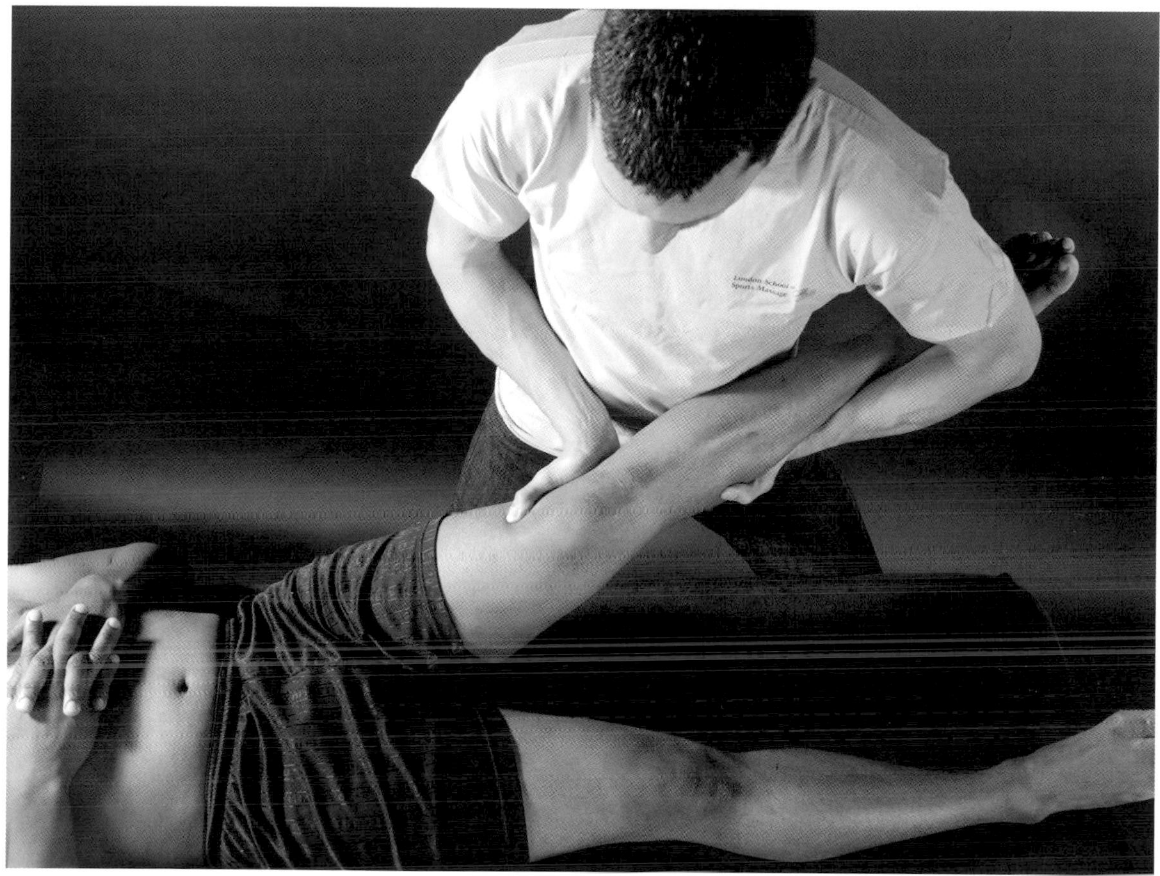

Photo 63. Considerable pressure can be applied to the side of the knee to stretch and test the collateral ligament on the other side. It is important to have good firm control of the whole limb to do this.

joint should be moved into different positions to access other parts of the articulating bone surfaces and reach deeper tissue. The therapist should also move to different positions around the couch to access the joint from other angles and directions. Client feedback can be very useful as they can sometimes help direct the therapist towards the exact point of the problem.

Where scar tissue or fibrous adhesions are found around the joint, deeper friction should be applied slowly to see if it causes pain. Deep friction should be applied to directly treat the tissues and then the joint should be re-tested. If there is an improvement, more friction treatment can be applied to good effect. Sometimes as one area of scar tissue is released it heightens awareness of other areas, and the client often feels that the pain has 'moved'. The same procedure should then be continued on these other sites. *(See photos 64 and 65 overleaf.)*

Some painful and chronic joint conditions are caused by nothing more than a very small mass of scar tissue in a critical place for the joint's function. Good palpation is the best way of finding this, and deep friction is an easy and effective way to release the scar tissue. The real skill, however, is usually in finding it.

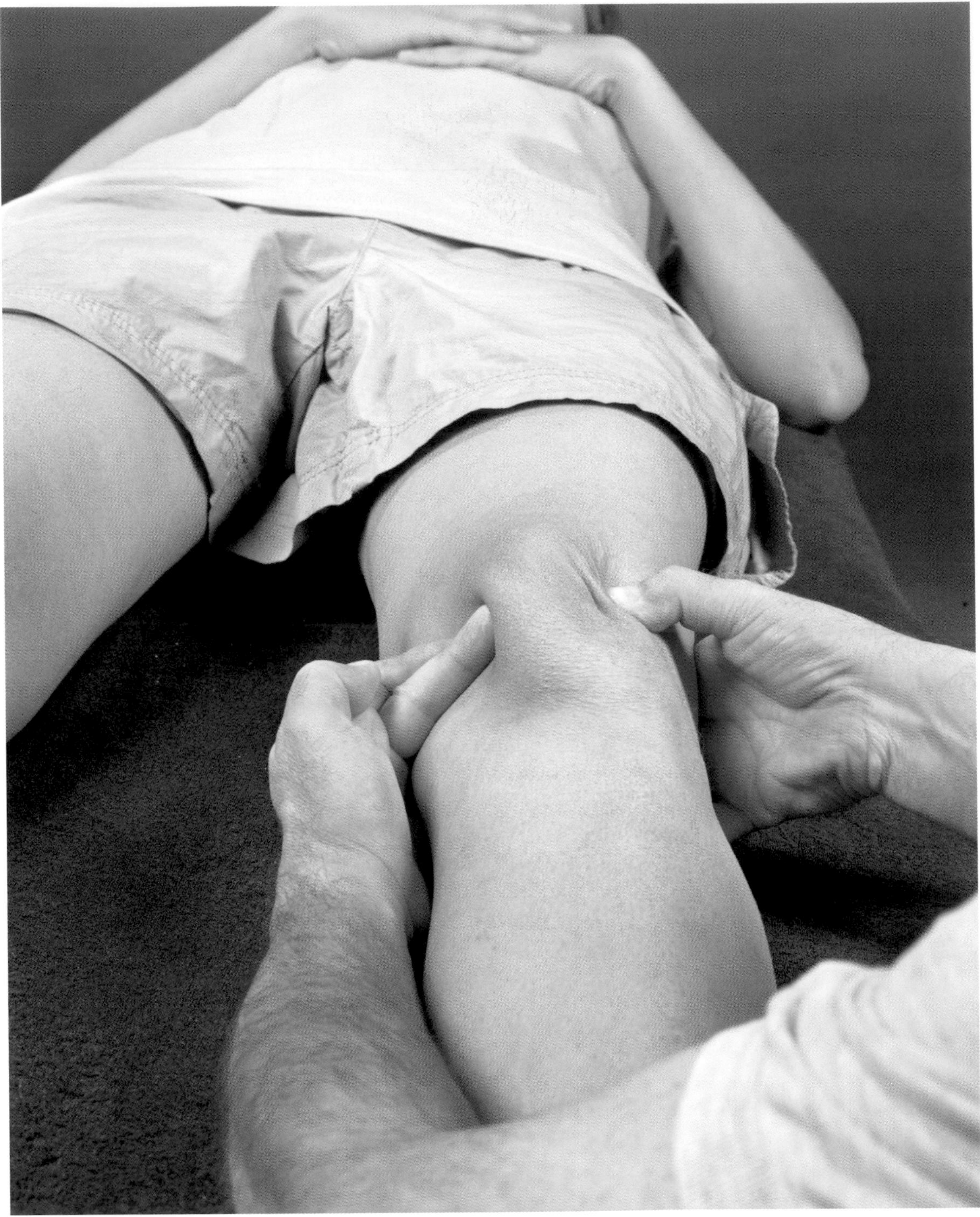

Photo 64. The leg is fully extended (without a cushion under the knee) so the quadriceps are shortened and relaxed. The patella can then be pushed to one side and palpation and friction can be applied down onto the condyle on one side, and the fingers of the other hand can work upwards and treat the tissues under the patella there.

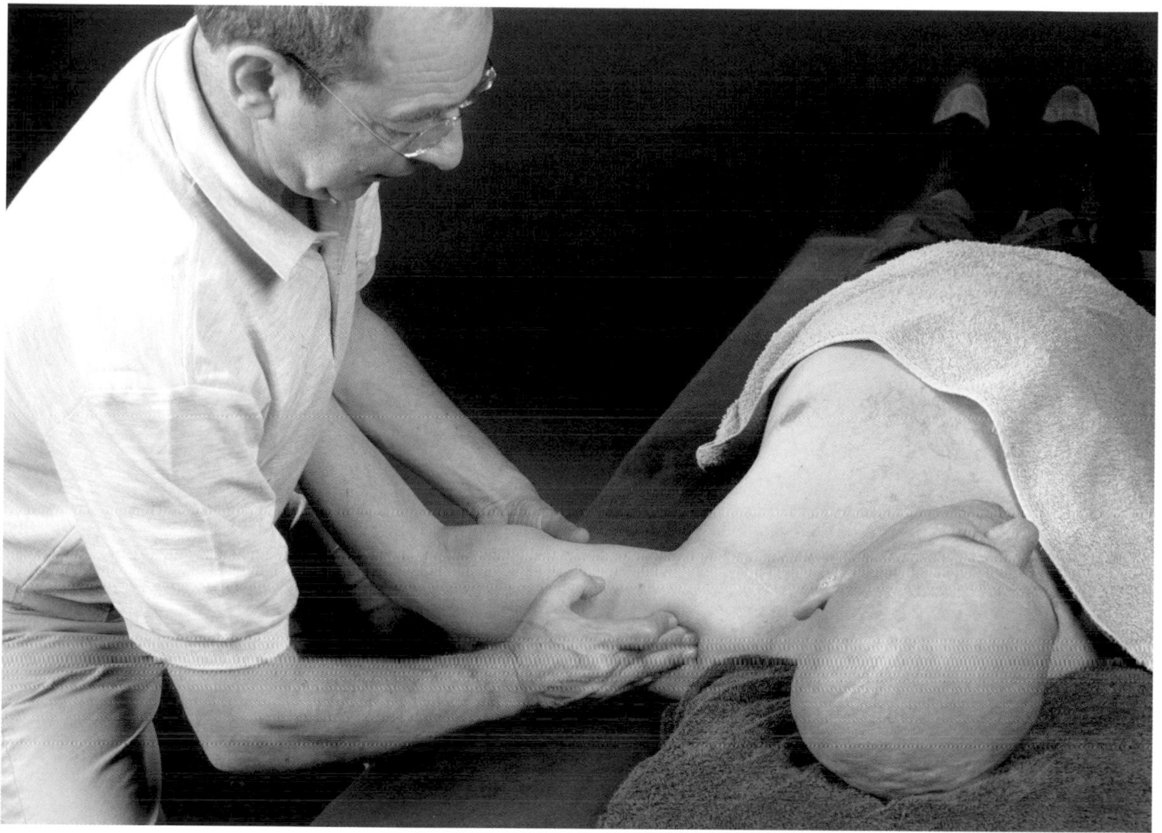

Photo 65. With one hand supporting the arm and passively moving the joint, the other hand is used to palpate the joint structures and apply friction where necessary.

Prosthetic (artificial) joints

It is possible to assess the function of the muscles associated with a prosthetic joint but this should only be carried out within a comfortable range of movement and it must not be tested to the end of its range. This is because it is not human tissue with a nerve supply so any potentially damaging over-pressure on the structures will not cause pain and warn the therapist that it could be harmful. Deep friction applied carefully around the artificial joint structures in a neutral position is an effective way of reducing any scar tissue in the local soft tissues and allow it to move more freely. Care must be taken when stretching the associated muscles not to stress any artificial joint structures at the end of their capable range.

The Arm

The shoulder

The shoulder needs to be considered in two parts. The shoulder girdle is formed by the clavicle and scapula, which can elevate and depress and protract and retract. At the distal end of this structure is the glenohumeral joint, which has a ball and socket that allows almost limitless movement in all ranges. It is essential to assess both parts separately because a

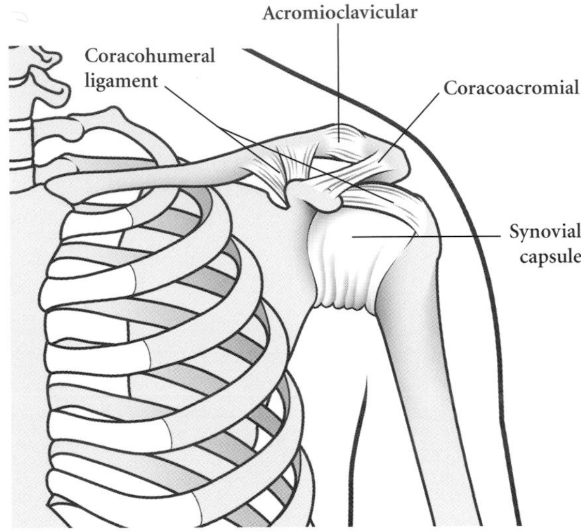

Fig. 70. Shoulder joint ligaments (anterior)

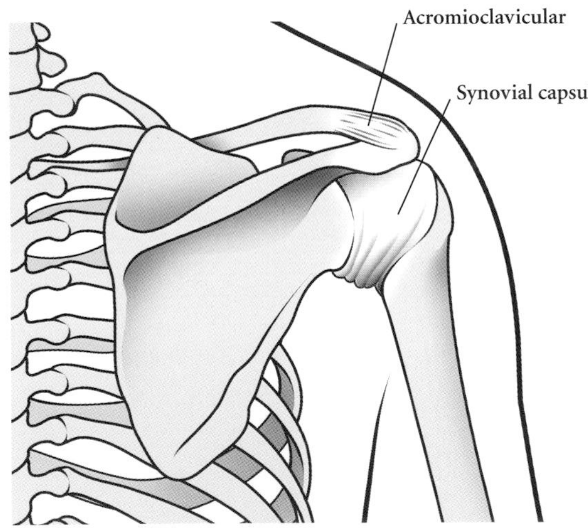

Fig. 71. Shoulder joint ligaments (posterior)

restriction in one can lead to a painful overuse problem in the other as it has to overcome the deficiency. *(See figs. 70 and 71.)*

Function and alignment of the **shoulder girdle** is often affected by postural issues because many sedentary occupations encourage the shoulder girdles to protract forward. The scapulae do not attach directly to the skeleton, and their position is maintained by the surrounding muscles. They can easily glide laterally away from the spine to allow protraction, but if they stay that way for long periods the rhomboid muscles eventually become lengthened whilst the serratus anterior and pectoralis minor become shorter. Protracted shoulders do not usually cause painful conditions directly but significantly affect the function of the glenohumeral joint and often lead to problems there.

With the client in a side-lying position, it is possible to move the shoulder girdle passively in all directions to assess any restrictions. This is also an ideal position to apply soft tissue techniques. *(See photo 66.)*

The **acromioclavicular** joint is bound together with short, strong ligaments which allow very little movement. These can get damaged in traumatic accidents, especially when the arm is used to stop a fall. The upward force through the humerus pushes on the acromion process and separates it from the clavicle, tearing the ligaments between them.

Most joint movements will cause considerable pain, and there may be a deformity at the joint with the clavicle appearing higher. Palpation will identify this as the exact source of pain. If ligament damage is very minor then rest and soft tissue treatment may be sufficient, but anything more serious may require surgical repair.

The **glenohumeral** joint is an incredibly mobile ball and socket joint, and to achieve such free movement it is not bound together with

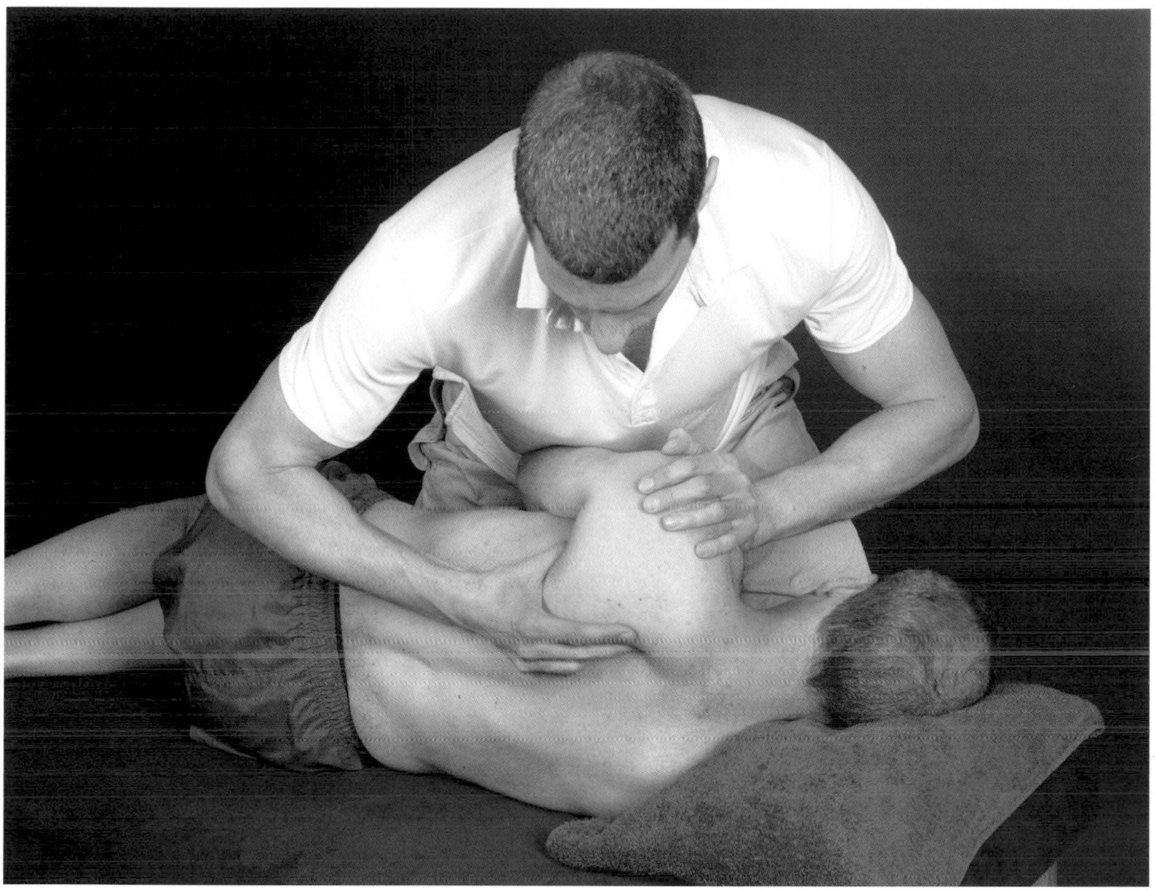

Photo 66. In the side-lying position, the shoulder girdle can be moved in all directions.

strong tight ligaments like most other joints. Instead, it has only a strengthened **synovial capsule** to control its end of range. The joint can get **dislocated** in traumatic incidents, and this causes considerable damage to the capsule and rotator cuff muscles. These require a lot of treatment and rehabilitation in the post-acute phase to help good recovery after orthopaedic realignment.

The scapula only forms a very shallow socket and it has an outer rim of fibro-cartilage (labrum) which creates the glenoid cavity for the head of the humerus to fit into. This means that at the end of range, the neck of the humerus engages with a softer cartilage rim rather than making a hard bone-to-bone contact. The labrum can get damaged in traumatic injuries (**labrum tear**), but because it is a very dense tissue with a limited blood supply it does not heal well and often requires surgical repair.

The stability and function of the glenohumeral joint is achieved by the **rotator cuff muscles**, and their dysfunction is always the cause or the consequence of any injury to this joint. The posterior muscles (supraspinatus and infraspinatus, teres minor) are easy to access for treatment, but the subscapularis is very important too. Although this muscle is rarely the source of pain, it is often tight and causes pain inside the joint where it attaches to the humerus.

Chronic overuse in the rotator cuff muscles

is common, with postural misalignment the usual cause. Over time, this can lead to a build-up of scar tissue and the tendons can thicken or become frayed. There is very little space within the joint, especially underneath the acromion process, so any scar tissue or thickening can cause the tissues to get pinched and trapped between the bones as the joint moves. This **impingement syndrome** causes sudden sharp pain only when the joint is moved in particular positions. It takes thorough palpation to locate the scar tissue and apply friction techniques to try to break this down. It is only possible to do this where the problem can be reached and if it is too far in beneath the acromion process it may require surgical repair.

As well as the rotator cuff muscles, all other muscles attaching to the scapula, clavicle and humerus should be considered as they all play a part in shoulder function. The **coracobrachialis** in particular is often the hidden problem in shoulder injuries and should always be assessed.

Biceps tendonitis can be a common cause of anterior shoulder joint pain in people with protracted shoulders, especially if they do a repetitive exercise like swimming. It occurs when the heads of the biceps rub against the bone as it passes through the bicipital groove of the humerus, and pain is felt when the client attempts to flex their shoulder. It may be caused by tension in the muscle and massage can help remedy this, but the postural shoulder alignment issue usually needs to be addressed for long-term results. Recovery tends to be rather slow because it is hard to rest this joint sufficiently, and secondary problems soon develop in the deltoid and rotator cuff muscles as they increase tension in an effort to protect the joint by holding it still.

The bursae under the acromion process and under the deltoid can become inflamed (**bursitis**) in overuse and joint misalignment situations. In mild cases, massage can be beneficial but, as the condition can be caused by friction and pressure, deep techniques could increase the inflammation. It should recover with rest providing the aggravating factors are corrected.

Adhesive capsulitis (frozen shoulder)

This occurs when a fold in the synovial capsule sticks (adheres) together when the joint is in a closed position, and it causes severe pain and restriction in all joint movements. The common test is to see if the client can bring their arm up behind their back, which will be severely restricted or impossible to do.

But muscular injury could cause the same symptoms so a further test needs to be carried out. If the therapist passively abducts the shoulder joint by moving the arm the scapula should remain still as the joint abducts to 90 degrees. But if the capsule is adhered, it will prevent the joint from abducting and so instead the scapula abducts and moves outwards along with the arm movement.

The capsule is difficult to reach and the adhesion does not usually respond to normal manual therapy techniques either. The condition does naturally release eventually but this can sometimes take many months, and in some long-term cases surgical release or manipulation under anaesthetic is required.

Although it is a capsular problem, the rotator cuff muscles are soon affected through restricted use and this adds to the joint's dysfunction. Usually the capsule releases naturally after a time but by then the muscles may replicate all the symptoms because they become set into the dysfunctional pattern. It may still be thought of as a **frozen shoulder** but, in this situation, soft tissue techniques to the associated muscles can produce incredibly good results.

The elbow

By far the most common type of elbow injury is muscular, with '**Tennis Elbow**' being the term commonly used to describe pain at the radial side and less commonly, '**Golfer's Elbow**' on the ulna side. But no two cases are ever quite the same, so it is better to assess all the muscles and tendons thoroughly, and treat the client's specific symptoms rather than follow any predetermined procedure. These conditions usually respond very well to soft tissue techniques and stretching, but unless the cause of the overuse is identified and corrected it will probably return.

Many muscles attach to the bony prominences at the joint, and repetitive powerful contraction can put stress on these points. This can cause inflammation (**tenoperiostitis**) and severe joint pain when the muscle contracts. It is essential to treat the muscles to reduce the tension on the attachment, but stretching techniques should be avoided in the early stage because this can pull on the attachment and aggravate the problem.

Scar tissue around the olecranon process can restrict joint extension or may impinge on the ulna nerve and lead to neural symptoms in the hand (**ulnar neuritis**). This may cause pain and restriction on full extension, especially with over-pressure. Good palpation usually identifies this, and deep friction techniques can be an effective way of breaking it down. Repetitive pressure on the point of the elbow can lead to **olecranon bursitis**, which needs rest rather than massage to help it recover.

The wrist

The functional relationship between the wrist and elbow is inseparable and both should be assessed. Some of the wrist extensor muscles also flex the elbow, so it is important to make sure the elbow is locked in full extension before assessing their range at the wrist.

The wrist is made up of many gliding joints, with the radius and ulna articulating with the carpal bones through a complex network of small ligaments. Together they enable a good range of flexion and extension and sideways movements. Rotational movements are created through a gliding joint between the radius and ulna. To enable good mobility in the wrist, it is not restricted by thick strong ligaments and relies more on muscle strength to control this.

The wrist can get easily sprained when putting the hand out to stop a fall. The muscles of the forearm are not strong enough to control the wrist against such a heavy loading so the joint can easily be forced beyond its normal range. The small ligaments between the carpal bones can get torn and bone damage is also likely. A build-up of scar tissue, if not properly treated at the time, can lead to chronic long-term restriction in the joint.

Other repetitive overuse factors like operating handheld machines or tools can also cause a build-up of scar tissue in and around the many joints. Restricted movement in the wrist may not cause painful symptoms there but can lead to problems developing in the elbow or shoulder joint as this often has to overwork to compensate for the deficiency.

On the palmer side of the wrist, the nerves and tendons pass beneath the flexor retinaculum and through the carpal tunnel. If this becomes constricted with inflammation, scar tissue and adhesions it can lead to pain and neural symptoms in the hand (**carpal tunnel syndrome**). Massage treatment to the forearm muscles and tendons with friction around the carpal tunnel and passive stretching across it can help relieve mild conditions but worse cases may need a surgical release procedure.

The fingers

The fingers all contain hinge joints which flex and extend. There are no muscles in the fingers, only the tendons coming from the strong muscles in the forearm. There is great strength from large muscles on the palmer side to flex the fingers but much less on the dorsal side for extension. The range of movement in extension is limited by the bones and if the flexor muscles are relaxed and the joint is forced into extension they can easily suffer damage.

The small collateral ligaments at the sides of the joints prevent any abduction/adduction and they will get sprained if the joint is forced sideways. Passive movements to attempt to abduct/adduct the joint will identify this, and friction massage can usually treat the ligament effectively in the post-acute phase.

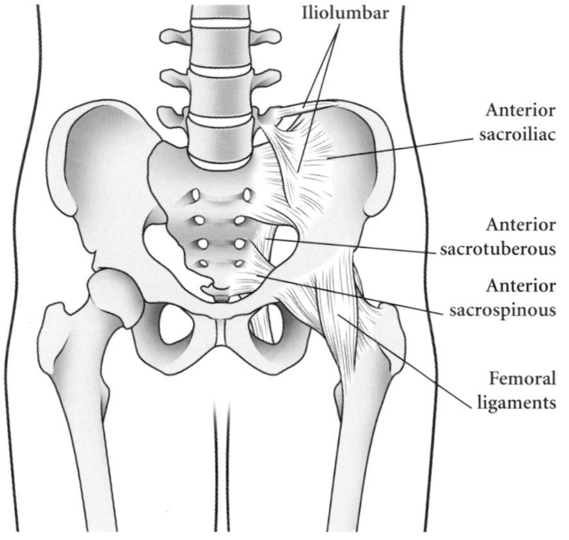

Fig. 72. Sacroiliac and hip joint ligaments (anterior)

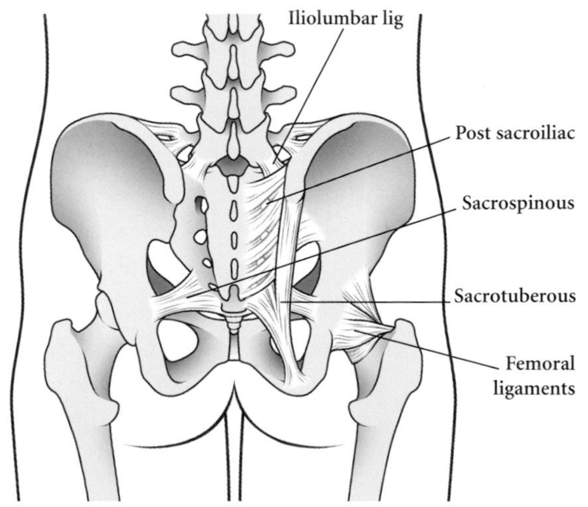

Fig. 73. Sacroiliac and hip joint ligaments (posterior)

The Leg

The function of the hip, knee and ankle joints are all interrelated and an initial assessment should be made of all three working together. This can be done by having the client do squatting movements on one leg. The forward-lunge movement is also a very good way of observing the balance, stability and alignment of the joints. This can reveal issues in other joints which may not be causing the client any noticeable problems but could be significant.

The hip

The hip is a very strong joint with a large ball at the head of the femur fitting deeply into the acetabulum and thick ligaments binding it all together. Injuries affecting the joint structures are not common because it is so strong, but poor alignment, repetitive heavy use and overweight issues lead to a wearing away of the articular cartilage inside the joint. This can develop into osteoarthritis, for which joint replacement is often the only eventual remedy. *(See figs. 72 and 73.)*

The most common cause of hip pain is muscular. There are many strong muscles involved in hip function, and repetitive powerful activities as well as postural misalignment and instability can affect any of them. Although only one or two muscles may be the primary cause of the trouble, the dysfunctional patterns they create will affect others so they all need to be assessed with active, resistive and passive movements as well as palpation.

The whole region should be thoroughly treated with massage in prone, side-lying and supine positions to identify and treat specific areas of tension and tissue damage. More advanced soft tissue techniques can be used to good effect to restore normal length and tone in the affected muscles. *(See photo 67.)*

The knee

Most minor knee injuries are caused by muscular issues. Imbalances between the knee flexors and extensors adversely stress the joint and can lead to knee pain even though the tissue problem is in the muscles some distance away from the joint.

Imbalances across the quadriceps can develop, with the vastus lateralis commonly being overdeveloped or hypertonic and the medialis underdeveloped and becoming neutrally weak and inhibited. This causes the patella to be drawn laterally instead of gliding evenly between the condyles when the joint

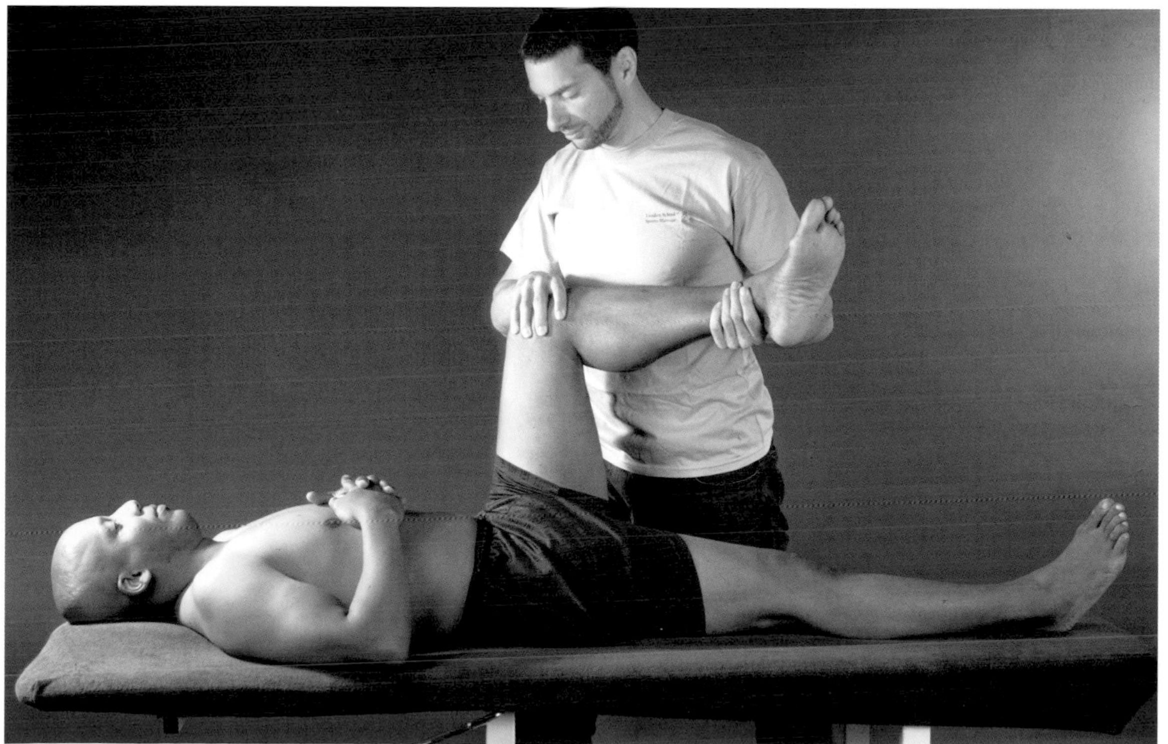

Photo 67. Supporting the leg, the hip joint can be passively moved to assess its range.

moves. The bones can then rub together and the tissues become inflamed.

Previous accidents or injuries which cause superficial damage to the knee may seem to recovery quickly and are soon forgotten. But they can leave some residual scar tissue which may lead to functional problems later on. Individually, they may be quite trivial, but collectively a few such injuries over many years can begin to compromise knee function. The joint needs to be thoroughly palpated in different positions to try to find these small sites of scarring, and friction can be used to good effect to break them down. *(See fig. 74.)*

The collateral ligaments

These ligaments on either side of the knee joint prevent adduction/abduction and can get sprained if forced in these directions. As they can be easily reached with friction techniques, they do respond well to treatment if damage is minimal, but more serious damage should be referred.

When the knee is fully extended, the femur and tibia lock together and the joint is very strong. When flexed, the bones unlock so the joint can slightly rotate, but it is far less stable in this position. The inner joint structures (cruciate ligaments and menisci) are vulnerable to any forced twisting action or side-impact, especially if it is weight-bearing at the time.

Cruciate ligaments

These two ligaments cross between the femur and tibia inside the joint in anterior and posterior directions. They prevent the tibia being displaced forwards or backwards, and they can get damaged if the joint is forced this way. With the knee flexed, moving the tibia passively backwards and forwards beneath the femur will cause pain if one or more of these ligaments is damaged. If there is a complete rupture, there may be little or no pain but excessive movement when compared with the other knee. It is impossible to reach these ligaments with manual techniques, and they must be referred.

Meniscus

These are two fibrocartilage discs which fit between the femoral and tibial condyles; they fill the space and make a good fit with a smooth surface for the condyles to glide on. But they are vulnerable to injury if the joint gets twisted or suffers side impact when the knee is flexed and weight-bearing. Joint misalignment can also cause meniscal damage through uneven wear. In minor cases, pain is only felt with certain movements but the joint may sometimes lock up or give way.

The menisci are very dense structures with a poor blood supply and so do not recover well if they get damaged. Massage techniques can only reach the very outer edges of the menisci, so is not really a viable treatment option and it commonly requires surgical repair. Some clients with sedentary lifestyles may find this only a minor inconvenience which they can accept, but more serious cases need to be dealt with early. A damaged meniscus can become an irritant that rubs away at the articular cartilage protecting the bone and this can lead to osteoarthritis.

Baker's cyst occurs when a swelling or herniation of the popliteal bursa causes a fluid sack to form at the back of the joint. This can be felt and seen quite easily as a distinct round swelling in the back of the knee. This needs to be seen by a medical practitioner and will usually be aspirated to remove the fluid.

Ankle

The ankle sprain is common because it is fully weight-bearing and often subjected to sudden

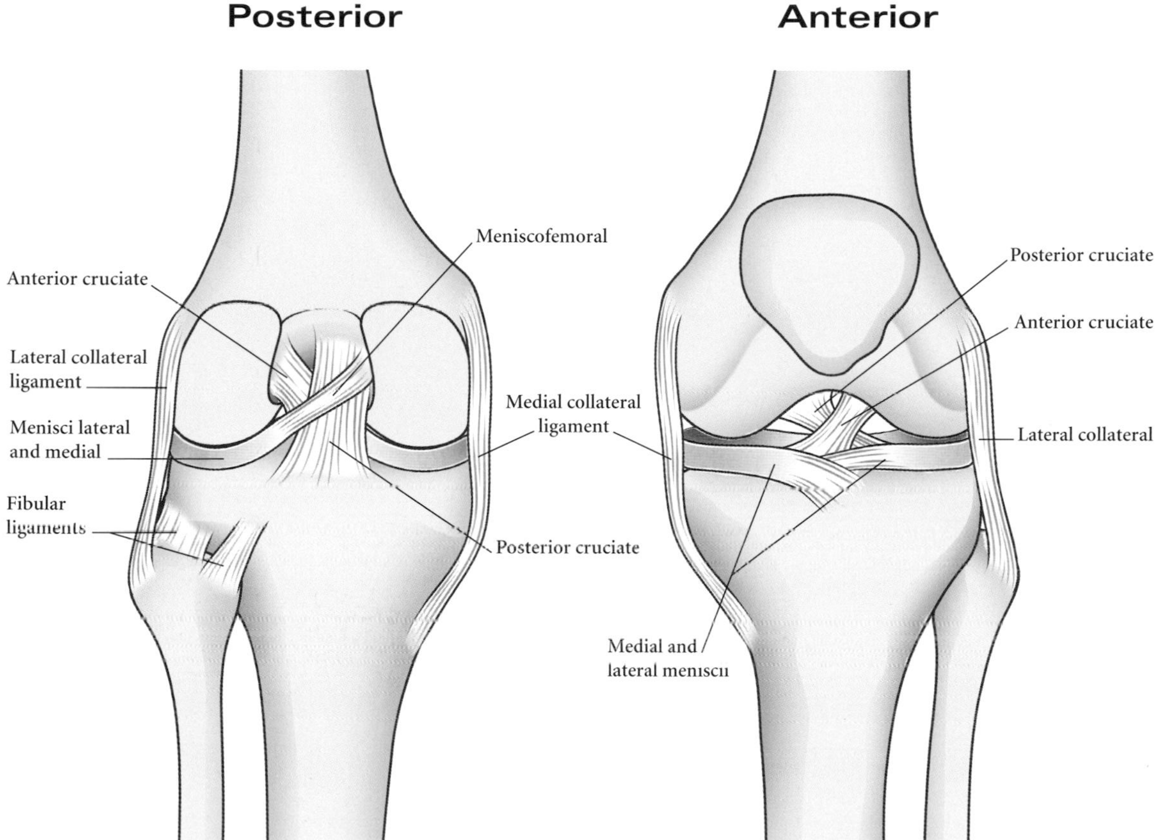

Fig. 74. Knee joint ligaments

sideways movements when landing on uneven surfaces. Such incidents invariably damage the lateral ligaments as the joint is easily forced outwards (inverting the foot), but it is quite rare for it to be forced in the other way.

Poor proprioception is often an underlying factor, and this is much more common in modern urban societies. Constantly walking on smooth, flat, man-made surfaces means we no longer require the same degree of neuromuscular skill to make the rapid adjustments needed to cope with walking on uneven ground. If the muscles are less able to respond instantly to random variations in foot-plant, the joint can easily be forced too far when suddenly and forcefully required to do this.

Proprioception exercises should always be an essential part of rehabilitation for any ankle joint injury, because this often deteriorates through lack of use during recovery. Clients sometimes report that they keep spraining the same ankle and this is usually because of poor (or no) proprioceptive rehabilitation after the first incident. Repeated sprains may eventually make the ligaments lengthen permanently, so they are no longer able to support the joint properly. This ligament laxity makes it more likely that bone damage may occur if they go over on the joint again and better muscular control through proprioception exercises are even more important to try to prevent this.

6 Massage

Over very many years, there has been overwhelming anecdotal evidence that massage has a wide range of benefits and that is why it has flourished for so long. Vast numbers of therapists and their clients are convinced of this, but is there scientific evidence to support it?

There have been research projects carried out to look at the benefits of massage on people with particular conditions, or in particular situations like sports performance. Some have compared groups who received massage treatment with those who did not. Others have compared massage with other treatment methods in dealing with the same conditions. But despite some good efforts, none (so far) have shown conclusive proof of any great significant benefits.

This is not surprising because there are inherent problems when attempting to carry out research into the effects of massage. For test purposes you need to use a standard unit of 'treatment' which would need to be made up of a set number of strokes at a set speed and a set pressure, etc. But this is not real massage where the therapist constantly and intuitively changes these in response to the condition of the client's tissues. No two therapists could reproduce exactly the same standard treatment and nor can a single therapist keep repeating it exactly the same way each time the test was carried out.

It is also impossible to do a 'blind' trial because the test groups will undoubtedly know if they have received a real massage treatment or not, and this must affect the results. One normally wants to eliminate any placebo effects in scientific studies but, because massage is so uniquely 'hands-on', those human factors are an integral part of the massage treatment. Any so-called 'placebo' effect should be somehow included in the research as a valid and relevant factor.

The criteria used to measure the effectiveness of massage are also difficult to determine. Massage seems to be a general panacea which can achieve a number of different benefits according to the particular needs of the client. Someone with tight muscles may have better flexibility after treatment. If a client feels stressed they may feel a lot more relaxed afterwards. A client with high blood pressure may find this has lowered as a result of massage. An athlete suffering symptoms of fatigue may feel a significant improvement in recovery and the prevention of injury in the long term.

The benefits of massage are numerous and in many ways can depend on the needs of the client at the time. It is a 'holistic' therapy which works on many levels by influencing several systems of the body. And its whole is even greater than the sum of its parts. Isolating one single factor as the measure of its effectiveness is very limited and proves little.

But even without research to guide us, massage therapy is widely used and has spread into many areas of healthcare because it does appear to have great beneficial effects.

The Effects of Effleurage and Petrissage Strokes on Blood Circulation

For centuries, massage therapists have made assumptions about the physiological effects of massage. The main supposition has been that strokes like effleurage and petrissage help pump the blood around the body. Because the blood contains all the ingredients the cells need for their health, repair and development, increasing the blood flow to them must be beneficial. But this explanation is too simplistic because overall blood flow around the body is actually determined by the heart, and massage has little direct effect on this.

The pressure and movement of these strokes does, however, have a significant effect on the micro-circulation. They utilise the natural blood flow and force it in volume and under greater pressure through local areas of the micro-circulation. Increasing the local circulation this way helps flush any muscle waste out of the area and stimulate osmosis (the exchange of chemicals on a cellular level). This aids the metabolic processes, improves recovery and helps maintain or improve the health of the tissues.

The volume and pressure of the blood being forced through the interstitial membranes can open up the pores within them and help fluids pass through more easily. This will improve recovery from trauma and fatigue and can have a more long-term effect by improving the interstitial permeability.

Massage also improves the flow of lymph and helps reduce levels of fluid in edema areas. But this can only be achieved by using very light gentle stokes that work carefully towards the lymph nodes.

The Effects of Friction Techniques on Scar Tissue and Adhesions

The formation of scar tissue is the essential first stage of the healing process, and it should be broken down by phagocyte cells in the blood at the end of the process. But such complete recovery is rare and some scar tissue usually remains. This is particularly the case with soft tissue trauma where there is often a lot of bleeding into the surrounding tissues. In the early recovery stage, as well as binding damaged fibres together this scar tissue can form adhesions which stick healthy fibres together in the surrounding area. The fibres need to glide freely alongside one another to function and any adhesion between them will prevent this happening.

Friction and deep effleurage strokes applied across the fibres are believed to break the adhesive bonds between them, and longitudinal strokes can help realign them as they repair. Although this is only an assumption, it does seem to explain what the therapist can actually feel happening in the tissues. Small masses of hard tissue can be felt within the soft tissues where there has been a past trauma, and they usually become softer and smaller after friction and deep stroking techniques have been applied. Although we may have believed this is done by agitating the fibres to break the adhesive bonds between them, it is more likely to be the effect these techniques have on the fascia around the fibres that causes these changes.

The Effects of Massage on the Soft Tissues

It's all in the fascia!

Therapists normally feel that the tissues are softer and more pliable at the end of a massage treatment, and the client feels that they are looser and more flexible too. This suggests that there must be some physiological change in the soft tissues which has caused this. We could consider how massage may affect the muscles, tendons, ligaments or joint capsules as separate structures, but to do so would miss the one single element which runs through them all: the fascia.

The deep fascia forms a single continual membrane which envelops and connects all the tissues of the body. It not only surrounds the muscle as a whole but also every part within it, right down to the individual fibres and fibrils.

And it continues beyond the muscle to form the tendon, becomes the periosteum where it reaches the bone, and the synovial capsule and ligaments at the joint.

If a muscle is held in a shortened position or is underused, the fibres do not get good regular use gliding alongside each other. Without this movement, the fascia around the fibres start to bind together on a microscopic level making the muscle stiff and inelastic.

General massage techniques may not work specifically along the fascial bands, but they do move and stretch the tissues in all directions. This breaks the bonds between the fascial layers within the muscle. As well as loosening the area, these strokes help rehydrate the fascia, which makes the whole muscle more healthy and elastic.

The superficial layer of fascia underneath the skin surrounds the whole body and can be a restricting factor in movement if it is dehydrated or becomes set in a shortened position. This layer is continually being treated whenever attempting to reach the underlying muscles. Areas of superficial fascial tension will be released along with the muscles and it will also improve its hydration.

The Effects of Massage on the Nervous System

The physical effect of massage on the tissues themselves does not fully explain why changes in muscle tension can appear to be so instant. It is the nervous system that controls muscle tension, and massage can have a significant effect on this level.

The mechanoreceptors in the soft tissues send sensory information to the central nervous system and this has a reflex effect on the motor nerves that maintain muscle tone. Because their role is to react to stimulation and stress within the tissues they will equally respond to the right type of stimulation applied through massage techniques. The smooth rhythmical stroking has a very calming effect on these mechanoreceptors, and this will have a relaxing effect on muscle tone.

As part of the autonomic nervous system, this calming effect on the mechanoreceptors can also influence other body systems and have a much wider influence. Towards the end of a massage treatment, a client's stomach is often heard to rumble because their digestive system has been stimulated. This can be explained by a more general autonomic response. Soothing mechanoreceptors in the soft tissues can have a calming effect on the sympathetic nervous system that reciprocally stimulates the parasympathetic nervous system which influences the digestive system.

Stimulation of the mechanoreceptors in the soft tissues may also induce an autonomic reflex effect on the receptors within the arteries and veins and improve blood flow that way too.

Techniques and Methods

Performing massage is physically demanding and, just as it is with any sport, efficient techniques and good posture are essential. Although some therapists suffer overuse injuries caused by their work, this is usually due to poor techniques, working posture or using a treatment couch at an inefficient height.

Students and new therapists normally start off doing only a few treatments a week, and at this low level any poor techniques or postural issues may not reveal themselves. Bad habits can easily be allowed to develop in this way, so great care must be taken right from the start to ensure safe techniques are perfected for the future.

Therapists are all different shapes and sizes and have their own physical strengths and weaknesses so there are no techniques that will exactly suit everyone. Precisely copying a technique from another therapist can feel slightly awkward or uncomfortable, and it should be altered to make it more smooth and effortless.

Basic Techniques

There are only four basic techniques in massage:

- **Effleurage:** Stroking techniques of varying lengths applied in longitudinal and transverse directions to the tissue fibres. They can be applied broadly with the whole hand, fist or forearm; or more specifically with fingers, thumb, knuckle or elbow. They pump blood through the micro-circulation as well as loosening and helping to realign the fibres.
- **Petrissage:** Rhythmical squeezing techniques usually performed with both hands. They can be applied to large areas using the whole hand or smaller areas using just the fingers. They also stimulate blood flow through the micro-circulation and loosen the fibres.
- **Friction:** Short, deep friction movements applied to small areas of tissue through the tips of the fingers, thumb, knuckle or elbow. They have a localised effect on circulation but are primarily used to break down scar tissue and adhesions between the fibres.
- **Tapotement:** Rhythmical percussion strokes applied with fingers, cupped hands or loosely held fists. They are primarily used to stimulate and increase muscle tone and can be very effective in pre-event sports situations. If percussion strokes are applied slowly, they can be very relaxing but other massage techniques are usually better at achieving this.

There is an infinite variety of ways that each of these can be performed and therapists can come up with any number of different names for their own particular styles and methods. But they are all just variations within these four basic techniques. There is no limit to the number of different ways a therapist can use their hands and arms to treat the soft tissues, and therapists should always keep trying new ways.

Deep and Superficial Massage

Deep massage and superficial massage are not separate types of treatment; therapists must combine both styles. Just because a client is a large, strong male does not mean he only needs deep heavy massage, and nor does a slight female client necessarily require only superficial massage.

Any good treatment must involve a blend of deep and superficial techniques. The lighter strokes can relax and prepare the tissues before the deeper techniques are applied. The very deepest techniques should be applied for only the shortest time and then followed by more superficial strokes to relax the tissues and flush them through with fresh arterial blood. Working deeply for too long will irritate the client and can cause tissue damage, but going back to the area to apply deep techniques 'little and often' can prevent this.

No Set Routines

Therapists should never follow set treatment routines, because no two clients will ever have the same needs. A single client will not always require the same treatment, and each leg will be different. Every treatment must be uniquely suited to the individual needs of the client at the time.

If the client is having a full body massage treatment but has some painful symptoms in their right leg, the therapist should start there before treating the left leg. Then return to the right leg again before treating the back. And then treat the right leg again before the client turns over. This way the problem area is treated several times.

Couch Height and the Efficient Use of Body-weight

The most important thing to get right is the height of the treatment couch. It must be low enough to allow the therapist to lean down over the client with straight arms. When the elbow is straight, the bones of the upper and lower arm are in line and the force is easily transmitted down through this shaft with very little effort. But if the couch is too high, the therapist has to bend their elbows and then the arm muscles

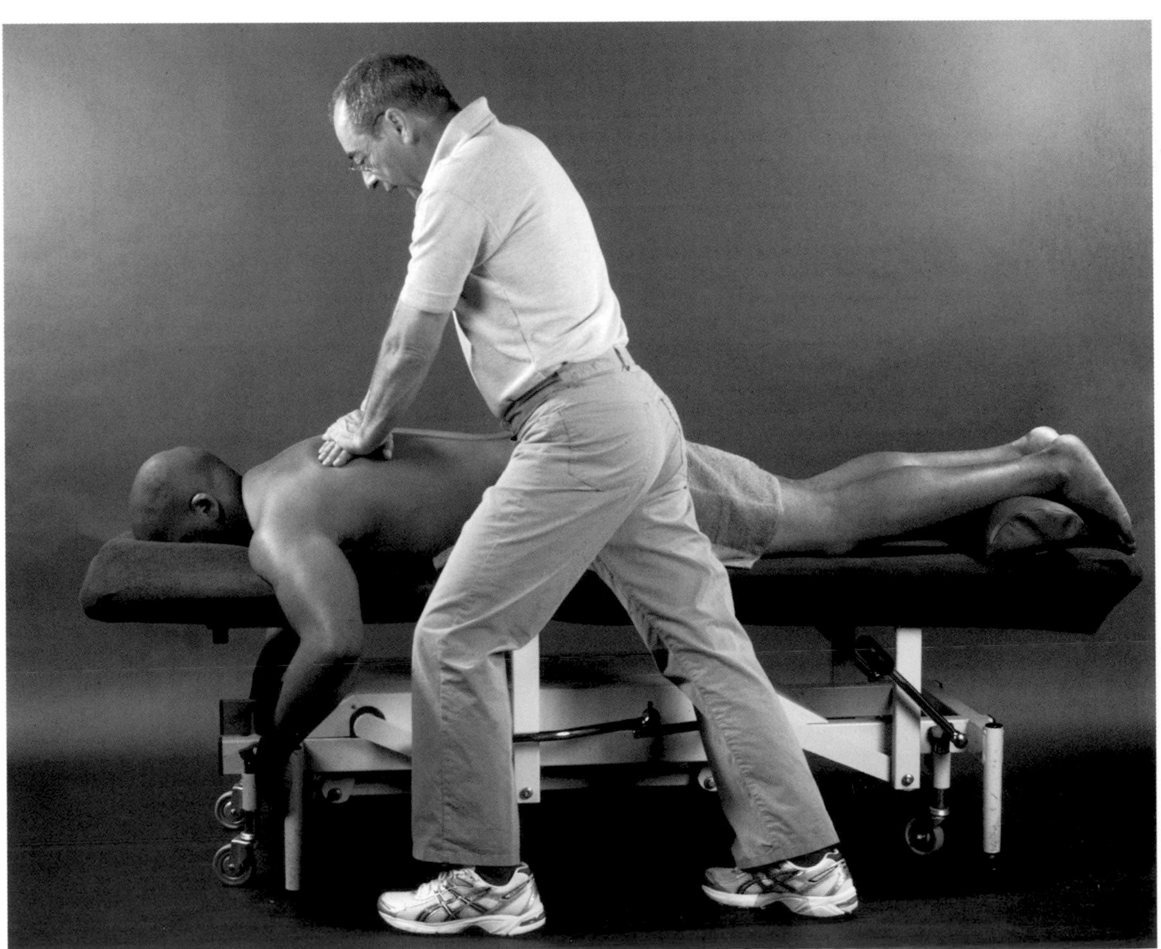

Photos 68 and 69. The treatment couch needs to be low enough to enable the therapist to apply their body-weight through straight arms.

have to work hard to transmit the force through to the client. *(See photos 68 and 69.)*

The height of the couch can depend on the size of the client as much as the height of the therapist. It will need to be lower when treating a big person and higher for a small one. It may need to be lower when treating the back but higher when doing the legs. Ideally the couch height should be adjusted during a treatment but hydraulic couches are the only ones that can do this. A fixed-height or portable couch will often be a compromise, and in this situation it is better to have it set slightly too low rather than too high. This is because it is more efficient to bend the knees and use the leg muscles more rather than overuse the arm muscles with a high couch.

With the gentler forms of massage, using a high couch and doing the strokes primarily with the arms may be adequate and this is the way it is often taught. For those therapists who are moving their careers on with deeper remedial massage, it is essential to change to a lower couch.

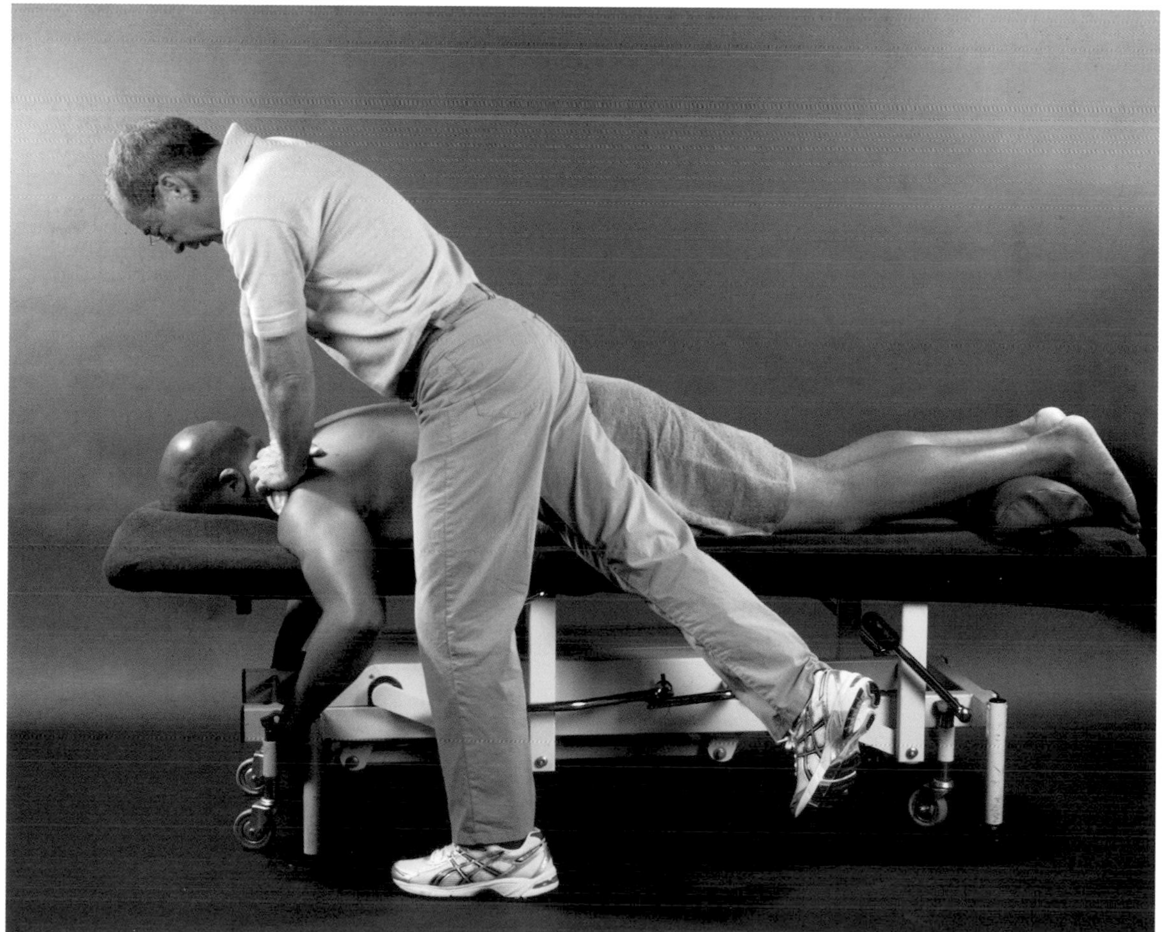

The Lunge

The most efficient way to apply a force is to lean down onto the client through straight arms using natural body-weight. And this can be turned into a massage stroke by simply using the legs to push along the client's body. The muscles in the legs are perfectly adapted to moving the body for many hours a day but the arm muscles are not. It is the legs performing this forward lunging action that is the most efficient force behind all massage strokes. *(See photos 70 and 71.)*

This basic lunging action forms the repetitive and rhythmical movement which should be maintained throughout the treatment. To change the direction of the stroke, the therapist should be constantly moving their feet to realign the hips to the new direction. The hips should always be squarely aligned so the legs can move the body forward in the right direction. Standing in a static position and twisting

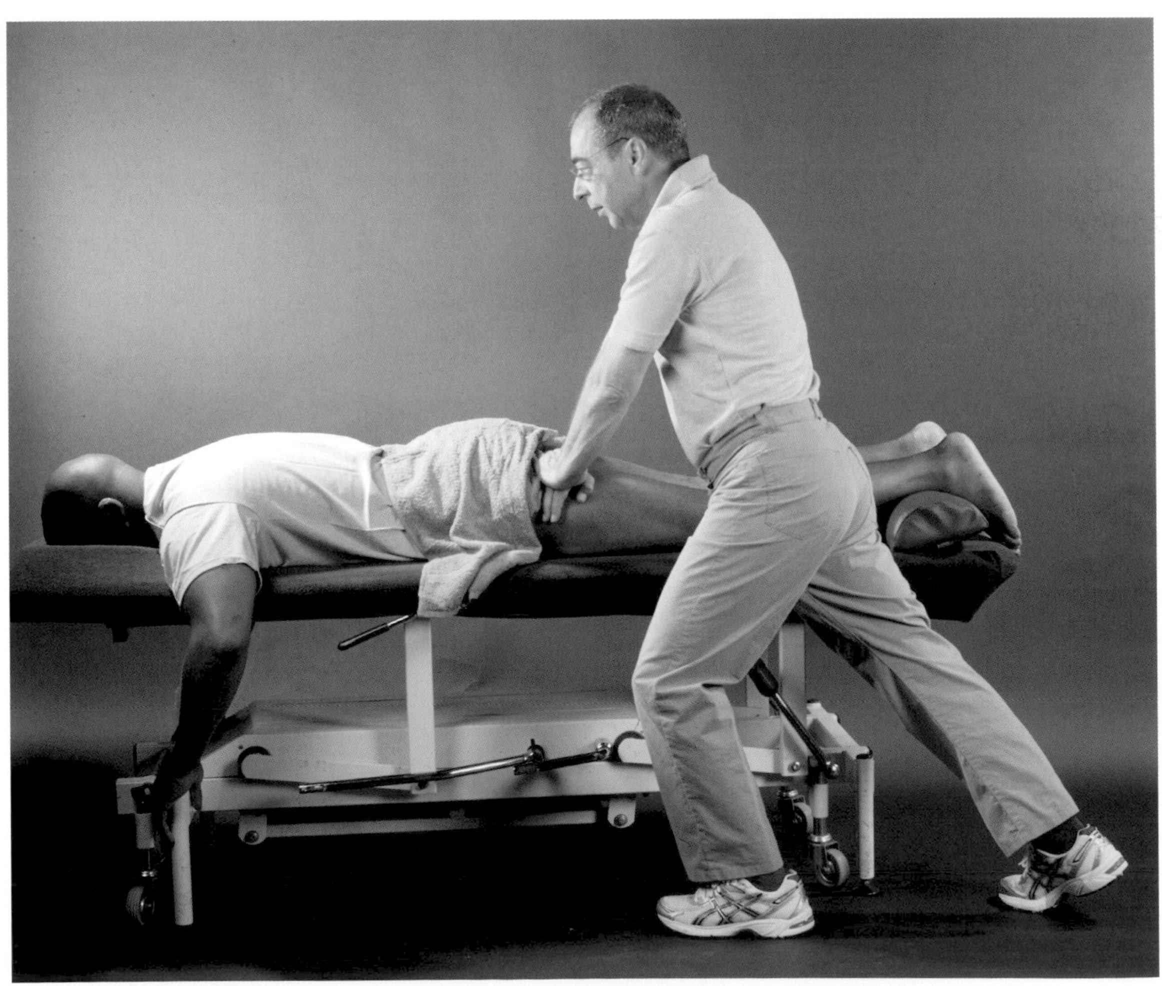

Photos 70 and 71. The 'lunge' is the most efficient way of using the therapist's body-weight and leg strength to generate the power behind any massage stroke.

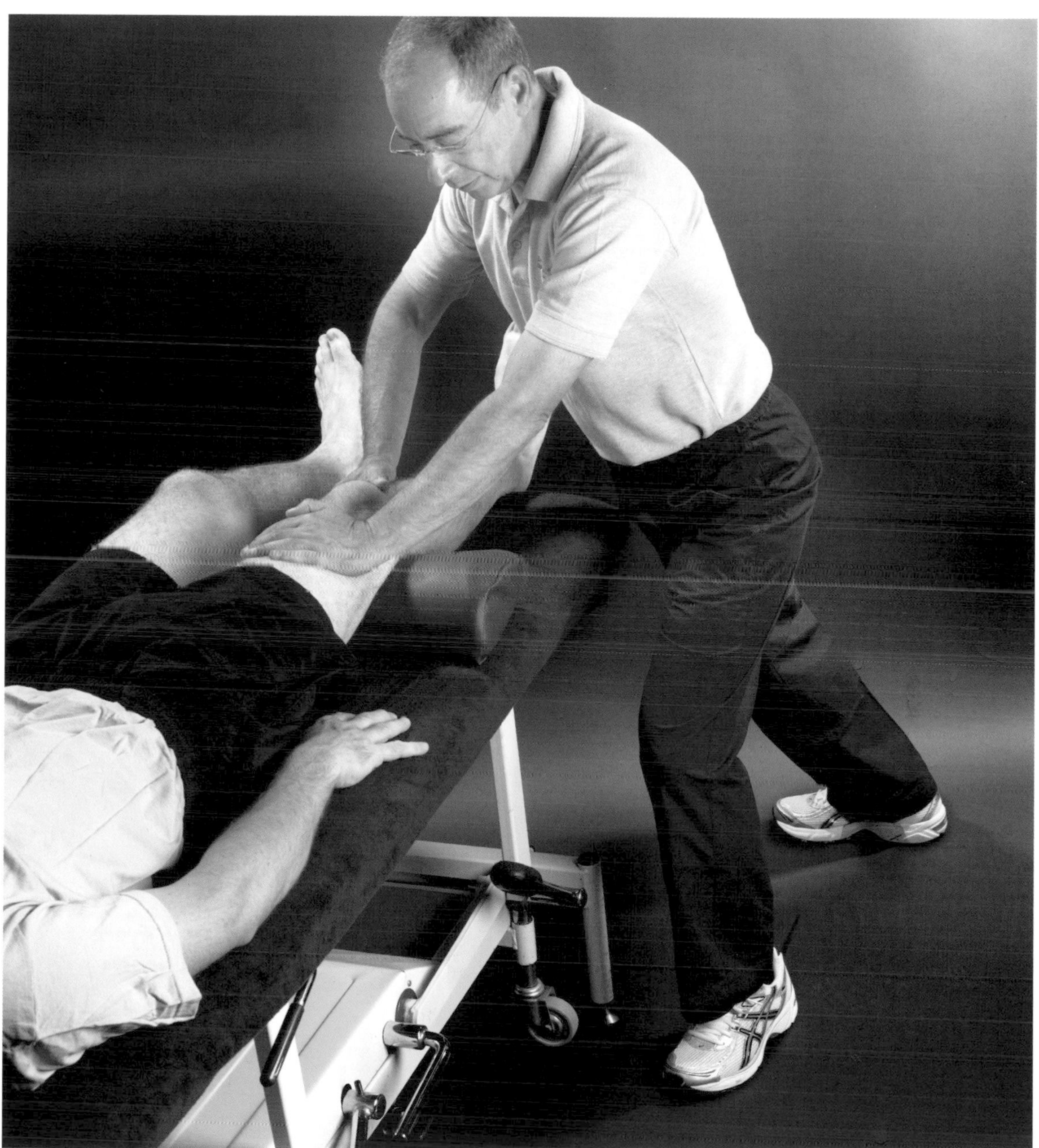

the torso instead is inefficient and unnecessarily stressful on the therapist's muscles and joints.

The depth and pressure of the lunging stroke can be varied by simply changing the hand position rather than using more or less effort. Applying the technique through both palms will spread the weight and work broadly through the superficial tissues. But exactly the same lunging stroke applied through a thumb or knuckle puts all the same force through a much smaller surface area which increases its pressure and depth enormously.

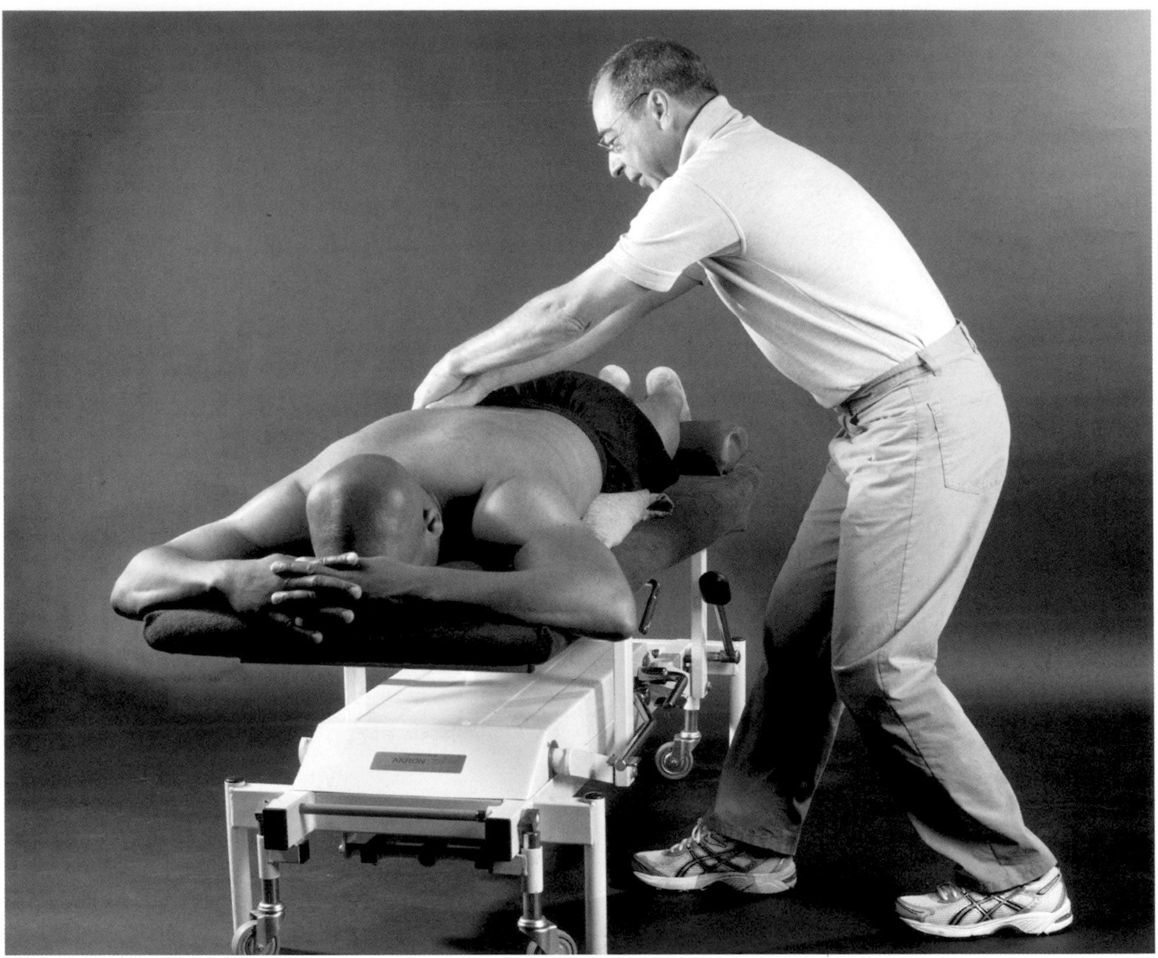

Photos 72, 73 and 74. The 'pull-back' stroke is very powerful and requires almost no effort to perform. This is particularly effective on the quadratus lumborum, latissimus dorsi and the upper trapezius.

Pull-back Strokes

The highly efficient lunge technique can also be reversed into an equally effective pull-back stroke. Here the therapist hooks their hands around the tissues across the body and, through straight arms, drops their body-weight back and downwards to effortlessly apply a very deep stroke. It is even possible to lock onto the muscle; lean back to apply body-weight and then use the legs rocking back and forth to achieve a very deep friction. *(See photos 72, 73 and 74.)*

Tai Chi

These lunging and pull-back strokes strongly resemble movements made in Tai Chi, and the similarity is significant. Tai Chi is a form of martial art which generates a great force with minimal effort and this is exactly what is needed when performing massage. If the lunging massage stroke is also a way of channelling Chi energy through the therapist to the client, this has to be a good thing. It also promotes the health and well-being of the therapist whilst

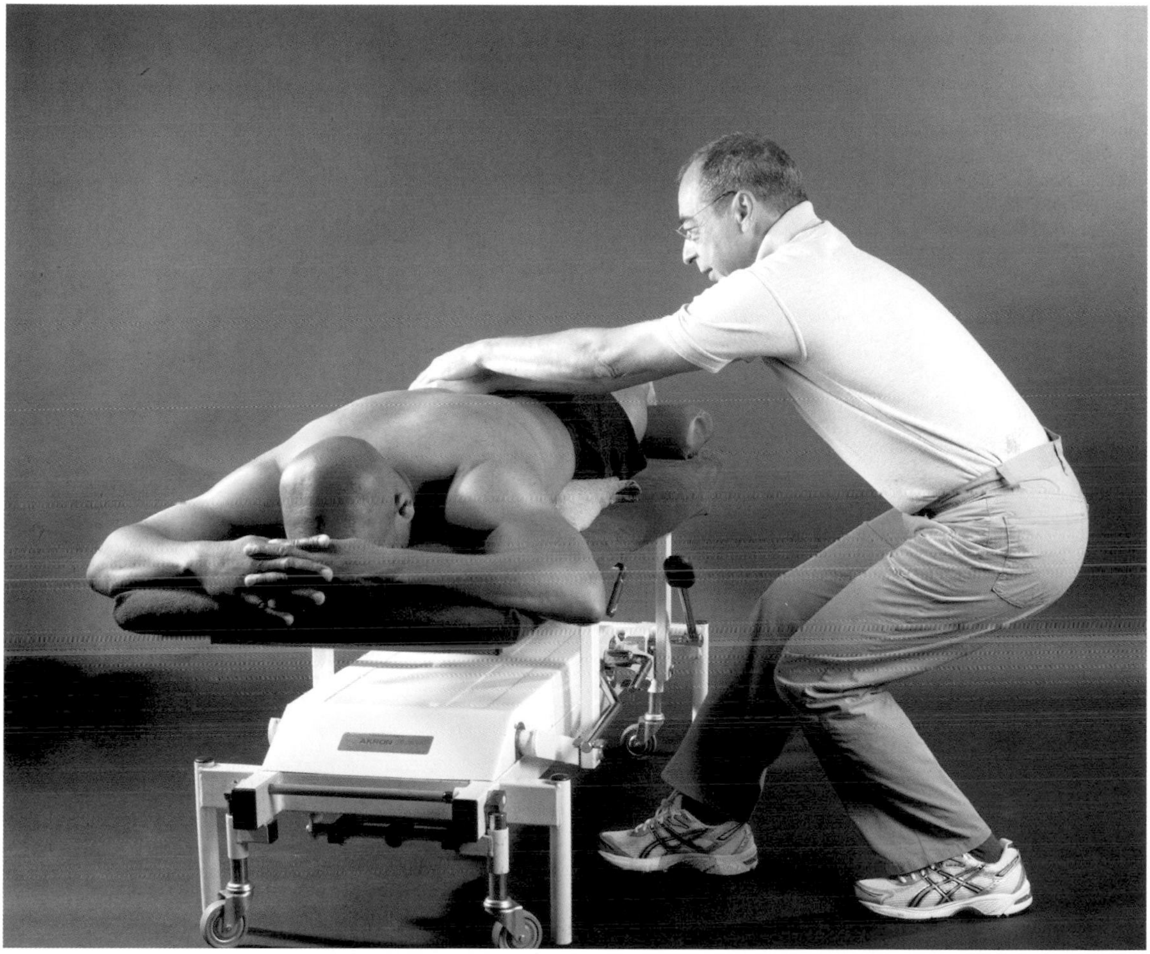

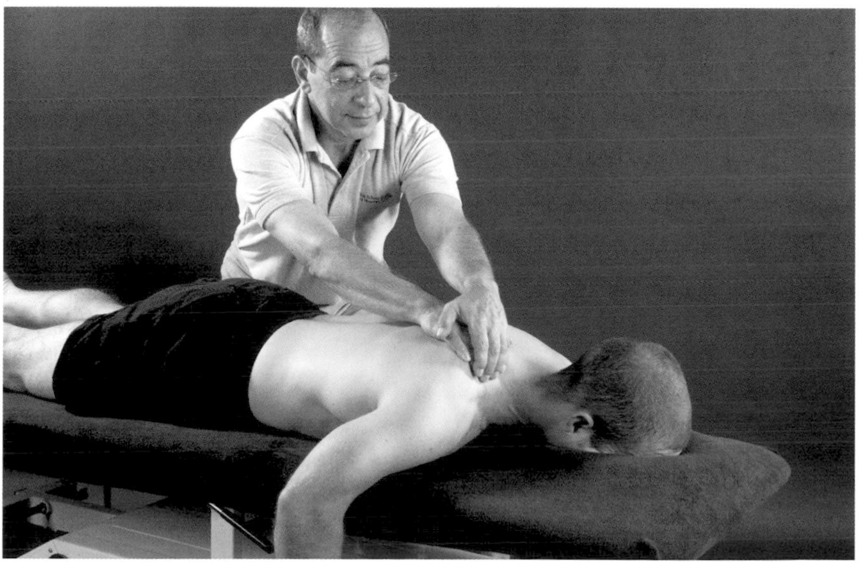

giving a treatment and is another reason why good therapists don't get so tired.

The Angle of Force

The depth and pressure of a massage stroke can be varied by altering its angle to the tissues. Applying the pressure at 90 degrees directly down into the tissues penetrates the deepest, but this can also squash the tissues hard against the underlying bones. This may cause considerable pain and even slight trauma, but the neuromuscular response to this pain can have a short-term relaxing effect. For this reason, some clients and therapists may wrongly think this type of deep painful massage is good.

Applying the pressure of the stroke at about 45 degrees to the tissues creates a 'bow-wave' in the tissues ahead of the stroke and a gentle stretch to the tissues behind it. By not squashing the tissues hard against the underlying bone, a greater directional force can be applied without causing pain. But when this stroke reaches an area of increased tissue tension or damage, the harder tissues will get squashed and cause pain. In this way pain is only felt where there is an issue to deal with, and the therapist can respond to this accordingly. (*See fig. 75.*)

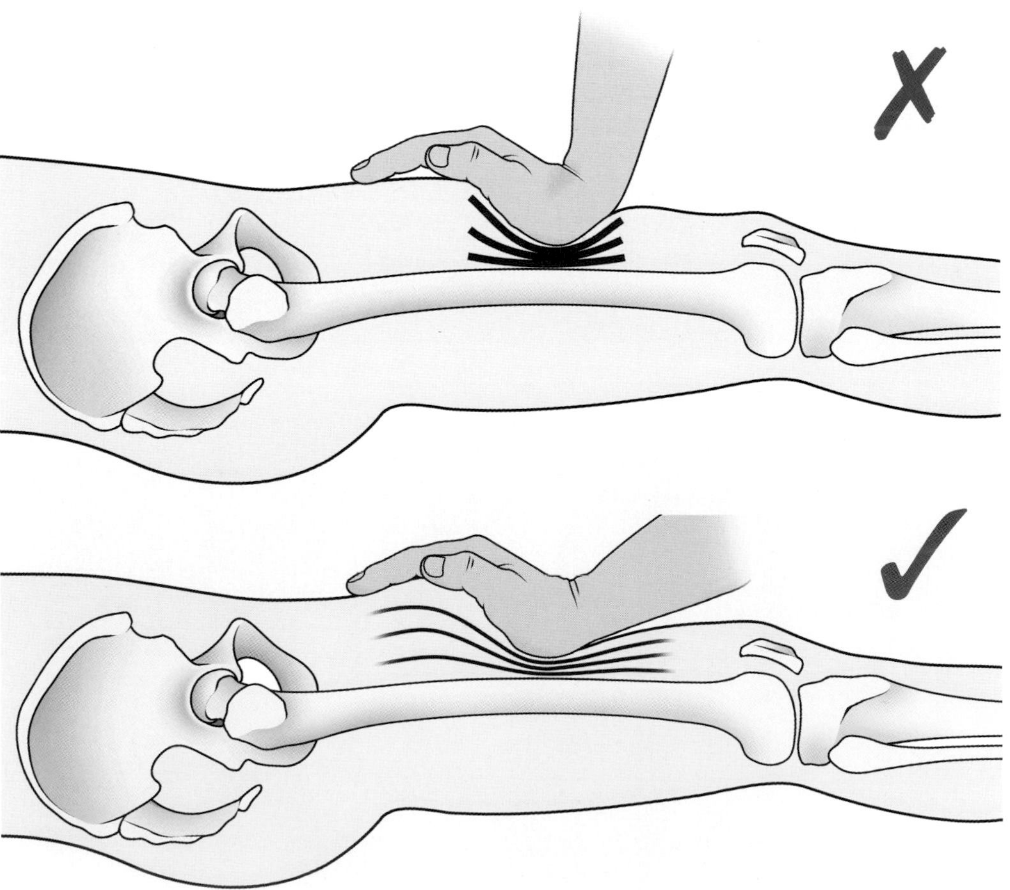

Fig. 75. General massage stroke.

Speed (the Deeper the Slower)

Fast deep strokes which blast their way through the tissues can cause a reflex contraction in the muscles as they try to resist a potentially harmful stimulus. This makes the stroke more painful because the tissues are fighting back against the stroke rather than relaxing into it. Fast strokes also tend to be more stimulating to the nervous system and increase muscle tone, which may not be helpful when trying to reach deeper layers.

Slow deep strokes give the nervous system time to anticipate the stroke so the tissues can relax into it rather than contract against it. A slow stroke also allows the healthy fibres time to slide out of the way so that it can safely move past them to reach the deeper tissues. Fast strokes which force their way through the healthy fibres may actually cause them some damage and could be the cause of post-treatment bruising. One very slow deep stroke can have a far better effect on releasing tissue tension then several minutes of fast vigorous stroking.

As well as being more effective, applying a slow stroke also gives the therapist more time to feel and assess the quality of the tissues, and fewer strokes mean less hard work too!

Combining Speed and Pressure

Working slowly and deeply has a more relaxing effect, and working fast and superficially can do the opposite by being more stimulating. By combining speed and pressure in different ways, it is possible to adapt a treatment to best suit the needs of the client. Even though the tissues may be relaxed after slow deep strokes at the beginning of a treatment, they may tense up again following deeper painful techniques. So slow, deep stokes should be repeated at regular intervals during a treatment to maintain good relaxation.

Fast, light and stimulating strokes are usually only performed towards the end of a treatment to prepare the client for their journey home, or in pre-event sports situations. But they can also play an important role when treating clients with some conditions where weakness and atrophy occur. Percussion (tapotement) techniques are the most stimulating and particularly useful on weak and inhibited muscles.

Safe Hand Positions

These are absolutely vital, but what is safe depends on the therapist. The degree of mobility in the wrists and hands can vary enormously from individual to individual, and techniques which are safe for one therapist could prove harmful to another. *(See photos 76, 77, 78 and 79 overleaf.)*

The basic principle with all techniques must be to protect the joints in the hands and wrists. To do this, they must be neutrally aligned when heavy pressure is applied through them. People with fairly rigid and immobile joints will do this naturally and are at a distinct advantage. But many people have a much higher degree of mobility in these joints and can naturally hyperextend their fingers and wrists. Putting heavy pressure through hyperextended joints stresses the articular bone surfaces and ligaments, and overuse damage to these can be difficult to resolve.

For those with hypermobile joints, it is safer to use the muscles in the forearm and hand to hold the joints in slightly flexed positions rather than relax them and put pressure

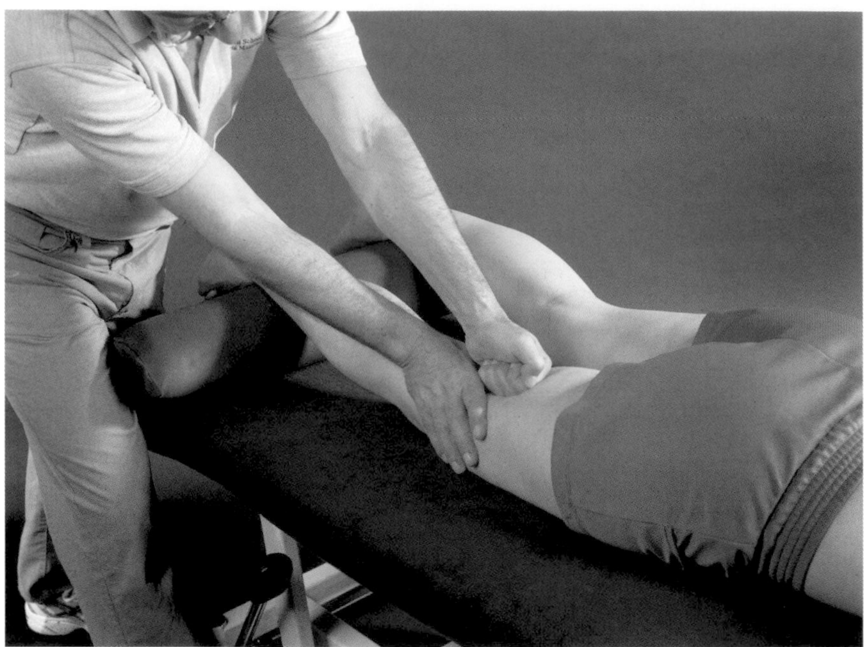

Photo 76. Using the fist guided by the other hand.

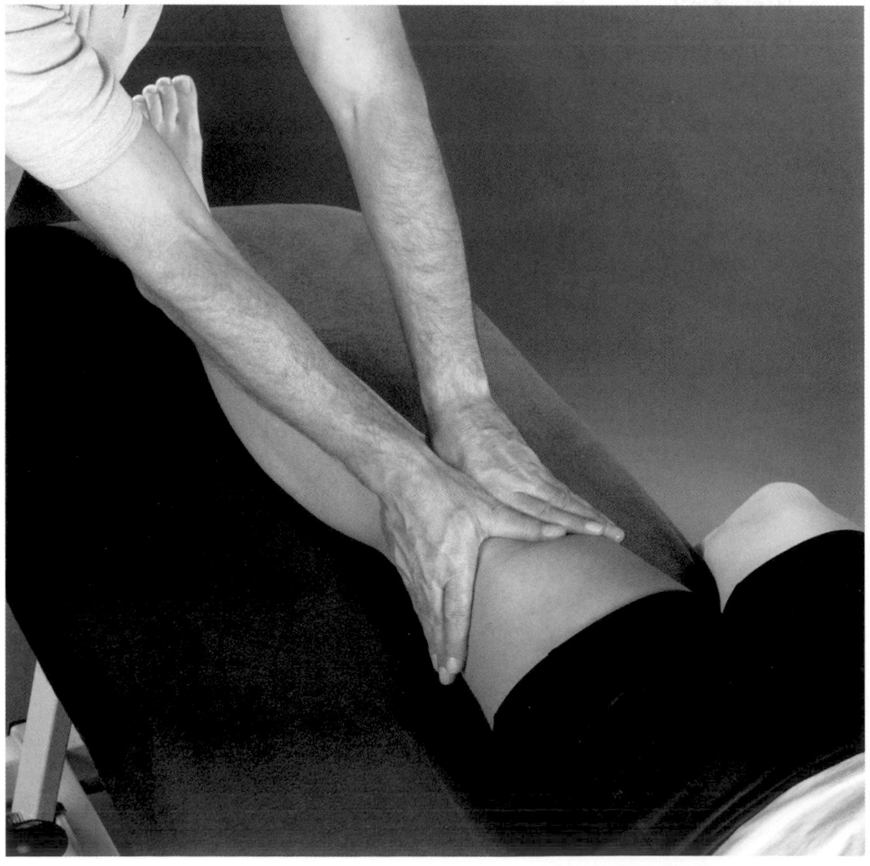

Photo 77. Using the hands in a way that protects all the fingers.

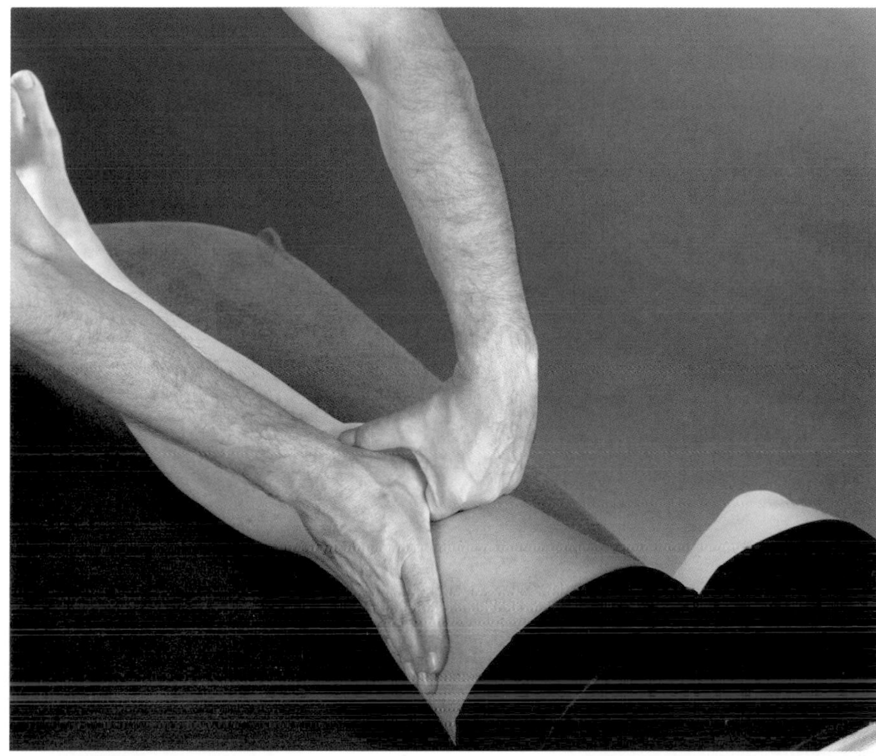

Photo 78. Wrapping a loose fist around the other thumb to apply deep strokes with the knuckles

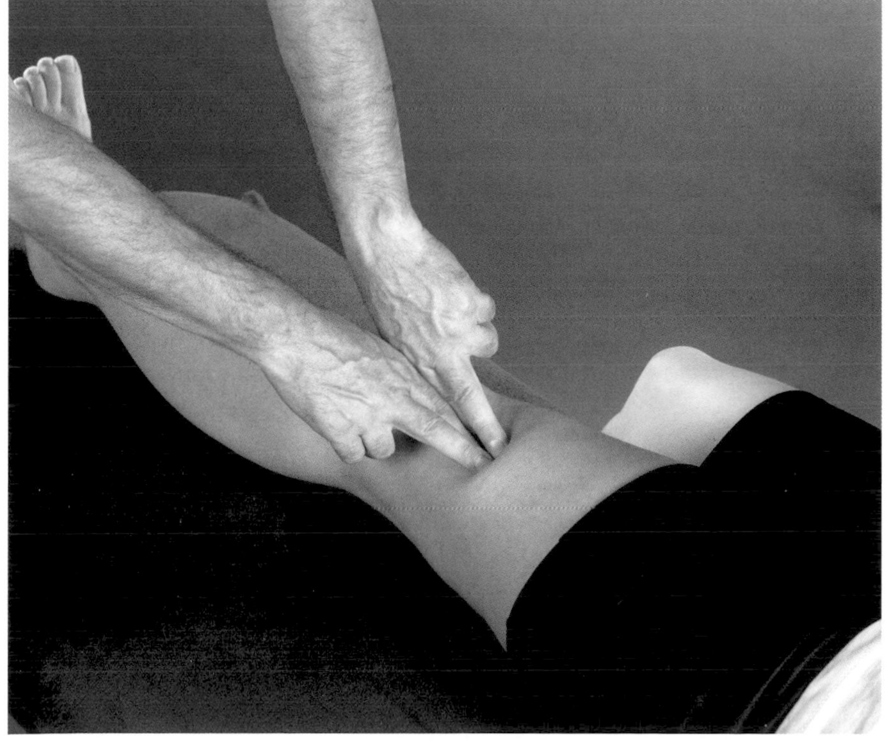

Photo 79. Using the fingers to protect each other to apply deep strokes between muscles.

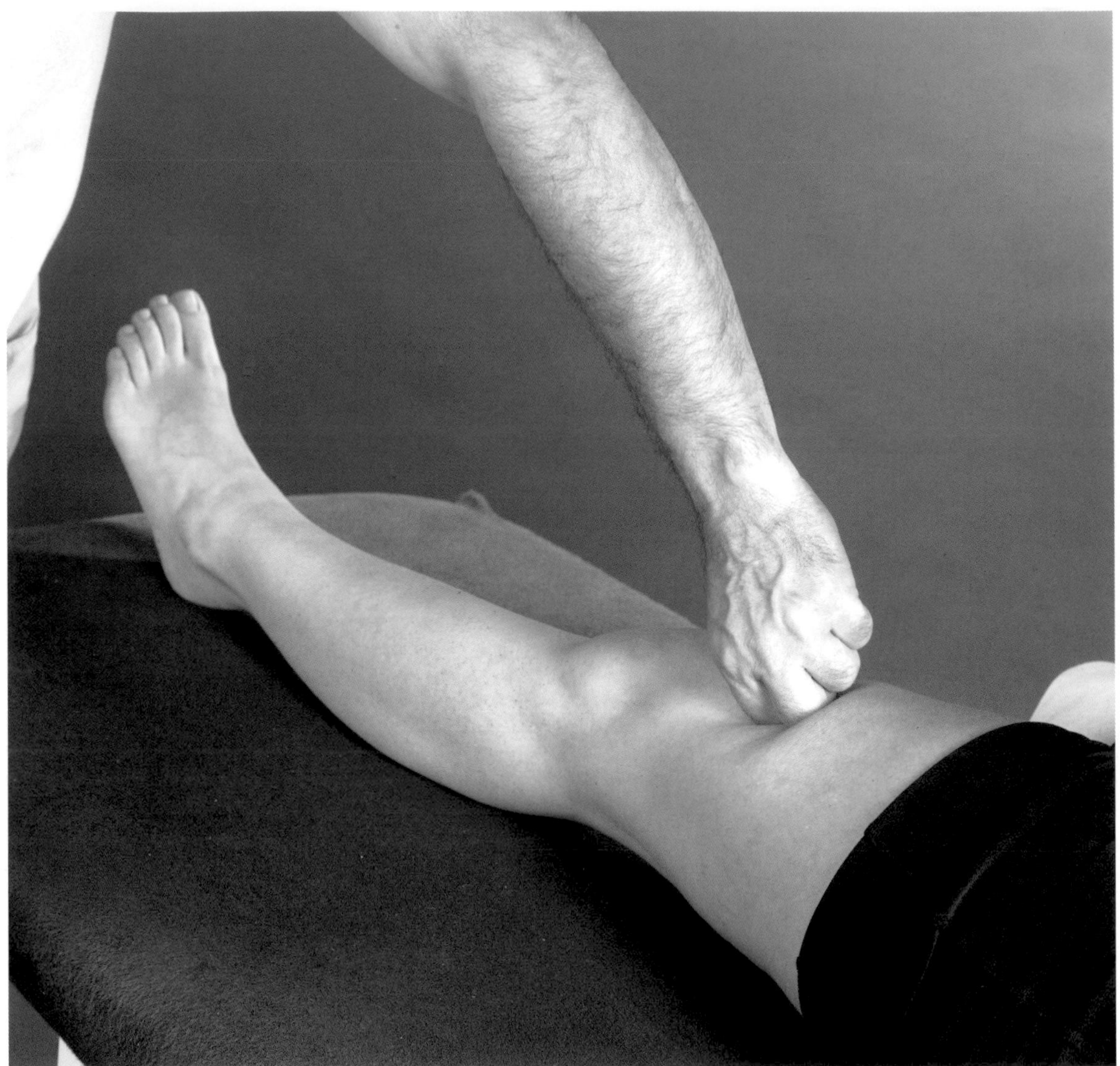

Photo 79. Using the knuckles.

through hyperextended joints. The worst thing this is likely to cause is mild overuse muscle strain which should easily be resolved with rest and self-treatment, but joint damage is much harder to recover from.

Therapists with hypermobile hands need to develop their own range of techniques which use knuckles, fists, forearms and elbows so they do not need to rely on their hands all the time. Although the hands have the greatest sensitivity, with practice a similar sense of feeling can be developed with these other body parts too. Even a therapist with strong rigid hands can have a particularly hard day and feel some overuse soreness as a result. By immediately switching to these non-hand techniques, they will quickly recover without having to stop work.

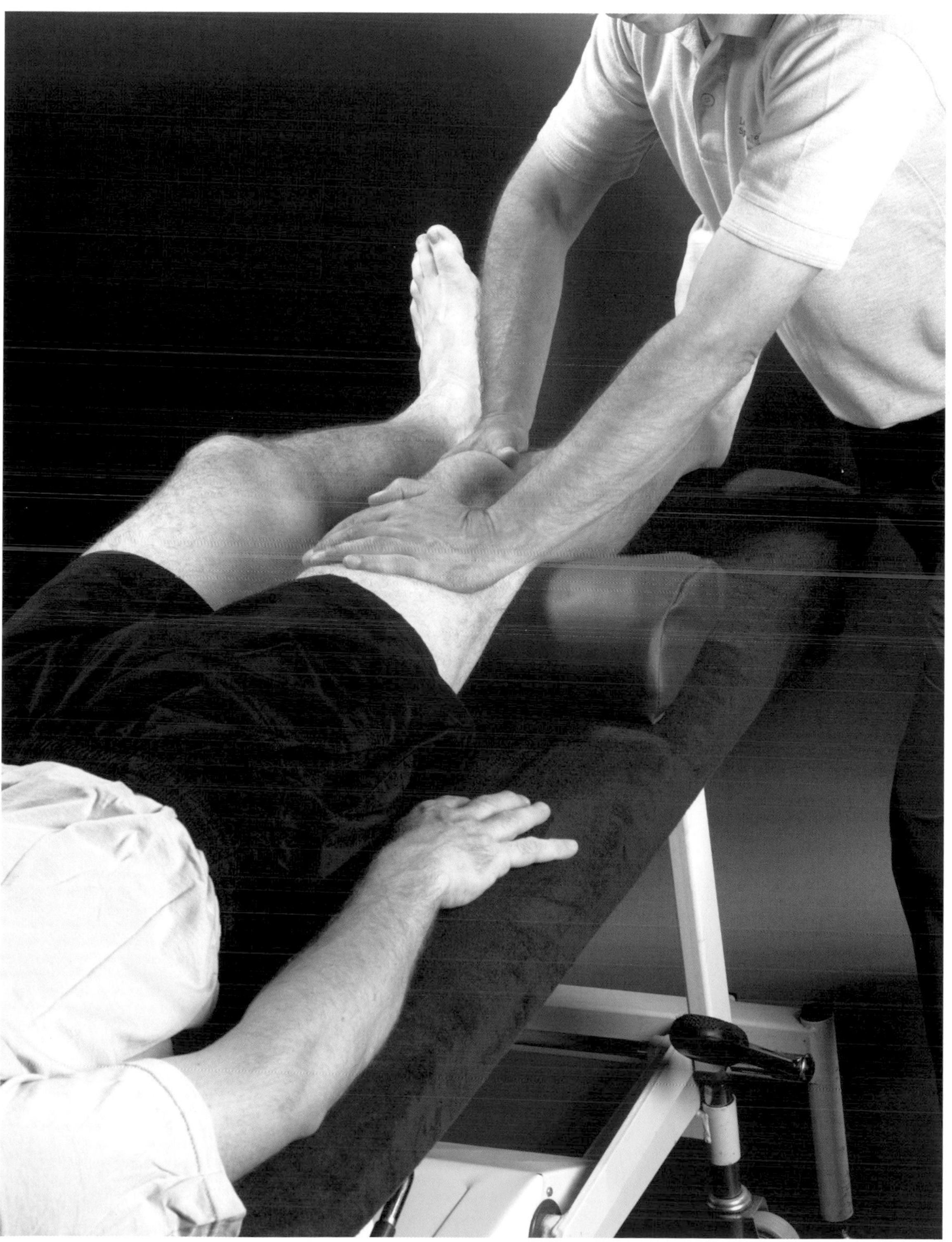

Photo 80. Using the heel of the hand.

Heel of the Palm

It is important to use the right tool for the right job. When applying broad heavy strokes through large areas of muscle tissue, the best tool is the heel of the palm. It forms a very good soft pad that can be used without any muscular force. Working heavily with the fingers stresses the joints and requires considerable strength from the small wrist flexor muscles in the forearm and can lead to overuse injuries. *(See photo 81.)*

The Protected Thumb

The thumb is a very strong tool which is heavily used in many massage techniques, and it must be protected against injury. The thumb should first be positioned at the beginning of the stroke and the rest of the hand should be comfortably aligned around it. The thumb then remains relaxed as the heel of the other hand presses down on it. The therapist's body-weight can be directed into the thumb without there being any stress on the joints or small muscles there. The thumb acts as a passive tool and, being relaxed, it has greater sensitivity even though heavy pressure is being applied through it. *(See photos 82 , 83 and 84.)*

Friction

Deep friction techniques may appear to only involve the use of the thumb or fingers, but if this were true it would be potentially

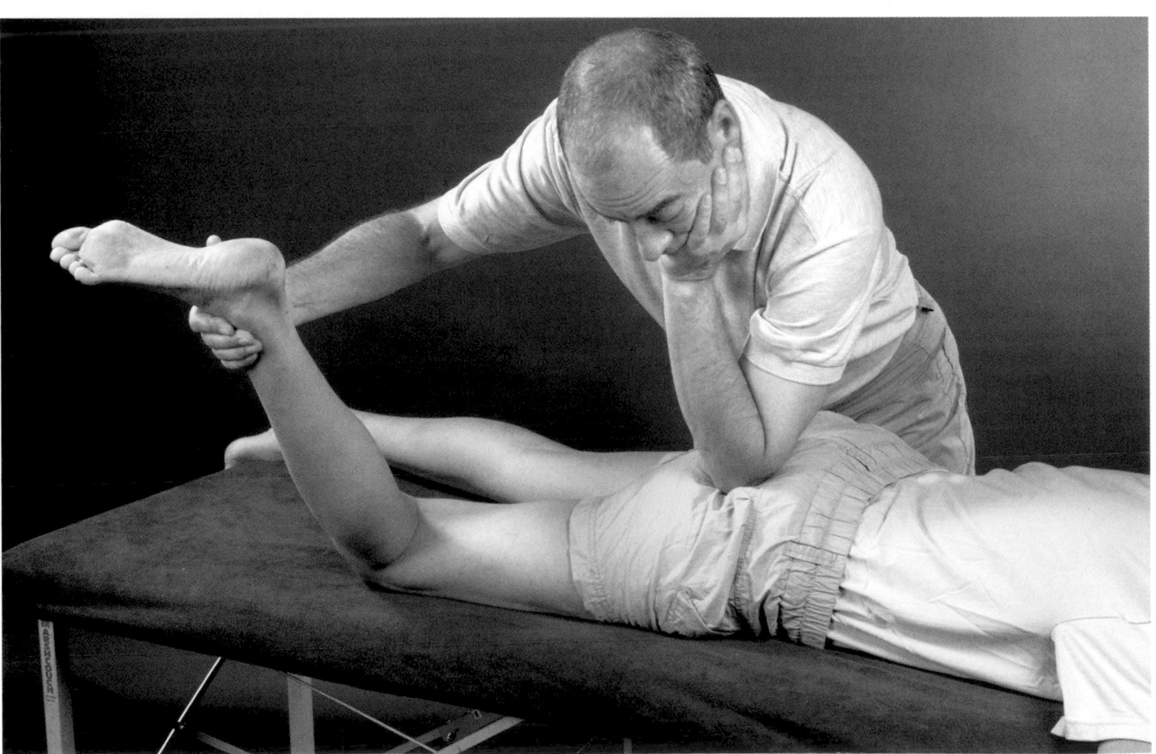

Photo 81. Deep techniques do not have to be hard work!

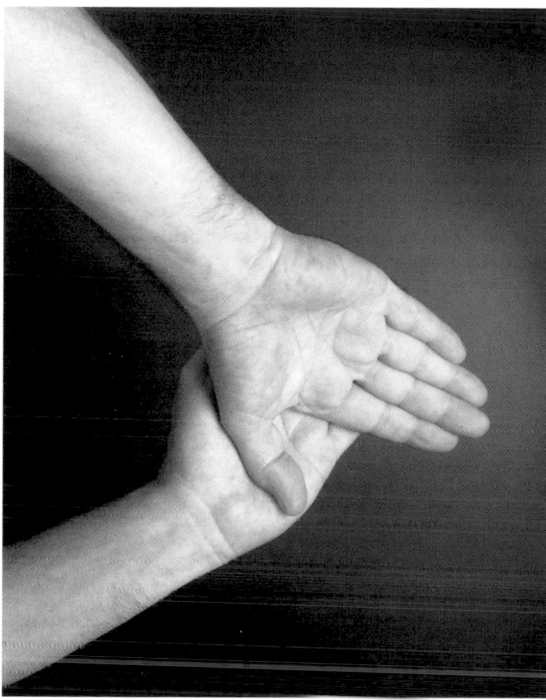

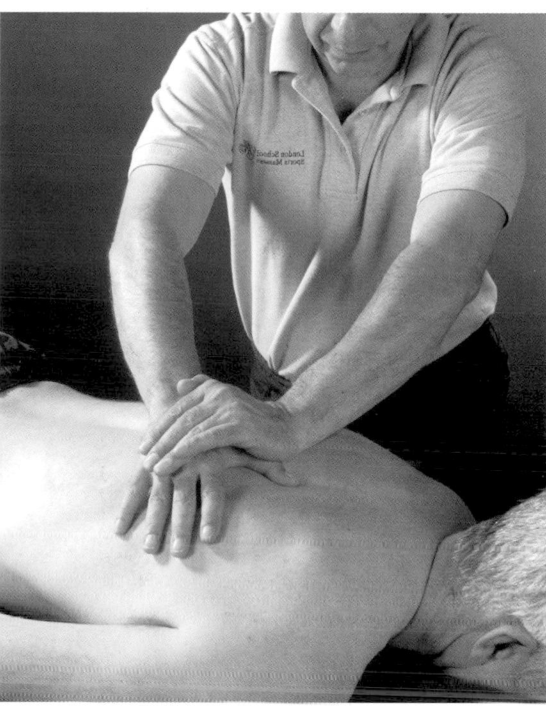

Photos. 82 and 83. The thumb is protected and relaxed but can be used to apply very deep strokes and friction.

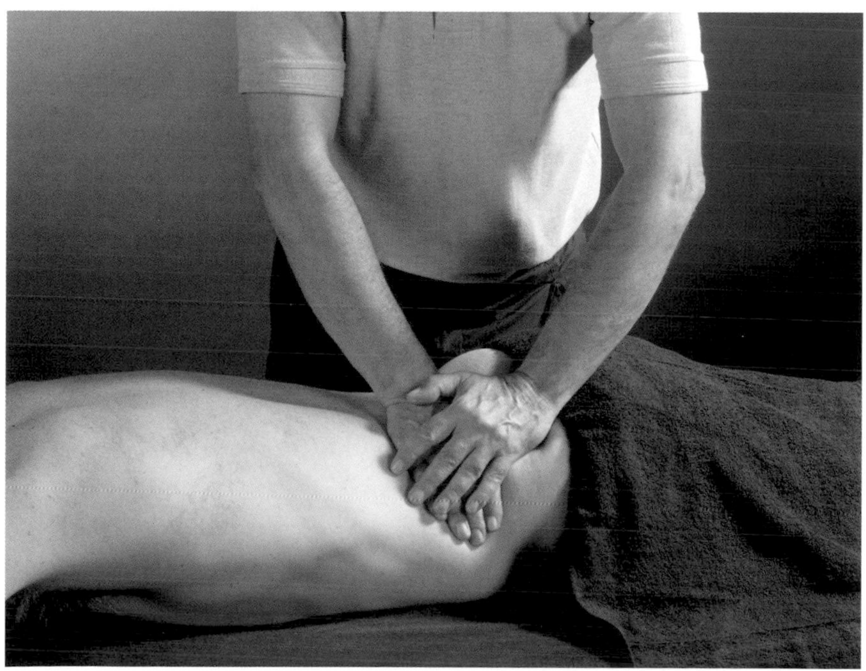

Photo 84. Great force can be applied with the top hand pushing strongly down on the passive thumb underneath it to safely apply the deepest strokes and friction.

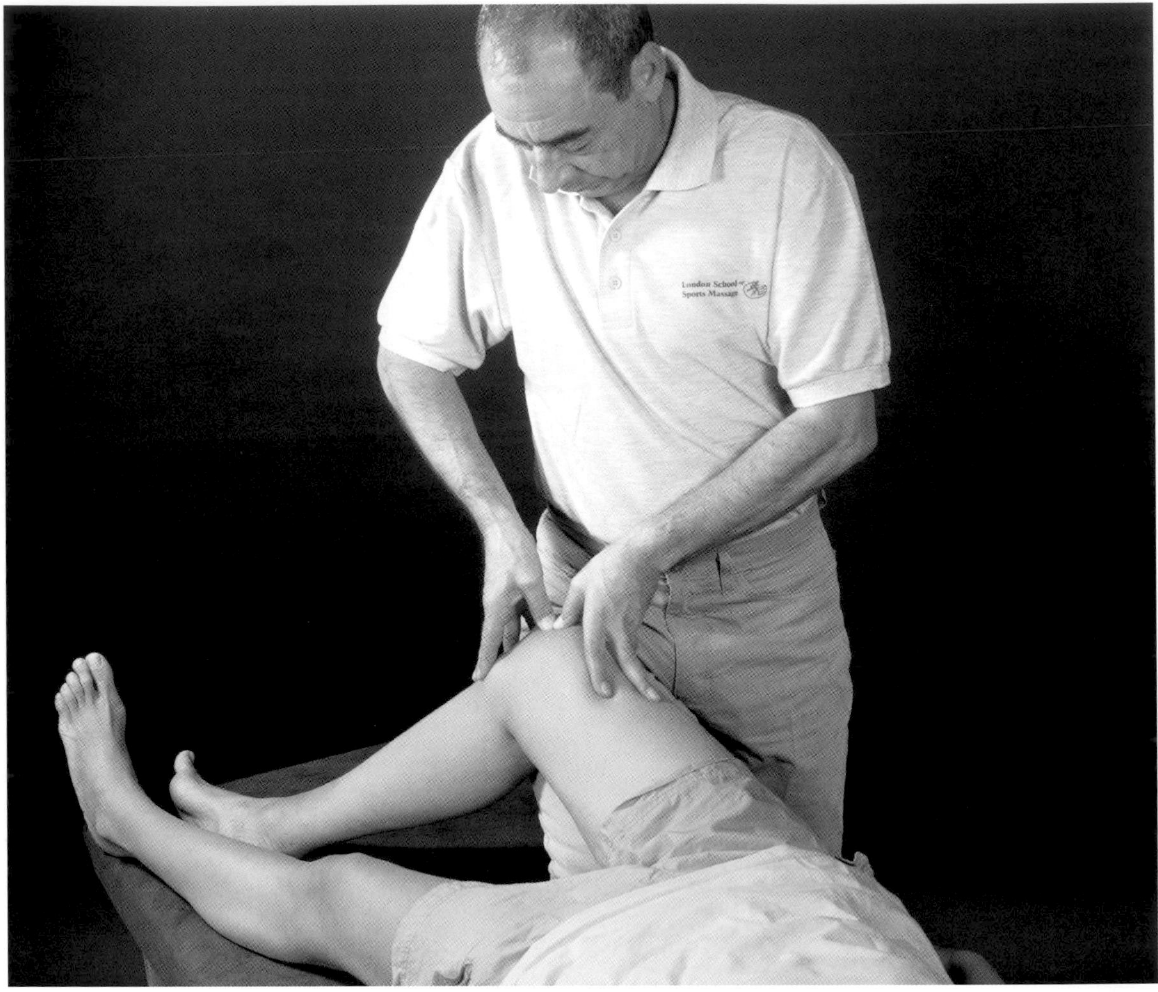

Photo 85. Friction can be applied with great force with the efficient use of body-weight and good support of the client's limb.

harmful. The same principles of protecting the thumb and fingers are even more important here because of the greater focused pressure involved. Therapists need to move into the best position possible so they can continue to use their body-weight to apply maximum force with minimum effort. When applying deep friction around joints it is often useful to support the client's limb on or against the therapist's body to get the best control. (*See photo 85.*)

To help thoroughly explore the tissues, the therapist can close their eyes and visualise the structures magnified 1,000 times. Although the fingers or thumb may make incredibly small slow deep movements, in the mind's eye they can be exploring caves, valleys and mountains.

Using the Couch for Support

The massage couch is a piece of equipment which can be used for more than just laying the client on. *(See photos 86, 87, 88, 89, 90 and 91.)* Kneeling or sitting on the couch is perfectly

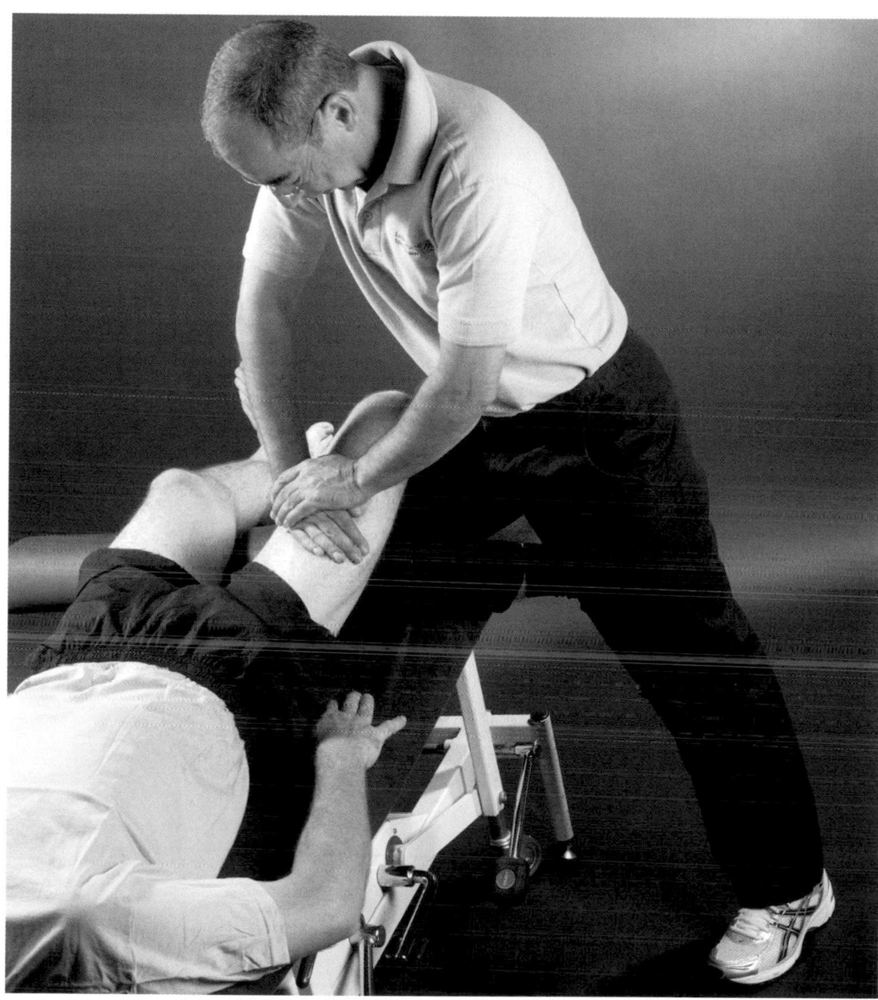

Photo 86. Kneeling on the couch and supporting the client's leg is very strong and efficient.

acceptable and offers many advantages both in terms of comfort and to gain better access to the tissues being treated.

Kneeling on the couch shifts the therapist's centre of gravity forward over the client and offers better postural support when working on areas like the neck or the lower leg when the client is lying prone. There are also very good working positions possible sitting on the side of the couch.

Lubricant

Deep massage strokes usually require slow controlled pressure, and a reasonable amount of grip on the skin is necessary to achieve this. Too much lubricant makes this difficult because the stroke slides too easily across the surface. Therapists should use only small amounts to allow a limited slip, but take on more at regular intervals when needed. Deep friction

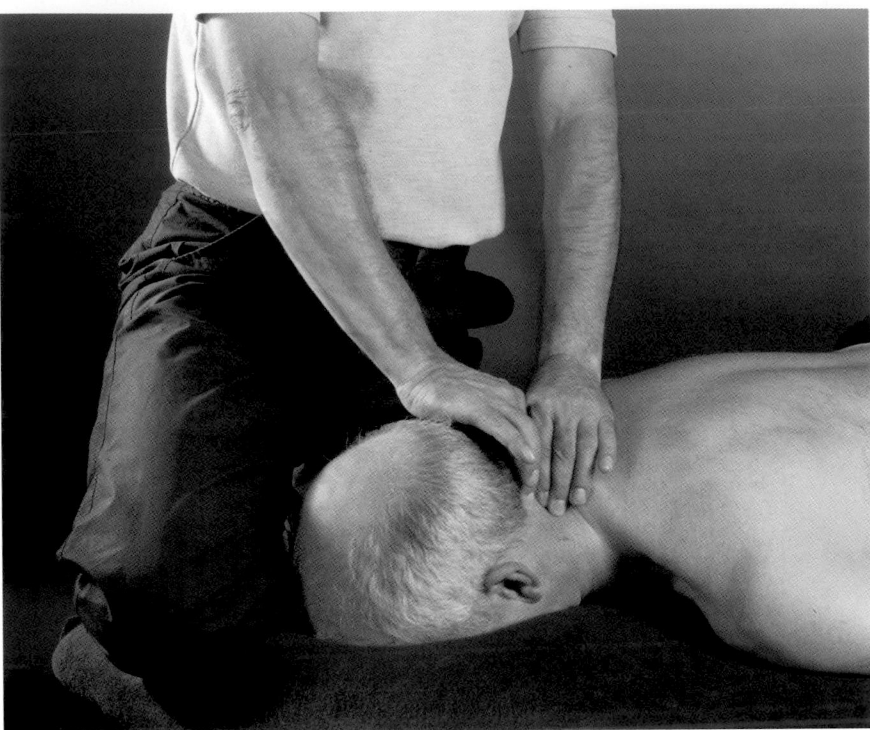

Photo 87. Kneeling as far across the couch as possible shifts the therapist's body-weight forward over the client and makes it much more efficient when applying deep techniques.

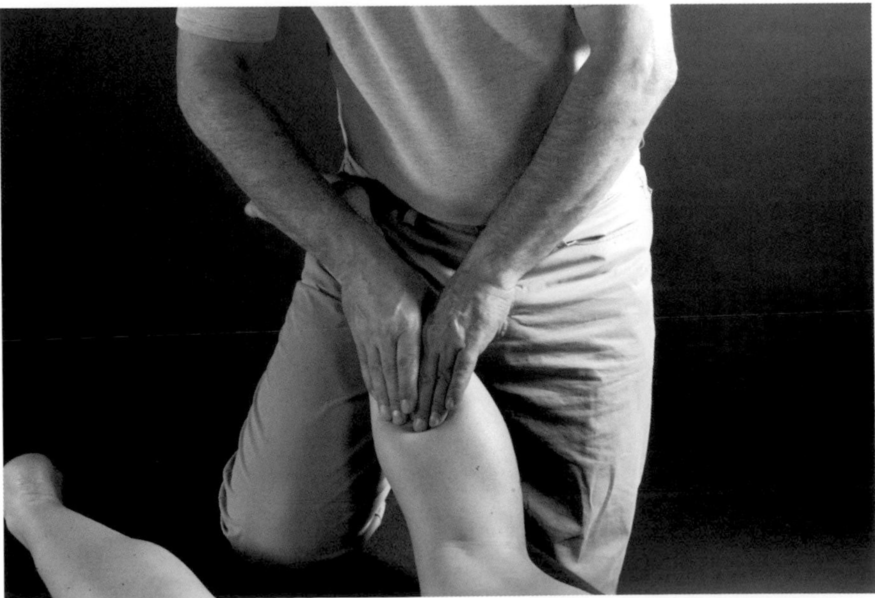

Photo 88. Supporting the client's lower leg on the therapist's thigh when kneeling on the couch enables the therapist to stand up straight and use their body-weight more efficiently.

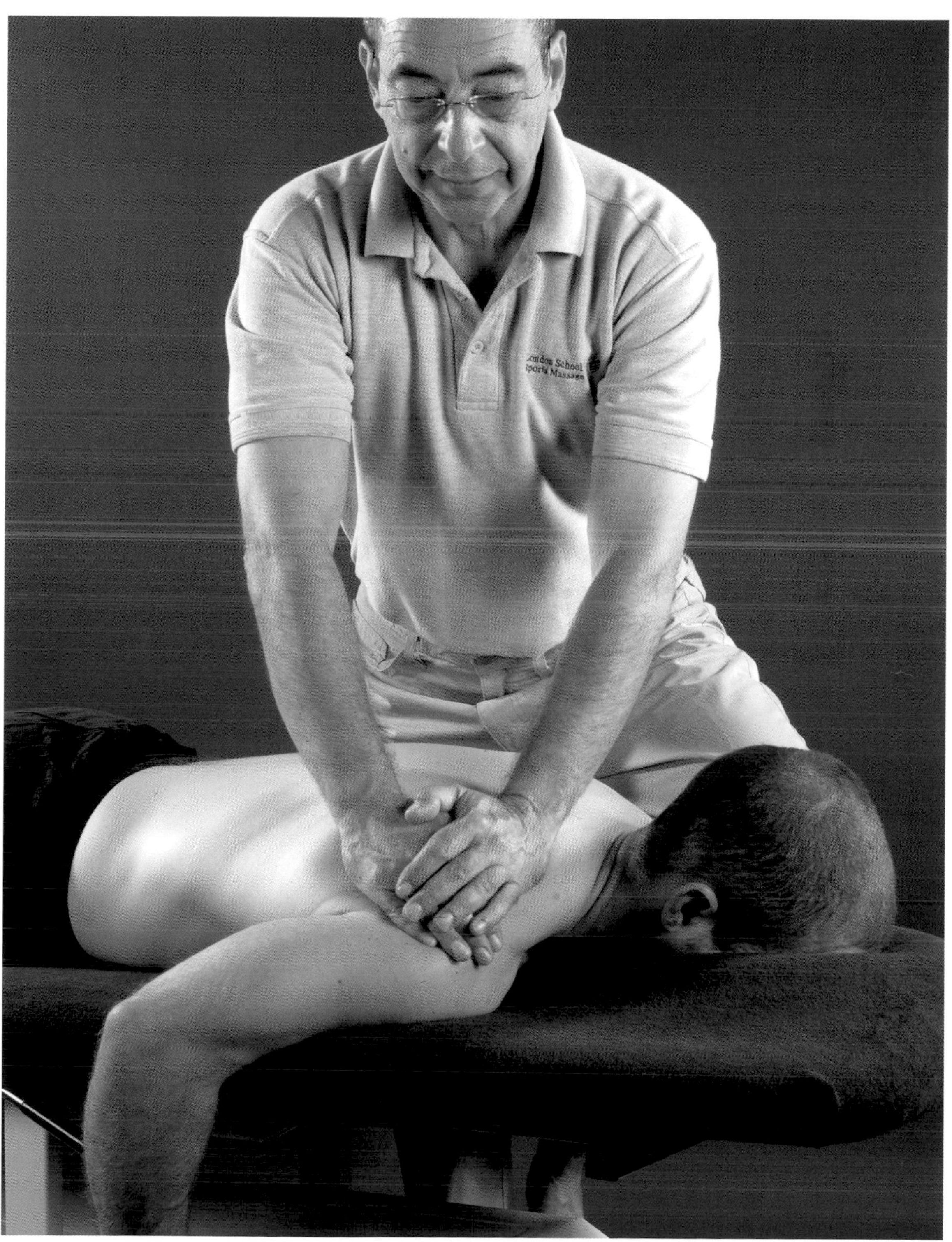

Photo 89. Kneeling on the couch and leaning across it is a very efficient way of applying pressure.

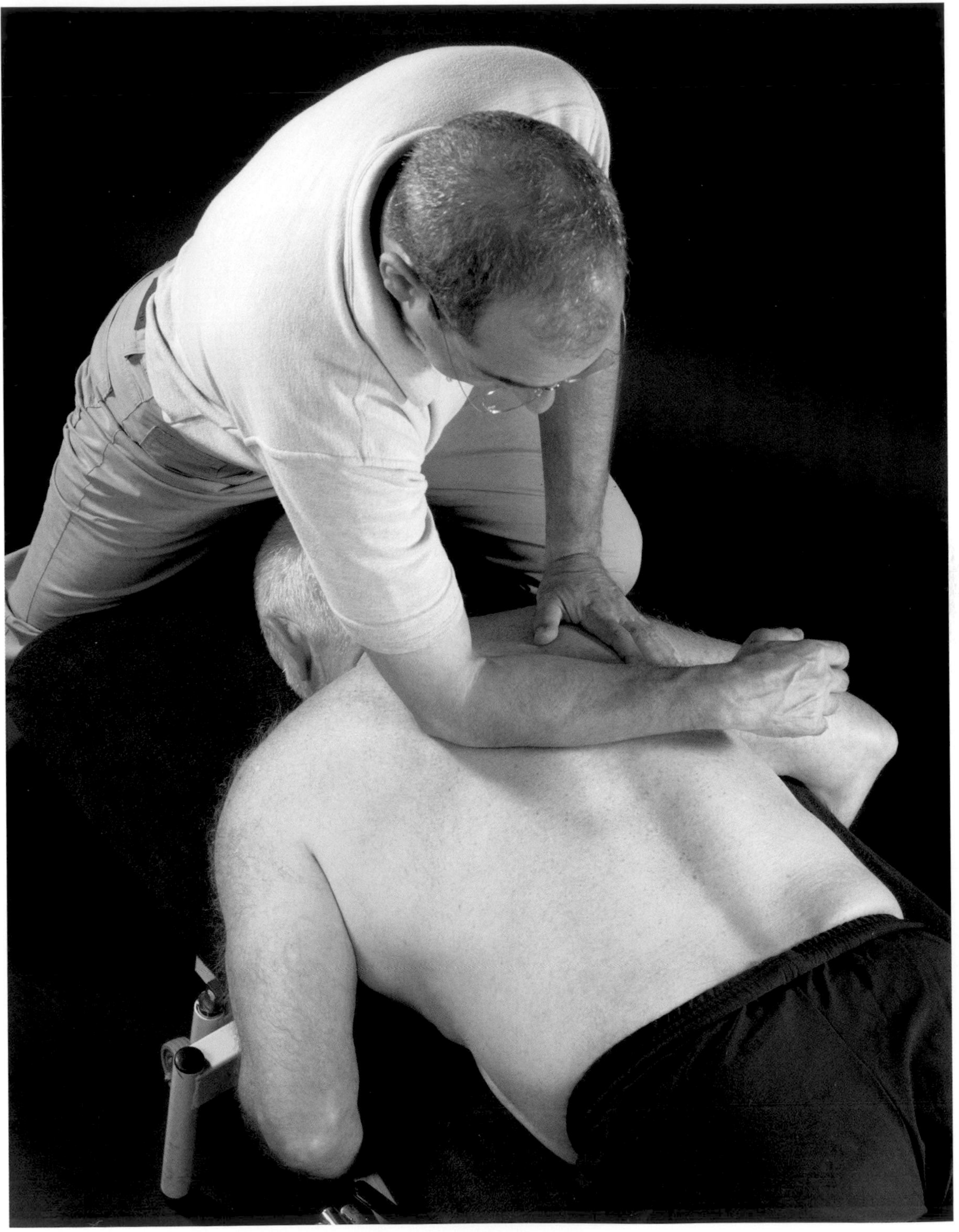

Photo 90. Kneeling across the head of the couch makes it much easier to treat the thoracic area.

techniques into small local areas are often easier to perform without any lubricant (or through a towel) because there is usually enough movement available through the superficial layers.

Moving the Client

Although prone and supine are the two common positions used to treat the client, the side-lying position is also very important and offers many advantages. The side-lying position provides excellent access to the muscles along the side of the body, shoulder and hip, and some of the more central deep muscles can also be reached better from the side. The side-lying position is the best way to treat pregnant women and can also be a safer position to treat clients who have had chest or abdominal surgery. *(See photo 91.)*

For the client to lie down or get up from the prone or supine positions requires a lot of core muscle activation and this can be harmful if these muscle are already injured. Sitting on the side of the couch and then lying down sideways, and doing the reverse to get up again, does not require such muscle activation and is safer in these situations.

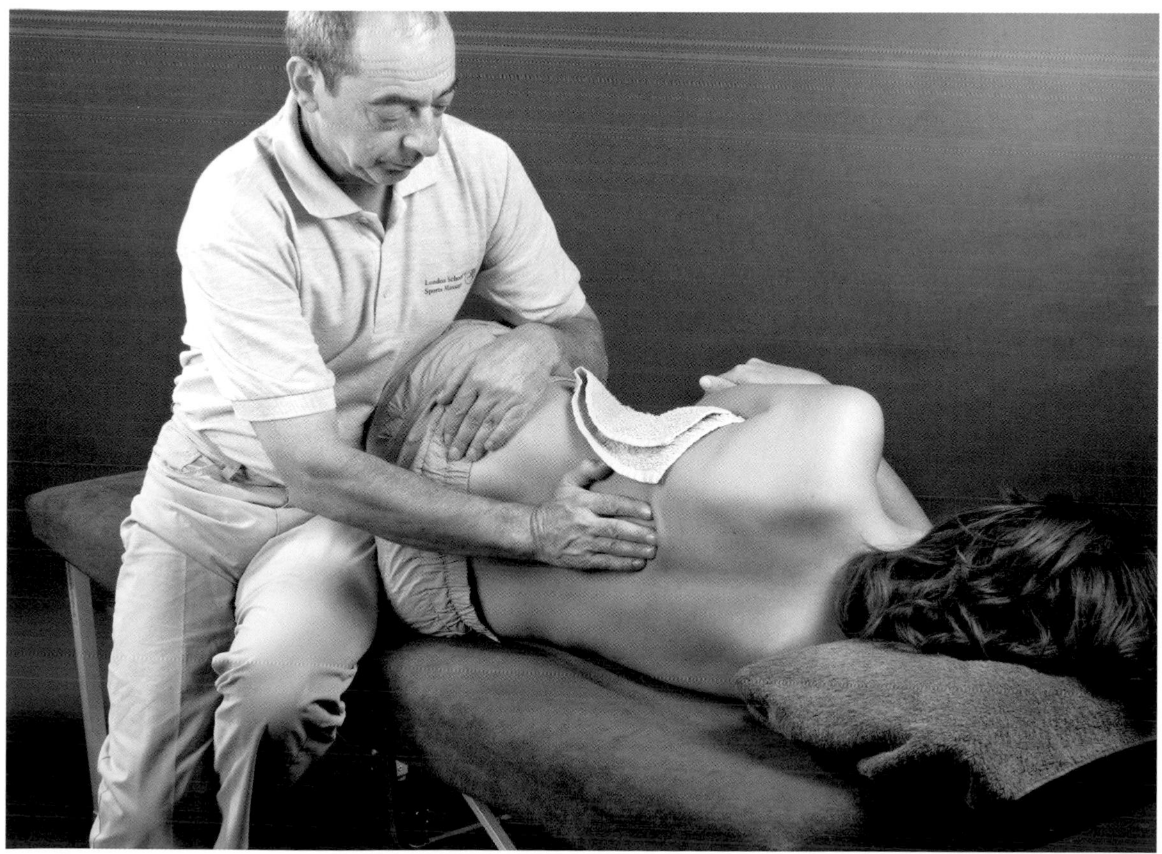

Photo 91. With the client side-lying, the therapist can sit on the couch, support the pelvis with one arm and use the other hand to apply strokes along the back. This is ideal for pregnant women and people who cannot lie in a prone position.

Moving Around the Couch

Whenever treating a problem in a particular area, it is better to try to approach it from as many different angles as possible. This gives the best all-round feel of the size, texture and shape of any tissue damage and helps find the best approaches to deal with it from. There is never one ideal way of reaching a muscle, and different clients with their different physical characteristics can present quite different challenges and possibilities. The therapist should keep moving around the couch and changing their working position constantly to find the best way to access the tissues.

Treating One Specific Area

When treating a specific problem area, it is not good to spend too long working deeply on it at any one time. Superficial strokes will soften the area first and help identify the location of the tissue problem. The pressure should gradually be increased with the very deepest techniques only being applied for about 30 seconds at a time before more superficial strokes are used to calm and relax the area again. It is then better to work away on another area for a few minutes before returning to repeat the procedure.

Spending too long working deeply on the same tissues could cause them slight trauma and lead to more residual pain for a day or two after treatment. Allowing the tissues a short recovery time during treatment can prevent this. Also, it is common to find a significant change in the tissues each time they are returned to. This is because the nervous system has a chance to adjust and relax in response to the treatment before more is done.

Clothes-On Treatment

There can be occasions when treating unclothed clients may not be appropriate:

- In public places like sports events.
- Working in cold conditions.
- Treating injured or disabled clients who have difficulties removing clothes.
- Clients who feel more comfortable keeping their clothes on for personal, religious or cultural reasons.

It is possible to give an equally good treatment through clothes when necessary, and this should be practised first so the therapist is proficient in working this way when the need arises.

Although conventional effleurage strokes cannot be applied through clothes, other methods can achieve a similar effect. Shorter strokes can be made by pressing into the tissues through clothing and using the elasticity of the superficial fascia to apply a stroke. Petrissage techniques can still be applied by squeezing the tissues through the clothes. All other massage and soft tissue techniques can be applied just as easily through clothing, and deep friction is often done better this way.

Floorwork

Although therapists hope to always work with a proper treatment couch there is a life outside the clinic and there will be times when they need to work without one. Using the floor rather than a soft bed is preferable, but a soft covering will help protect the therapist's knees. Having just one knee and the other foot on the floor enables a lunging action similar to when standing.

7

Excessive muscle tension (hypertonicity) is a common factor in a great many injury situations. Although this may be in part due to local tissue damage, the actual tone of a muscle is maintained and controlled by the nervous system. Basic manual therapy techniques aim to treat the local tissue damage, but to normalise muscle tone it is the nervous system that has to be influenced.

For centuries, manual therapists have found that a significant relaxation can result from applying very deep focused pressure for a sustained period into local areas of excessive soft tissue tension. A variety of therapies have evolved around this phenomenon, ranging from acupressure based on an Oriental philosophy to trigger-point therapies based on a Western approach. Although they may all show strong similarities in the way they are performed, the explanations of how they work can be very different.

Trigger and Reflex Points

If the entire surface of the body is palpated very thoroughly using exactly the same pressure all the time, some specific points will be found to produce more pain than others. Some of these points may also cause a referred pain pattern in other areas, and these are considered to be true trigger points; those that are only felt locally are usually called reflex points. If all these points are marked on a chart and the process is repeated on a large number of people, common points start to appear in the same place on most people. Charts that show these common trigger and reflex points closely match traditional Chinese acupuncture charts.

These trigger points do exist, and if the body is in a good physical and emotional state they all remain very calm. But if someone has health problems, is injured or is under stress some or all of their trigger points will become active and extra points will develop. But they will only become consciously aware of the heightened activity of these trigger points when deep pressure is applied to them.

Traditional trigger-point and acupressure techniques apply very deep pressure into these points. This is quite painful at first, but the pain eventually subsides and the tissues can spontaneously relax. This may be explained by the release of endorphins (natural opiates), which suppress the pain and relax the tissues. The strong focused pressure also squeezes all the blood out of the underlying tissues, which causes a local ischemic reaction. To try to keep the compressed tissues supplied with blood, the body pumps more into the area and then when the pressure is removed there is a far greater inflow. This sudden engorgement of blood aids healing and also relaxes the tissues.

But if these were the only reasons why neuromuscular techniques worked, it would be a simple matter of just pressing as hard as possible into trigger points, causing as much pain as possible to get the biggest release of tension. But such a brutal method does not work well at all, which suggests there may be more to it.

Changing Reflex Patterns

To see how NMT can reset reflex patterns, it is necessary to consider the cause of hypertonicity. A muscle which is injured or stressed will cause discomfort if it is stretched and lengthened. This sensation is transmitted along sensory nerves into the central nervous system which, through a reflex pathway, sends messages back along motor nerves to increase contraction and shorten the tissues. This takes the tension of the affected area so the discomfort goes away. Because this hypertonic state is now the new position of comfort, it becomes set by the neuromuscular system and becomes the new 'normal' level of tone. A neuromuscular technique needs to influence the reflex pathway to reset this correctly. It does not achieve this by simply causing pain; instead, it uses the painful trigger point as a gateway into the neuromuscular reflex system to effect a change.

The client only becomes consciously aware of the acutely tender trigger point when the therapist presses into it and makes it hurt. The first normal reaction to any painful stimulus would be to move out of the way and stop it happening, but in the unique environment of the clinic, the client does not do this. They overcome a natural reaction to avoid pain and instead they accept it and confront the issue. This in itself is a significant factor in the success of the technique.

If a person is subjected to painful pressure which they cannot escape from, their next natural reflex action would be to contract and harden the muscle, creating some 'armour' to resist the pressure and stop the pain. But the real skill in a neuromuscular technique is to apply the pressure in a sensitive and gradual way that enables the client to do the opposite and keep relaxed instead. By overcoming their normal neuromuscular reflex to contract they can reset the reflex pathway back to a normal level.

To further increase the effects, the therapist should pay attention to the client's breathing pattern. In response to pain, people may tend to hold their breath and in this situation they should be encouraged to breathe deeply instead. As well as reversing their normal reflex action, this can also focus their attention on the trigger point.

Finding Trigger Points

Acupuncture and trigger-point charts show the location of all the main points and therapists should become familiar with those that are commonly found to be active. But massage therapists can usually find them as they feel their way through the tissues whilst doing very deep slow massage and friction strokes. Where an area of increased soft tissue tension is found, the area should be explored very thoroughly to find the most painful tender point within it. Feedback from the client saying where they feel the most pain will further help.

Applying Neuromuscular Techniques

Traditional techniques apply passive pressure into a trigger point for up to about 90 seconds, and therapists can use whatever tool works best for them: thumb, knuckle or elbow usually. The most important thing is having the sensitivity to feel how the tissues are responding to the pressure being applied. Although at first therapists may think they have little feeling through their elbow, it is rich in sensory nerve endings and with practice the sensitivity there does develop well. *(See photos 93, 94, 95, 96, 97, 98 and 99 overleaf.)*

Once a trigger point has been located, the therapist needs to consider their posture and alignment before applying any deeper pressure. If the client has to relax as they receive the technique, it is equally important that the therapist is also fairly relaxed as they apply it. They should align themselves comfortably so deep pressure can be applied in a very controlled way using their body-weight. The most effective way to increase the pressure is when

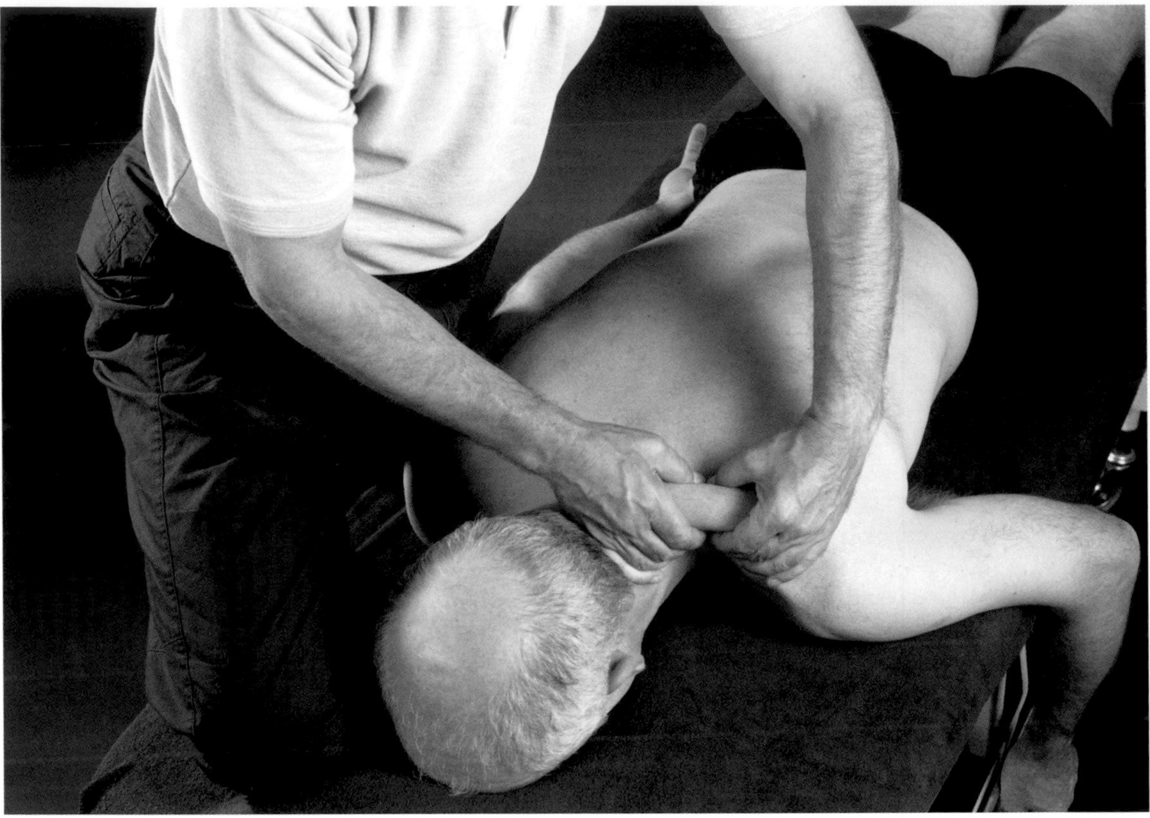

Photo 92. Using a 'pinch' technique to a trigger point in the upper trapezius.

the therapist only has to lean into the client and relax to do it.

Pressure must be applied gradually so the pain increases slowly, giving the client time to adjust to it and stay relaxed. If done too quickly, it is impossible for them to resist the reflex to contract and, although this may not be seen as a big muscle contraction, it happens on a much smaller scale around the trigger point itself. The therapist has to be able to sense any subtle increases in tissue tension and ease off the pressure when necessary to allow the client more time to relax before increasing it again.

The whole body slightly increases tension when breathing in and releases tension when breathing out. If the client is breathing deeply, the therapist can take advantage of this and increase pressure each time the client breathes out. It is even better if the therapist breathes in time with the client and both relax and exhale together as the pressure is increased.

Once the pressure is being applied as deeply as possible, with the client remaining relaxed but at the very limit of their pain tolerance, this should be maintained for up to 90 seconds. The client should report a reduction in pain during this time, and the therapist should feel a spontaneous relaxation take place in the tissues. The pressure is usually released fairly slowly at the end, but sometimes removing it suddenly can also have a good reflex effect.

As well as pressing into the trigger point

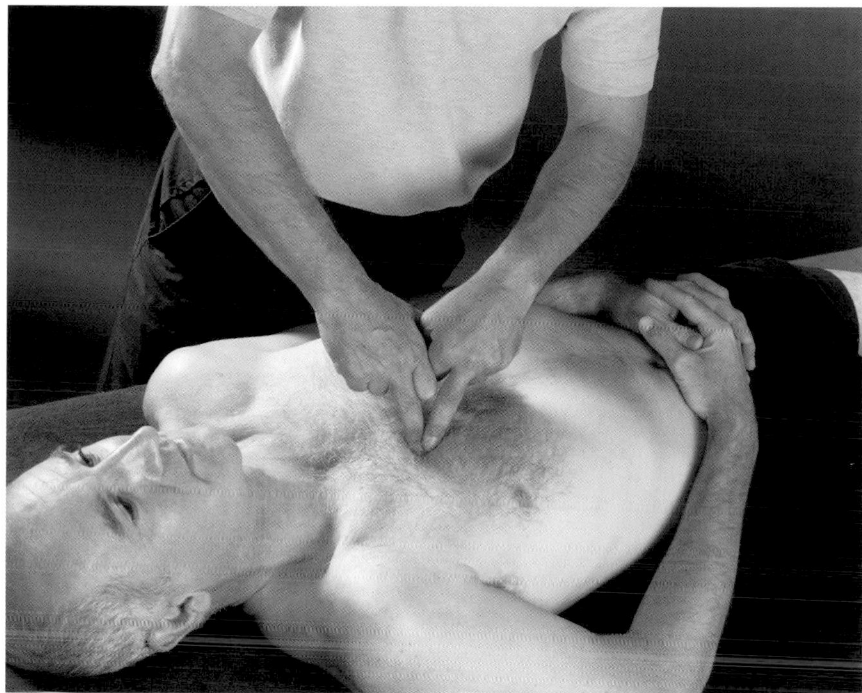

Photo 93. Neuromuscular Technique applied to the intercostal muscle.

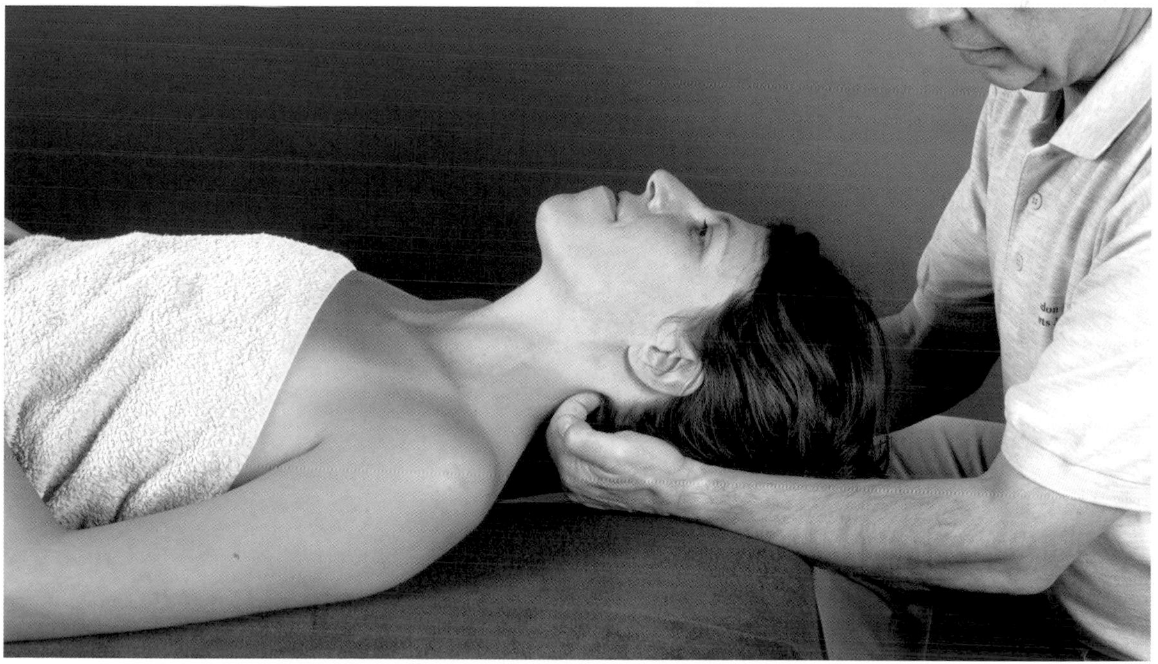

Photo 94. With the head resting in extension to relax the superficial muscles, a deep neuromuscular pressure can be applied with the fingers to trigger points along the occipital ridge and deep neck muscles.

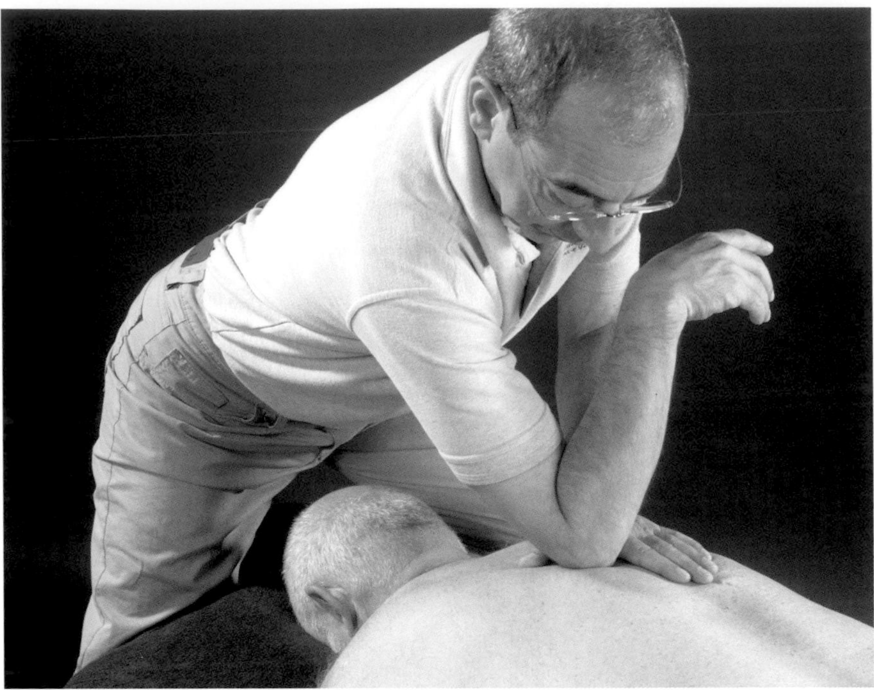

Photo 95. Using the elbow to apply a neuromuscular technique into the deep spinal muscles. Note the therapist's hand controlling the position and pressure of the elbow.

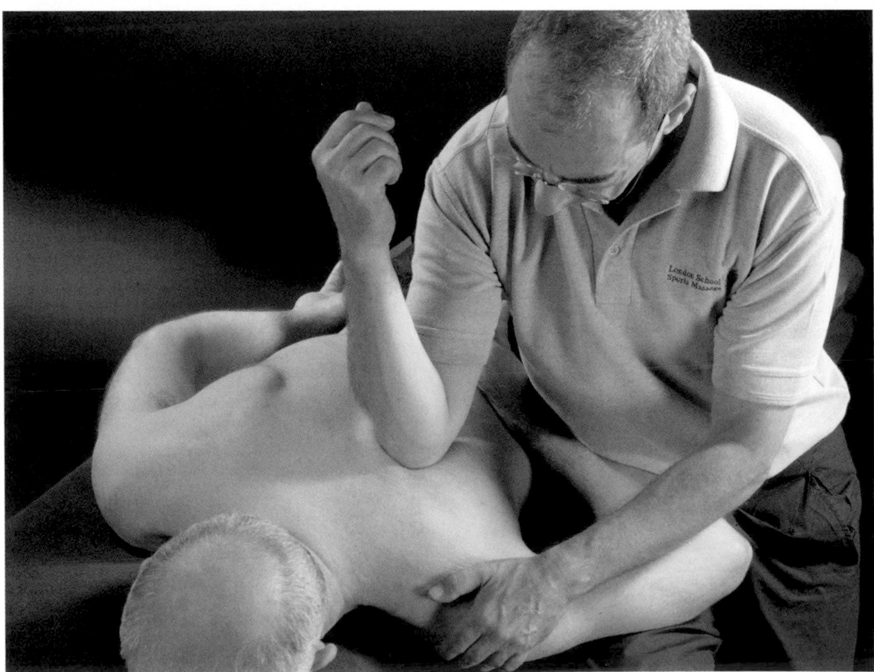

Photo 96. Using the elbow to treat trigger points along the medial border of the scapula.

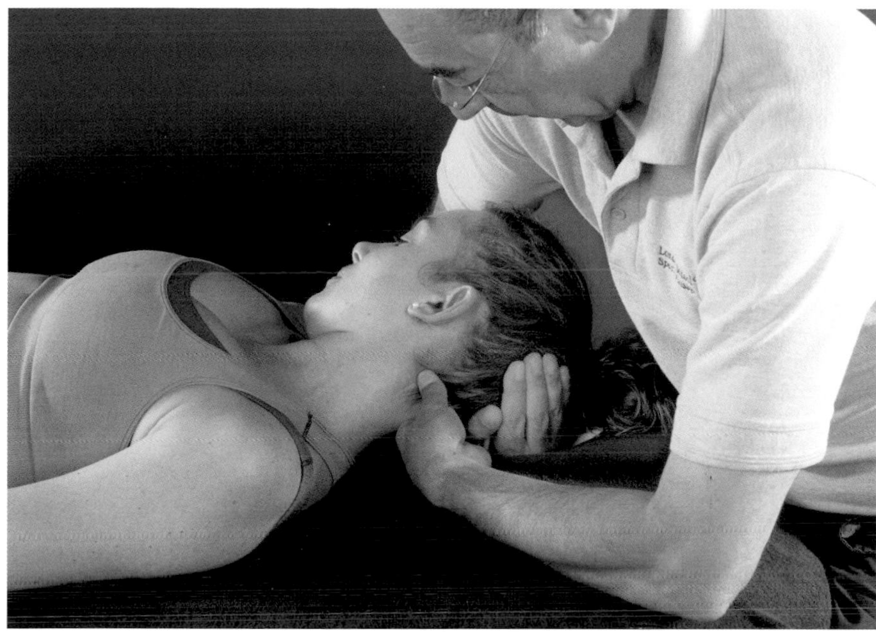

Photo 97. With the head firmly supported by the therapist's hand and arm, the thumb of the other hand can be used to treat trigger points around the mastoid process.

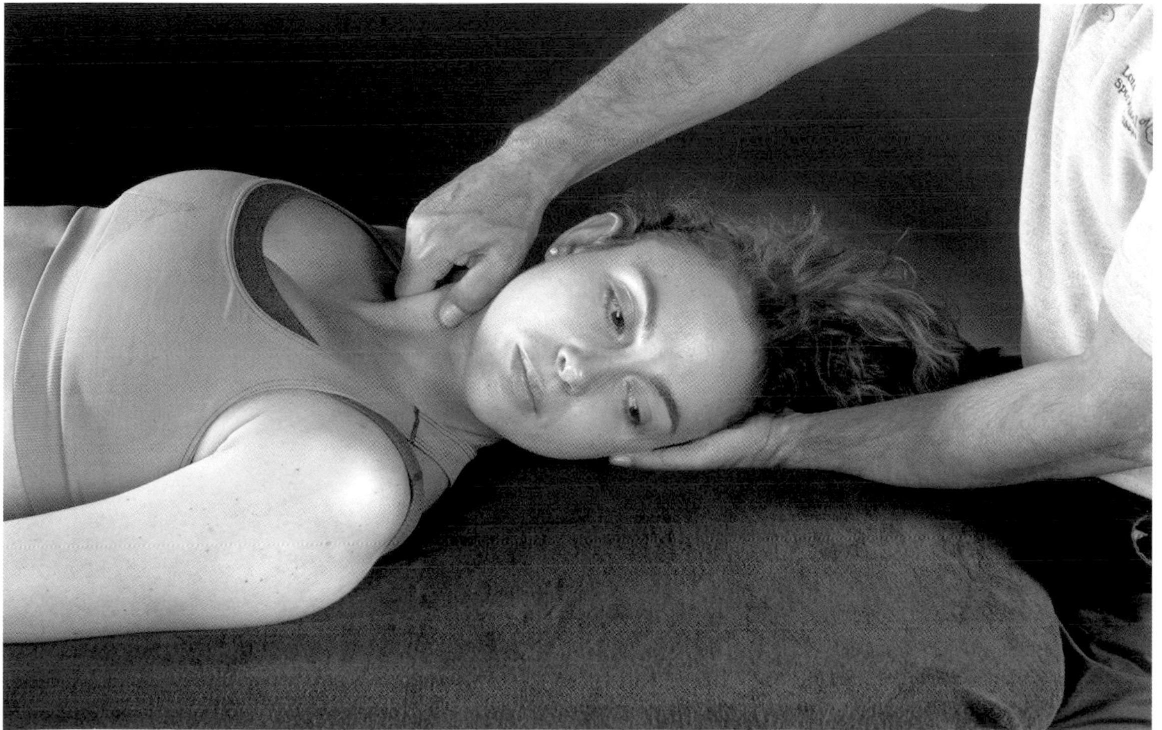

Photo 98. Using a 'pinch' technique to apply a neuromuscular technique to the sternocleidomastoid.

itself, it is also good to make contact with the client in other places too. If using the thumb to apply the technique, the fingers of that hand can form a bridge making contact with the surrounding area. Not only does this make the thumb more stable but any secondary contraction can also be felt through the fingertips.

When using the elbow, it helps to place the other hand around it. This enables the therapist to relax into applying pressure without the risk of their elbow slipping. The hand and elbow can also work together to carefully control pressure and apply slow frictional movements. It can help to have the other hand or arm resting gently on the client, and this can even be used to gently rock the client to help encourage good relaxation. The combination of feeling pain at the trigger point but gentleness at the same time is an unusual experience for the neuromuscular system and this can also help in resetting the reflex pathways.

Everything possible should be done to create a relaxed environment for the client so the therapist should make sure they are warm and work through a towel if necessary. Even the tone of the therapist's voice can help – calmness and constant reassurance adds to the overall effectiveness of the technique.

Traditional neuromuscular techniques involve treating just the trigger points without any movement, but the change in reflex pattern caused by relaxing into pain need not be restricted to these alone. Any very deep technique on non-acute tissue that causes pain has a neuromuscular potential. When applying very deep techniques which cause pain, the therapist must work slowly and sensitively so the client can resist the reflex to contract. The deeper the technique, the slower and more sensitive it has to be. One very deep, very slow stroke can achieve a far greater release of tension than five minutes of hard vigorous massage because it works on this more profound neuromuscular level.

The Effects of Neuromuscular Technique

Although it is an excellent way of normalising muscle tone, how long this effect lasts often depends on the causes and history of the problem. With chronic tension or where postural factors are involved, the effect may not last long unless other issues are also dealt with through treatment and remedial exercise. Neuromuscular techniques are rarely the answer to long-term problems on their own, but combined with others techniques and advice they are extremely useful.

It is natural for therapists to assume that there must be a musculoskeletal cause to musculoskeletal pain and injury, but this may not always be the case. Emotional factors can also affect posture and muscle tone and these can lead to painful soft tissue conditions. Neuromuscular techniques influence the whole nervous system and, although the aim may only be to release muscle tension, it may have far greater significance than anticipated.

Sometimes the client's tension is part of a deeper emotional defence mechanism and releasing this can be quite a disturbing experience for them.

It is not the role of the physical therapist to treat emotional conditions, but this may not be known until it becomes apparent from the client's reaction to NMT. Although it may not be the intention, the emotional outcomes occasionally caused by these techniques can be quite significant in helping a client confront and deal with these other issues as well.

Muscle Energy Technique is an umbrella term which covers a number of ways of using the energy of the client's contracting muscle, rather than the force of the therapist, to create a beneficial change. They were originally developed by osteopaths to correct joint function by restoring muscle balance, and were also a good way to release muscle tension in preparation for joint manipulation. But, as these are soft tissue techniques they have now been incorporated into the range of skills used in remedial massage therapy. And like so many other natural techniques, we can also see distinct elements of MET performed within some long-established traditional styles of massage and body work, too.

Although a muscle's energy is used in exercise to strengthen it, these MET techniques are primarily aimed at releasing excessive tension and restoring normal length and elasticity. They only work where there is a real restriction in the tissues and will not make muscles any longer or more elastic than they should normally be. The muscles to treat with MET are found by testing the range of joint movement to see, and feel, the muscles which are causing restriction. As well as treating large common muscle groups like the quadriceps or hamstrings, with skill and knowledge the techniques can be very specifically targeted to small muscles involved in quite intricate movements. They can also be applied to equal effect on groups of muscles working with functional movement pattern rather than just individual muscles.

The effects of MET can be quite dramatic, but to maintain the improvement in muscle length the client usually needs to carry out regular stretching exercises afterwards. The technique itself helps them in this by improving their self-awareness. Because they can clearly feel the tissues that are being lengthened when the technique is performed on them, they can aim to reproduce the same sensation when they practise it themselves.

As well as being incorporated into massage treatment, MET can be used as a standalone technique. But muscles do respond better if they have been well prepared with general massage first. Also, during a massage the therapist can identify where the specific areas of tension are, making it possible to target the technique more accurately.

If the client has arrived wearing loose casual clothing, it is more practical to do these techniques when they are dressed. It is easier if the therapist does not have to keep the client properly covered with towels at the same time. In this situation they should take a note of the areas they want to stretch and allow time to do them at the end when the client is dressed.

MET techniques involve moving the client and articulating their joints which requires very good client-handling skills along with some strength and agility. Clients can vary hugely in size and in their ranges of movement, so the therapist has to be versatile in finding the best methods to use on each one.

The Two Basic Principles behind MET

All MET techniques are based on the principals of **Post Isometric Relaxation** (PIR) and **Reciprocal Inhibition** (RI). These are two different phenomena that occur naturally through the neuromuscular system and both induce a temporary state of deeper relaxation in a muscle. In this relaxed state, the tight muscle can be more easily and safely stretched and lengthened.

Post Isometric Relaxation (PIR)

Following a period (about eight seconds) of mild isometric contraction, a muscle becomes inhibited and more relaxed for a short period of up to about five seconds afterwards. Whilst in this relaxed and inhibited state, it can be stretched to a new resting length.

Quite how this phenomenon occurs within the neuromuscular system may not be fully understood, but it would appear to happen through a reflex action. The Golgi tendon organs respond to the muscle contraction by stimulating the sensory nerve to the spinal cord. Here it creates a reflex inhibition through the motor nerves, which releases the muscle's tension. Although this seems logical, it would suggest that a more powerful contraction would achieve a greater relaxation. In practice, however, this is not the case, and a mild contraction achieves better results. Even though we may not yet understand exactly how PIR occurs, it is still a very effective device which we can, and must, use because it has such great treatment potential.

The PIR technique fixes a muscle in a lengthened position, and the client contracts this against a resistance. This is quite safe with muscles that are tight but otherwise strong and healthy. However, following recent acute trauma this could overload the repairing fibres and re-tear them, and this method is less safe.

Reciprocal Inhibition (RI)

When a muscle contracts, whichever muscle(s) oppose this action will automatically become inhibited and relax. This is a natural neural phenomenon which is essential for efficient movement. It means that when a muscle moves a joint it is not held back by adverse tension coming from muscles working in the opposite direction.

A tight muscle can be inhibited and stretched more easily by contracting the opposing muscle. Unlike PIR, this reaction is instant and as soon as the contraction stops so too does the reciprocal inhibition. With PIR the therapist can take a short time to ensure full relaxation before increasing the range, but with RI it must be done instantly.

With RI the client can stretch the muscle themselves through an active movement which makes it very safe. Their neuromuscular system will respond to any possible tissue damage and stop them before they stretch too far. So this is a much better technique to use if there has been a recent acute injury or when treating potentially critical areas like the neck.

If joint range is good the antagonist muscle may be in a very short position when the target muscle is stretched. If the client tries to contract a muscle which is already very shortened it can go into spasm, and RI should not be used in this situation.

The Barrier Position

Before looking at the different ways of using these two principles, it is important first to consider the 'Barrier' position, which is the common starting point for all applications of MET. It is the position at which a muscle is taken to a length where the first sensation of tightness can be felt by the client. This is the point at which the fascia is lengthened out but not actually stretched. It is easy to take a muscle into a stretch where therapist and client can feel a strong resistance, but with MET it is essential to find this much more subtle point of tensioning that comes some way before this.

Finding the Barrier accurately requires a good knowledge of the anatomy as well as good tactile skills. It takes time and practice before a therapist can feel it accurately, and client feedback is essential in helping achieve this. Even the very experienced therapist should still ask the client if they can feel the slight tension in the muscle because their mental attention also helps to make the technique work better.

As well as being an essential part of the MET techniques, therapists can use the Barrier position as a general assessment tool to identify the muscles which appear tight and restricted. This can be far more revealing than testing how far a muscle will fully stretch.

The Barrier position can vary enormously between individuals, either because of genetic make-up or because of the degree of tension in the affected muscles. A heavy rugby player may only get to 45 degrees of hip flexion before feeling the Barrier in his hamstring muscles, but a dancer may not feel it until she reaches

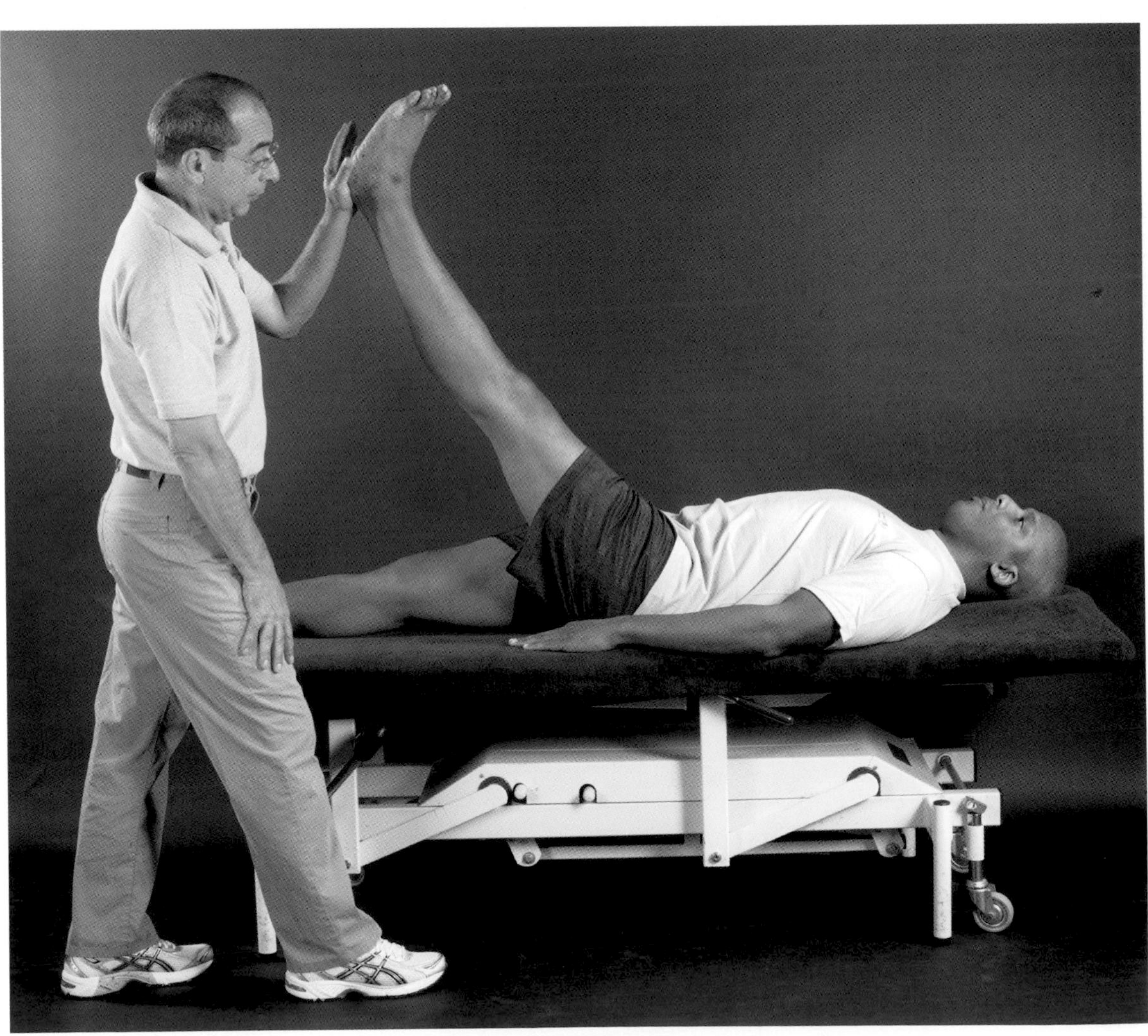

Photos 99 and 100. The natural Barrier position for a muscle (in this example, the hamstrings) can be very different with individual clients.

145 degrees. Therapists have to adapt their techniques to suit the range of movement the client is capable of, rather than rely on a standard position for each muscle. *(See photos 99 and 100.)*

It is important that only the target muscle is being lengthened, and care must be taken to make sure the rest of the body remains still and relaxed. Usually, as soon as other parts start to move, the Barrier has been reached and the fascia is starting to be stretched beyond it.

Proprioceptive Neuromuscular Facilitation (PNF)

The method called the 'PNF stretch' involves taking a muscle into a fairly full stretch first and then applying a strong PIR technique. This method works well on muscles which are tight but otherwise strong and healthy. It is widely used to good effect in the sports environment, but it is less useful in most remedial situations where weakness and injury is often involved.

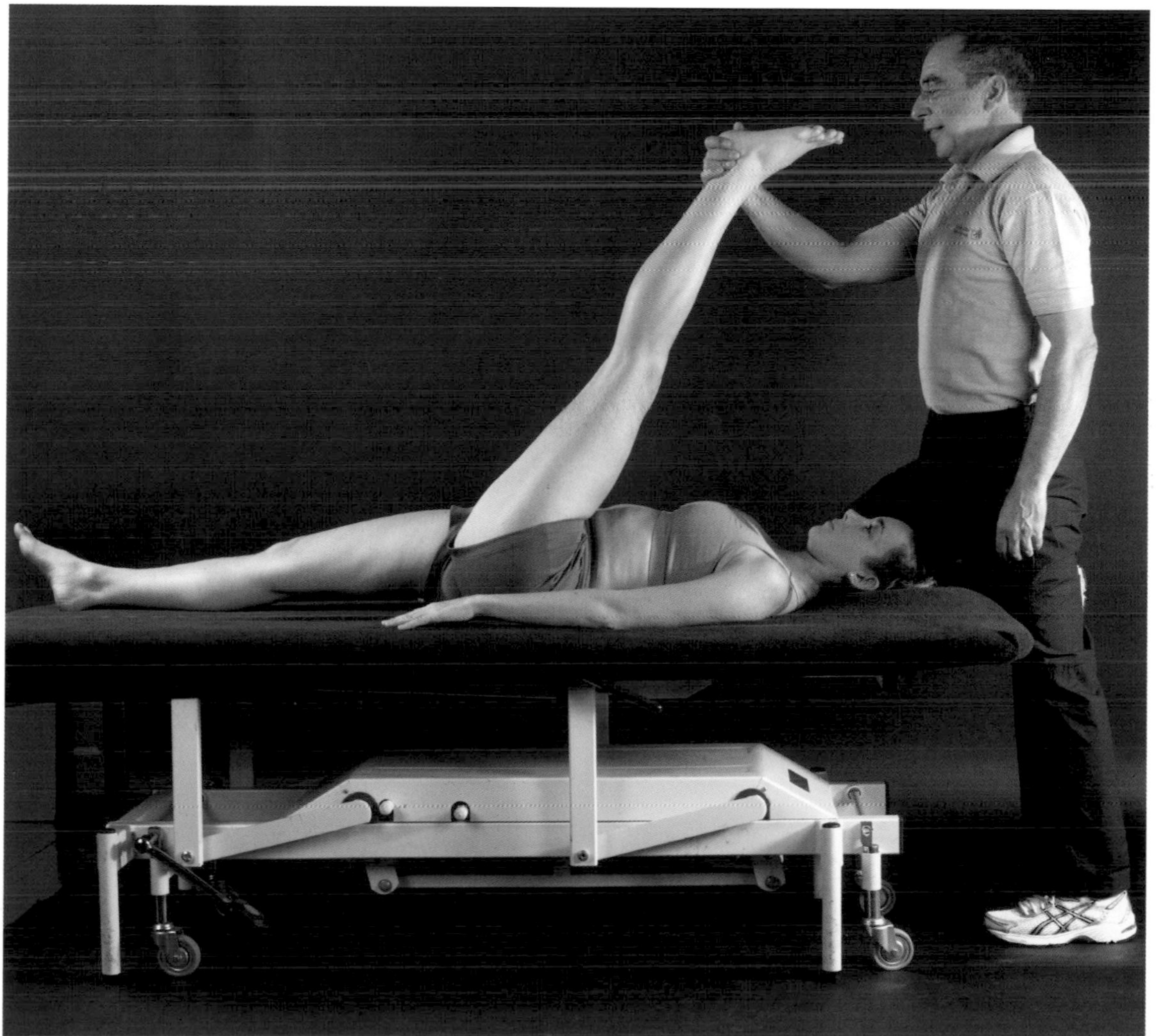

Positioning the Client

Therapists need to first consider the origins, insertions and actions of the muscle being treated so the client can be correctly aligned to make it easy to stretch. This often means moving the client out of the normal prone and supine positions on the couch, so good client handling skills are essential. The therapist also needs to be aligned correctly so they can support and move the client without unduly stressing themselves. During the technique, the client may have to apply a contraction against the therapist's resistance. Even though they only need to use a small amount of their strength, this can still be quite considerable in some cases. The therapist needs to anticipate this and be well positioned to control it properly.

Stretching

When stretching the muscle to a new Barrier, it is important to isolate it so no other area is moving. If other parts of the body begin to move, this means the muscle has reached its new Barrier or the stretch is not being controlled properly. To prevent any other parts moving, the therapist may need to fix them in position and if their hands are already occupied performing the technique they may have to do this with their shoulder or knee.

Communication

The client takes an active part in MET techniques and the therapist needs to communicate with them clearly. Although when learning these techniques we use proper anatomical terminology, this does not always work well with the client. Instead it is better to use everyday terms like 'press against my hand' or 'lift your leg towards the ceiling'.

It is also helpful to touch the muscle the client should contract and point in the direction they should move in at the same time as telling them what to do. This gives tactile, visual and audio direction, which makes them much more likely to comply correctly.

As relaxation is the key to MET, the tone of the therapist's voice can also be important. Rather than shout out firm instructions, a calm voice and softer words like 'press' instead of 'push' work better. There are several stages to an MET technique, and it is better to give one instruction at a time and not tax the client's memory with the whole list at the start. Some positions need to be held for several seconds and although some therapists actually count them out aloud this may not be the most relaxing method for the client.

Breathing

Breathing can also play a part in the overall relaxation process too. The body increases tension when breathing in and releases tension when breathing out. So the client can be instructed to take a deep breath in and then breathe out and relax at the same time to enhance the effect.

The Basic PIR Method

1. **Barrier:** Passively take the target muscle to the Barrier position and support it firmly and comfortably there. Ask the client for confirmation that they feel a very mild sensation of a stretch in the target muscle.

2. **Isometric contraction:** Have the client then contract the target muscle gently (10–20 per cent strength) for 6–8 seconds against a fixed resistance. This must be firm and solid because any shaking caused by an unstable resistance tends to spoil the result. In certain positions it is possible to use gravity as the resisting force, in which case ask the client to lift their limb up a few centimetres and hold it in that position to achieve the isometric contraction.

(A very useful tip: During this stage, ask the client if the mild feeling of stretch at the Barrier has reduced. If they say 'yes', this means the technique is being performed perfectly correctly. If it remains the same or increases it means that (a) the muscle is being held in a stretched position rather than at the Barrier, or (b) the client is contracting too forcefully, or (c) there may be a recent acute trauma in the target muscle making PIR inappropriate.)

3. **Relax:** Instruct the client to relax, and wait a second or two to ensure they have fully done so. A gentle shake of the limb or muscle usually helps achieve this better.
4. **Lengthen:** Slowly and passively stretch the muscle until a new Barrier position is felt.*
5. **Rest:** The new Barrier should ideally be held for about 20 seconds to allow the neuromuscular system to adapt to the new length.
6. **Repeat:** Many therapists tend to hold it for only about 5 seconds and then repeat the technique from this new Barrier. The technique can be repeated several times until no further progress is being made. When the final Barrier has been reached, this position must be held for at least 20 seconds.
7. **Return:** At the end of the technique, always passively return the muscle to its neutral resting anatomical position.

** If it is a chronic problem and the muscle is tight but otherwise strong, it can be stretched some way beyond the new Barrier where a stronger resistance is felt. Then return back to the Barrier to repeat the technique again. Following a recent trauma, PIR can be used but lengthened carefully only to the new Barrier position and not beyond it.*

Two Basic RI Methods

Reciprocal Inhibition is a more versatile tool, and here are just two main examples.

Method A

1. **Barrier:** Passively take the target muscle to the Barrier position and support it firmly and comfortably there. Ask the client for confirmation that they feel a very mild sensation of tension in the target muscle (same as with PIR).
2. **Isometric contraction:** Have the client contract the muscles which oppose the target muscle gently (10–20 per cent strength) for 6–8 seconds. This is usually done by placing a hand on the client in such a way that they can press against this to contract the correct muscle. In certain positions, it is possible to use gravity as the resisting force, in which case ask the client to lift the area up a few centimetres and hold it there to achieve the isometric contraction.
3. **Relax and stretch:** Instruct the client to relax and immediately lengthen the muscle smoothly to a new Barrier.
4. **Repeat:** After the muscle has relaxed fully in the new position, the method can be repeated several times until no further improvement is made.
5. **Return:** When the final Barrier has been reached, hold it there for at least 20 seconds

before passively returning the muscle to a neutral anatomical position.

Method B

1. **Barrier:** The client actively moves themselves to the Barrier position by contracting the opposing muscle. If you ask the client to move to their comfortable end of range without forcing they will naturally stop at the Barrier position. This is the safest way of reaching the Barrier, as the client's neuromuscular system will not allow them to go too far and cause injury.
2. **Rest:** Support the client in this position and allow them to relax fully for about 5 seconds, or more if necessary.
3. **Lengthen:** Instruct the client to actively increase the range further by contracting the opposing muscle again to a new Barrier position.
4. **Rest:** Support the client in this position and allow them to relax again.
5. **Repeat:** This can be repeated several times until no further improvements are made.
6. **Return:** When the final Barrier has been reached, hold it there for 20 seconds before passively returning the muscle to a neutral anatomical position.

RI in many ways is safer, as the client is in greater control and will not take themselves beyond the safe Barrier. And because they are functionally performing the movement to the new length, it helps re-educate the neuromuscular system. Also, because the client is doing most of the work, it is much easier for the therapist and this is a very important consideration when treating big heavy clients.

But RI has one key limitation: if the opposing muscle is already in a very short position when the target muscle is at the Barrier, attempting to contract it in this state could cause it to go into spasm. On its own, RI is best in cases of recent acute trauma, and in these situations the opposing muscle is rarely in a shortened position when the injured muscle reaches the Barrier. But RI can be put into more general use, and to far greater effect, when combined with PIR.

An example of combining PIR and RI

1. **Barrier:** Passively take the target muscle to the Barrier position (PIR), *or* have the client take themselves to the Barrier (RI), whichever is more practical or safe.
2. **Isometric contraction:** Have the client contract target muscle isometrically (PIR).
3. **Lengthen:** The client then actively increases the range to the new Barrier by contracting the opposing muscle (RI).

Combining the effects of PIR with the safety and functionality of RI is very effective, and it rarely needs to be done more than once to achieve the fullest result possible. But in many cases it can be difficult for the client to comply properly with the instructions to make all the different actions required. Therapists should first master the individual methods before trying to combine them.

The Practical Application of MET Techniques

Although many examples are shown in this book, there can be no definitive list of all the possible application of MET, because the variety and potential is limitless. MET could be described as a craft in itself with experienced therapists developing their own repertoire of preferred techniques based on what works best for them and their clients. The way a short therapist applies a technique on a tall client will be quite different to how a tall therapist will treat the same muscle on a short client. And with vastly different ranges of movement, the way you apply a technique to a gymnast would be quite unlike the way you would need to do it on a normal person. It is also useful with main muscle groups which commonly need stretching, to develop ways of applying the technique on clients in prone, supine and side-lying positions so it can easily be used in a variety of treatment situations. (*See photo 101.*)

In training and practice, we may become adept at applying MET techniques on a range of commonly affected muscles but there will be occasions where small, less familiar muscles

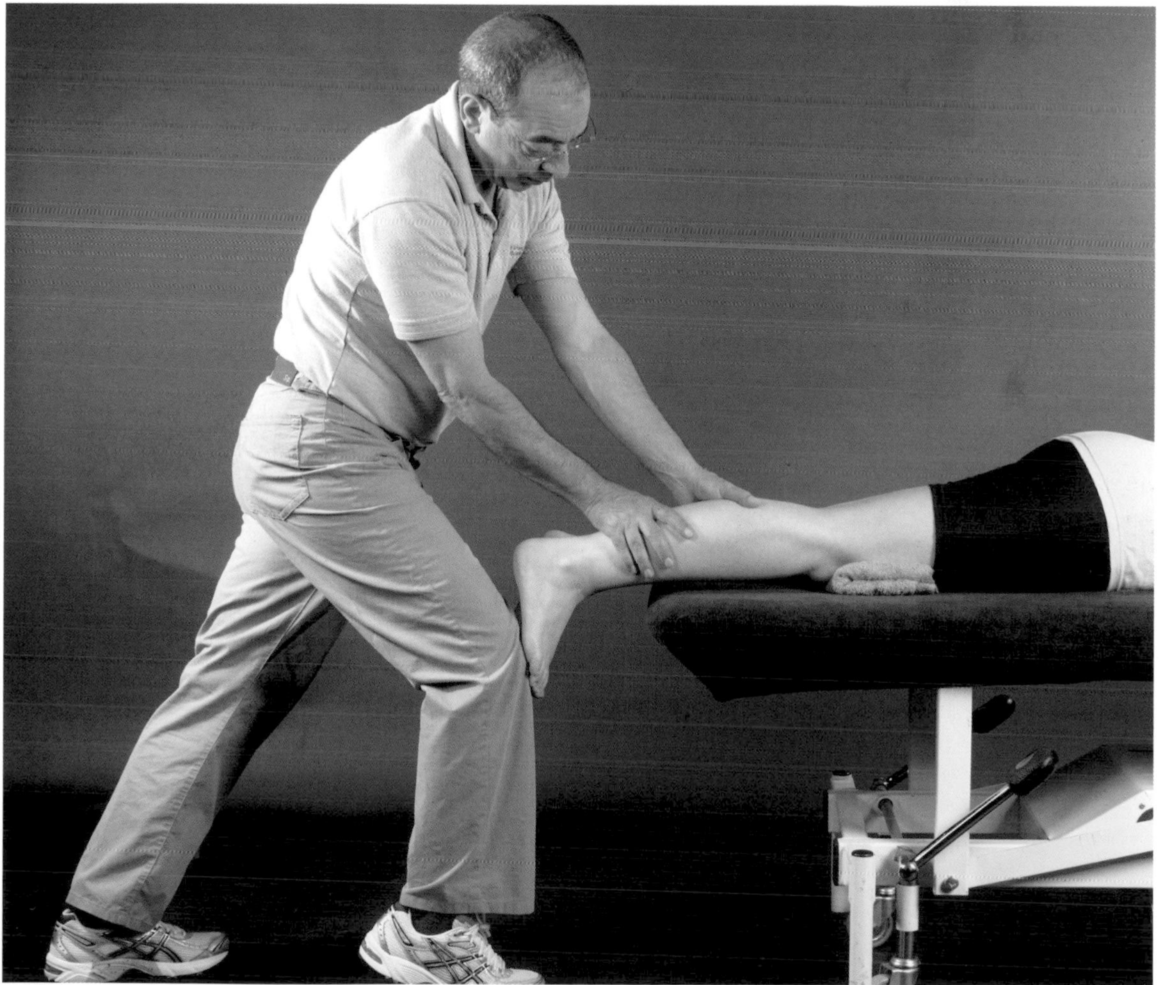

Photo 101. Treating the gastrocnemius in the prone position. Because the muscle crosses two joints, it is important that the knee is fully extended so only the ankle has to move to perform a stretch. This can be done by placing some padded support just above the knee and gently pressing the lower leg down. The client's foot is extended off the end of the couch, and the therapist can use their knee to push the ankle into dorsiflexion to perform an MET stretch.

need to be treated. Therapists should not feel they are restricted to just the techniques they have already practised. With knowledge of the particular origin, insertion and action, combined with the tactile skills to feel where the restrictions are, innovative ways can be found to treat almost any muscle with MET.

Instead of applying it to the individual muscles, whole areas of the body can be treated generally with MET. If a client is tight and restricted in their back as they rotate their torso for example, they can actively rotate into the position where they begin to feel the resistance, which will be the Barrier, and the therapist fixes them in that position. To apply PIR the client attempts to straighten back up against the therapist's resistance to isometrically contract the restricted muscles. RI can be applied by the client attempting to rotate further against a resistance to contract the antagonists.

The following photos show just a few examples of Barrier positions from which PIR and RI techniques can be performed. *(See photos 102–118.)*

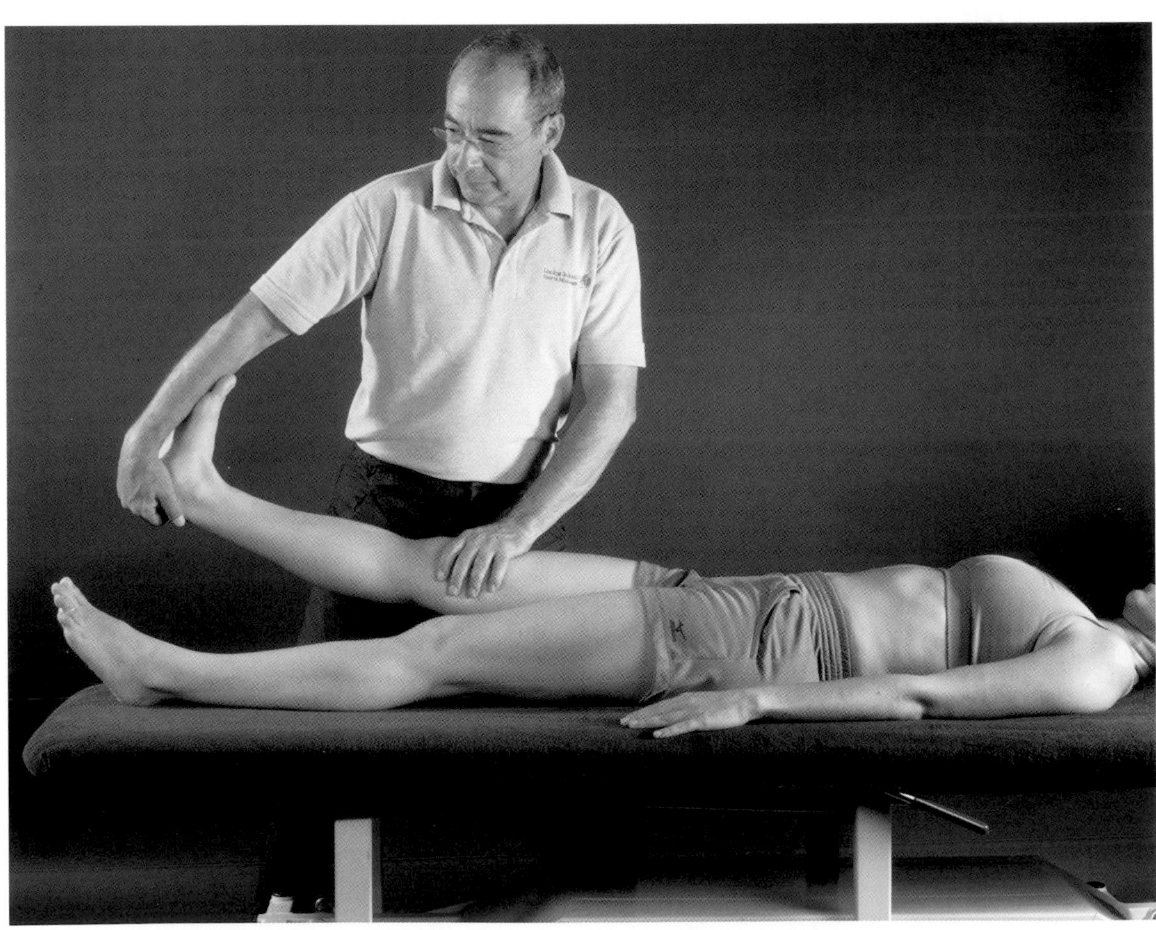

Photo 102. Treating the gastrocnemius in the supine position. Raising the ankle off the couch and gently pressing the knee down ensures it is fully extended. The therapist can then use their arm as a level to dorsiflex the ankle and perform the MET stretch.

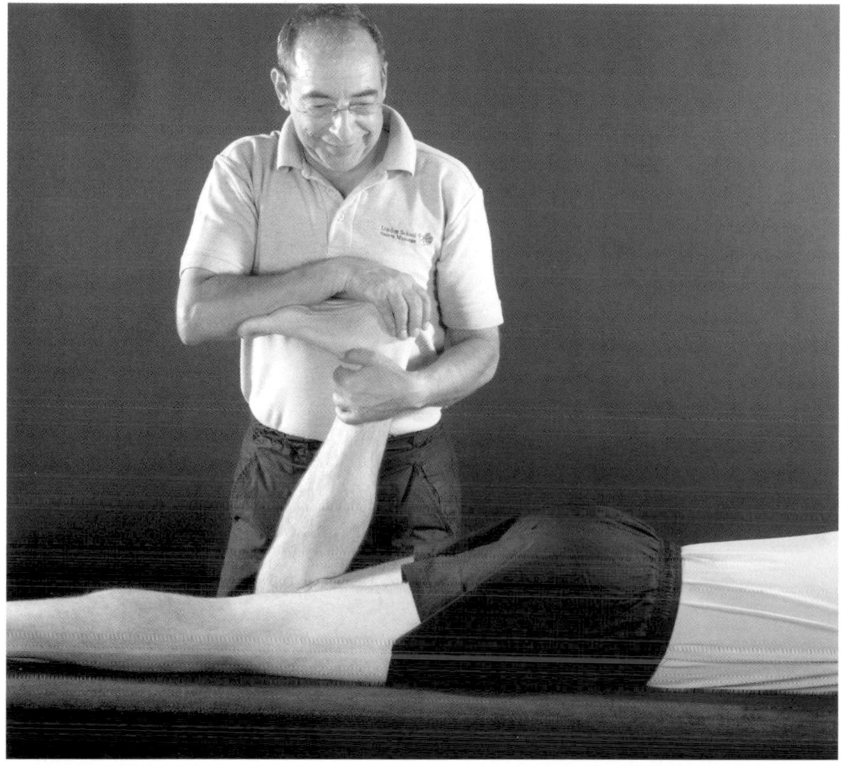

Photo 103. Treating the soleus in the prone position. The knee must be in a flexed position so the gastrocnemius is shortened and only the soleus will then be stretched when the ankle is dorsiflexed. Supporting the leg in this position, the therapist can use the forearm to press the forefoot down and apply the MET stretch.

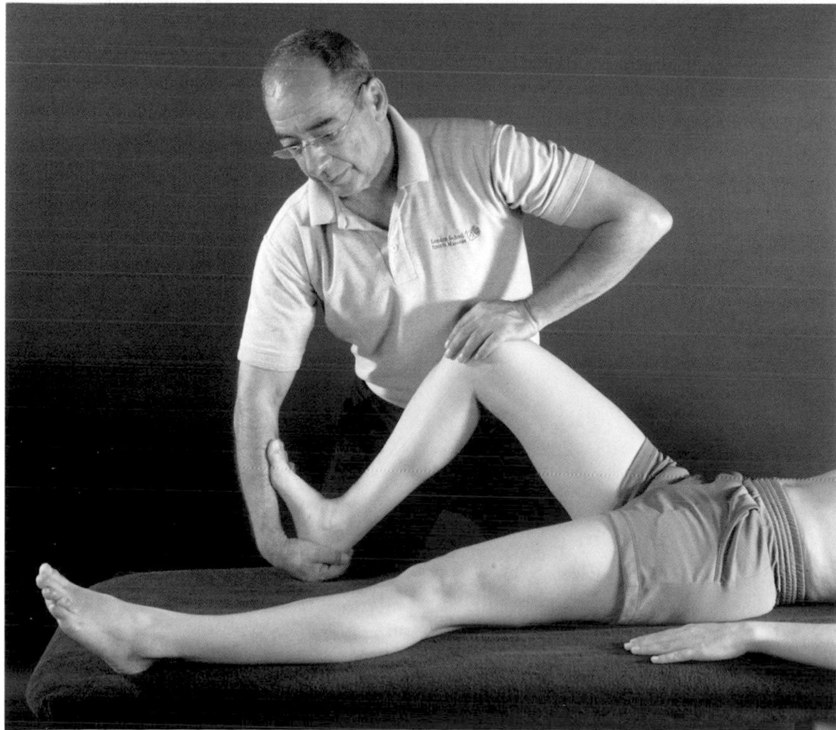

Photo 104. Treating the soleus in a supine position. With the knee flexed and supported with one hand, the therapist grasps the calcaneum bone strongly and uses the forearm as a level to apply the MET stretch.

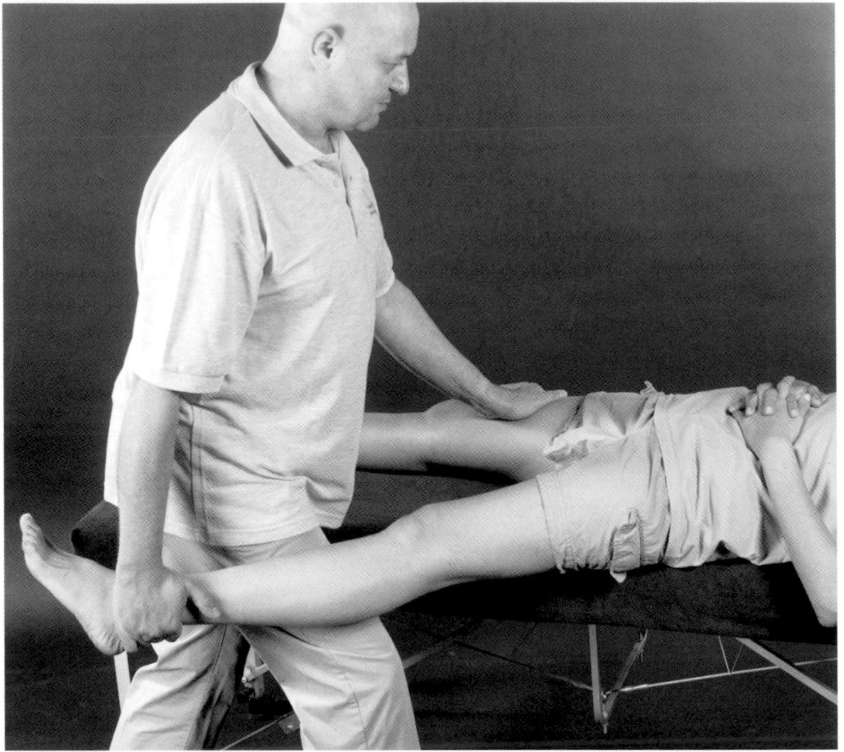

Photo 105. Treating the adductors. The therapist is applying a slight outward rotation on the left leg to prevent the client raising their left hip. The leg being stretched is supported on the therapist's thigh, and their hand is used to prevent any outward rotation taking place when the leg is abducted. The therapist can then use his legs to move the client and apply the MET stretch by increasing abduction.

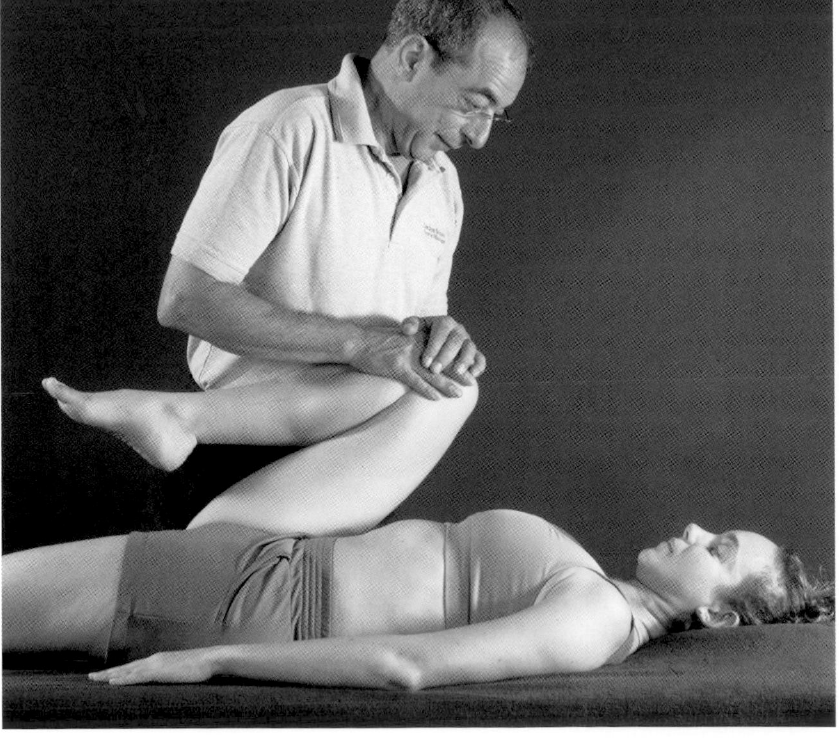

Photo 106. Treating the gluteus maximus. Pressing the knee down towards the shoulder on the same side of the body will effectively stretch the gluteus maximus.

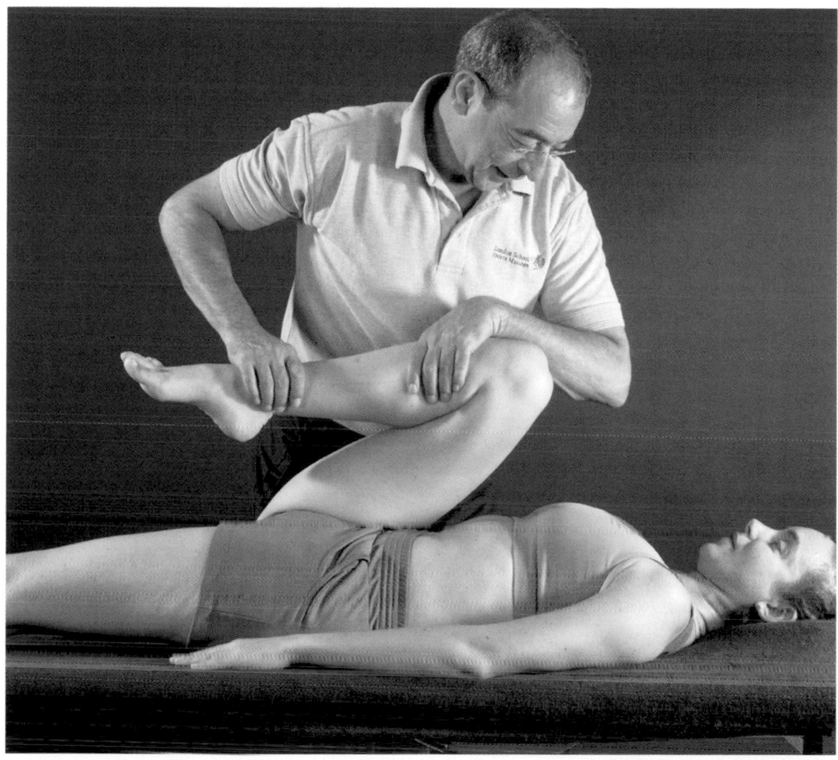

Photo 107. Treating the gluteus medius and minimus. Pressing the knee towards the shoulder on the other side of the body will stretch the gluteus medius and minimus.

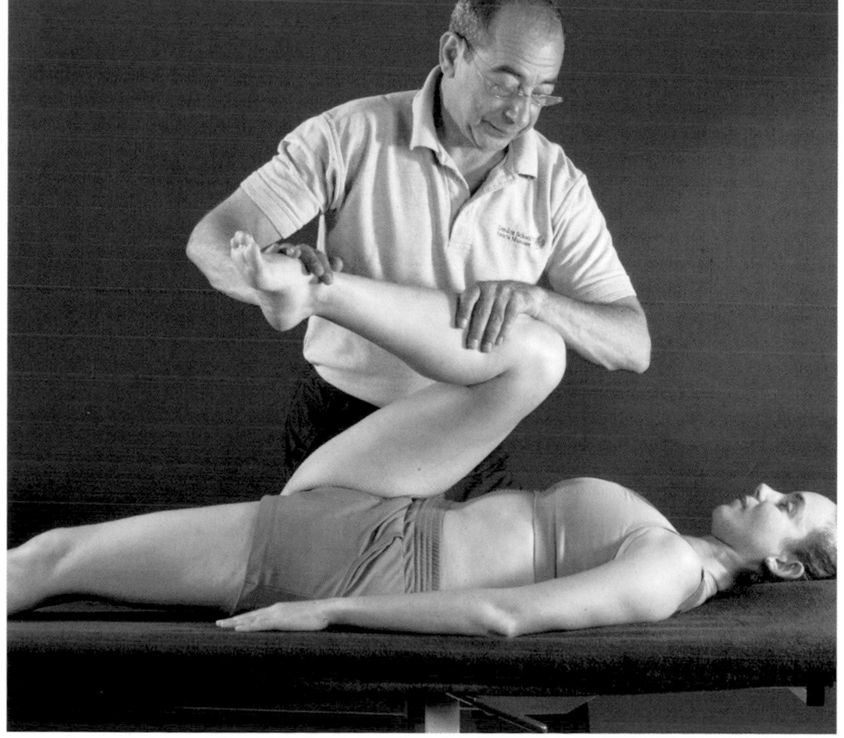

Photo 108. Treating the piriformis. When the hip is flexed beyond 60 degrees, it becomes an inward rotator, and from this position the muscle can be effectively stretched by outwardly rotating the hip. With the knee pressed down towards the shoulder on the opposite side of the body, the lower leg can be taken further across the body to outwardly rotate the hip and effectively perform an MET stretch on the piriformis.

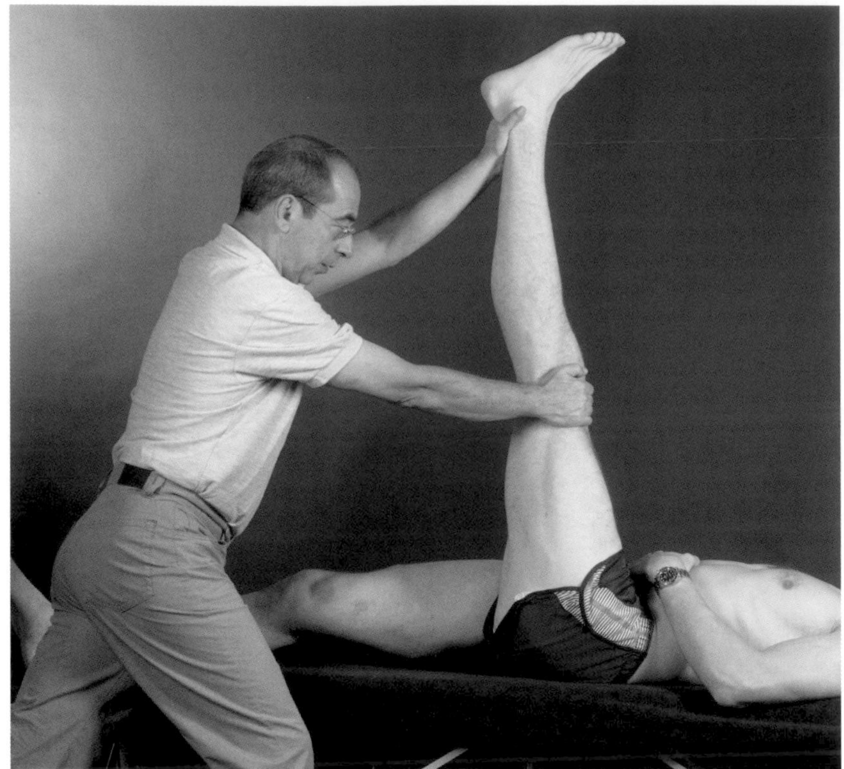

Photo 109. Treating the hamstrings. As the hamstrings cross two joints it is important to fix one, the knee, in full extension so only the hip needs to be moved to perform the stretch. This is done by pulling slightly on the knee and pushing slightly on the ankle. With the leg fixed in this straight alignment, the hip can be flexed to apply an MET stretch.

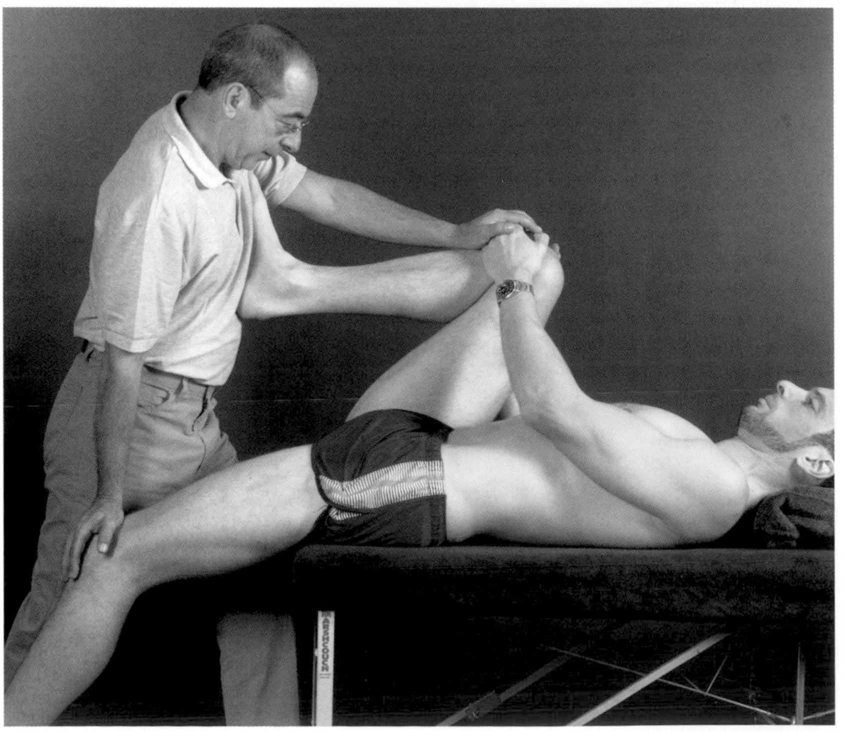

Photo 110. Treating the psoas, iliacus and rectus femoris. With one leg hanging off the couch, the other hip must be strongly supported in a flexed position to protect the client's lower back. The leg will naturally rest in the Barrier position, and the technique can be performed from there. The therapist can press the knee down to perform an MET stretch on the psoas and iliacus. To treat the rectus femoris, the knee must remain still and the therapist can flex the knee by pushing the lower leg with their foot or shin.

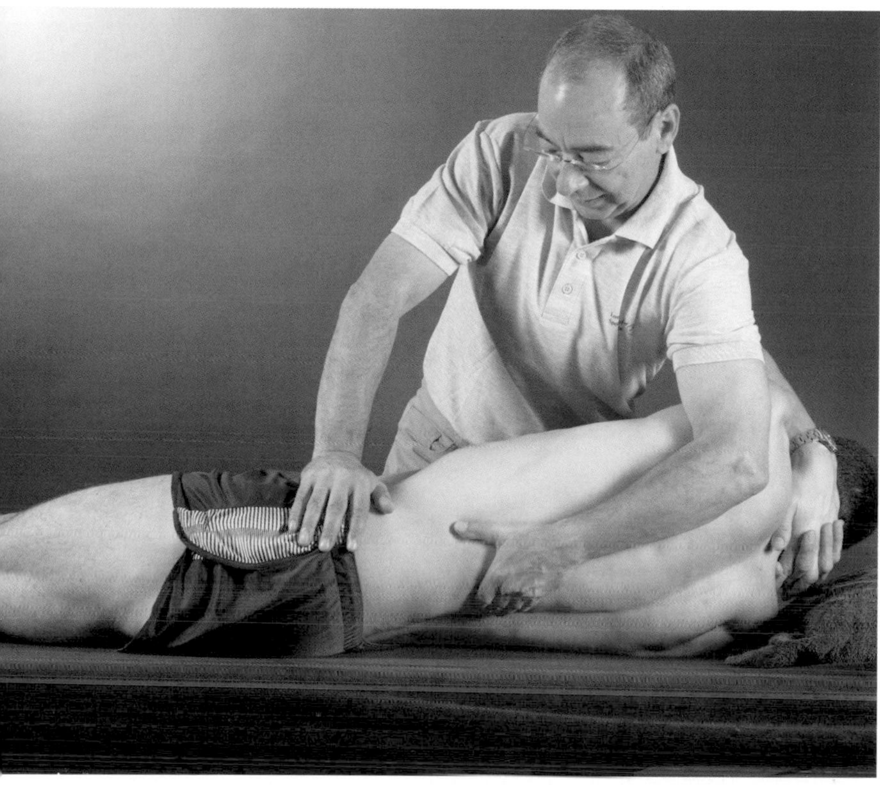

Photo 111. Treating the quadratus lumborum. The therapist uses one hand to fix down the ilium, and the other hand is placed over the bottom rib with the arm supporting the client's weight. By leaning back and pulling on the bottom rib, an MET stretch can be applied to the quadratus lumborum.

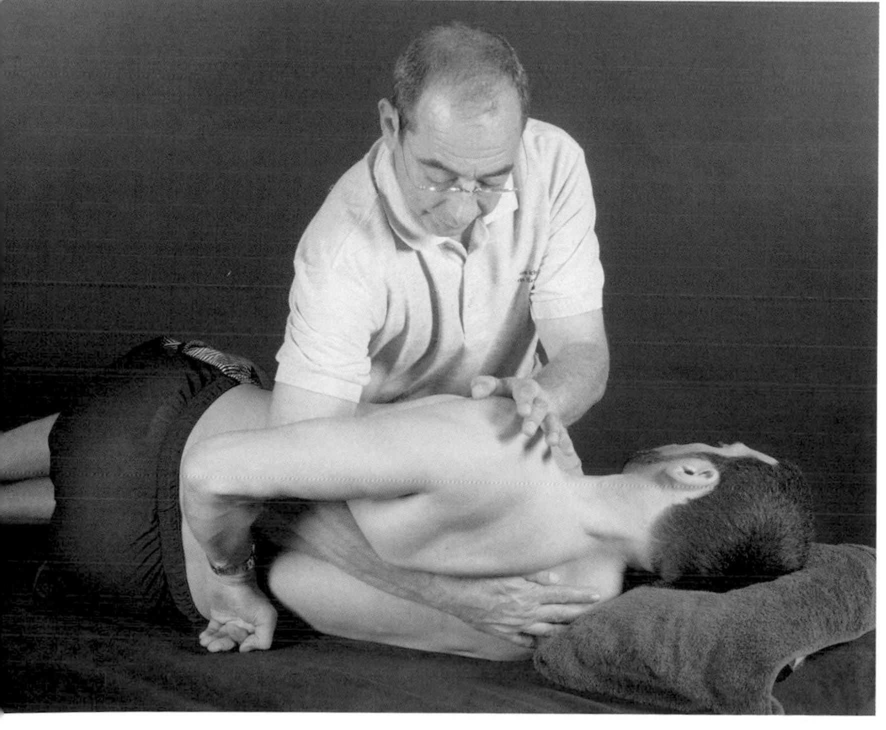

Photo 112. Treating the pectoralis minor. The therapist places one arm along the client's spine so the scapula is not restricted. The other hand is used to push the shoulder girdle and apply an MET stretch to the pectoralis minor.

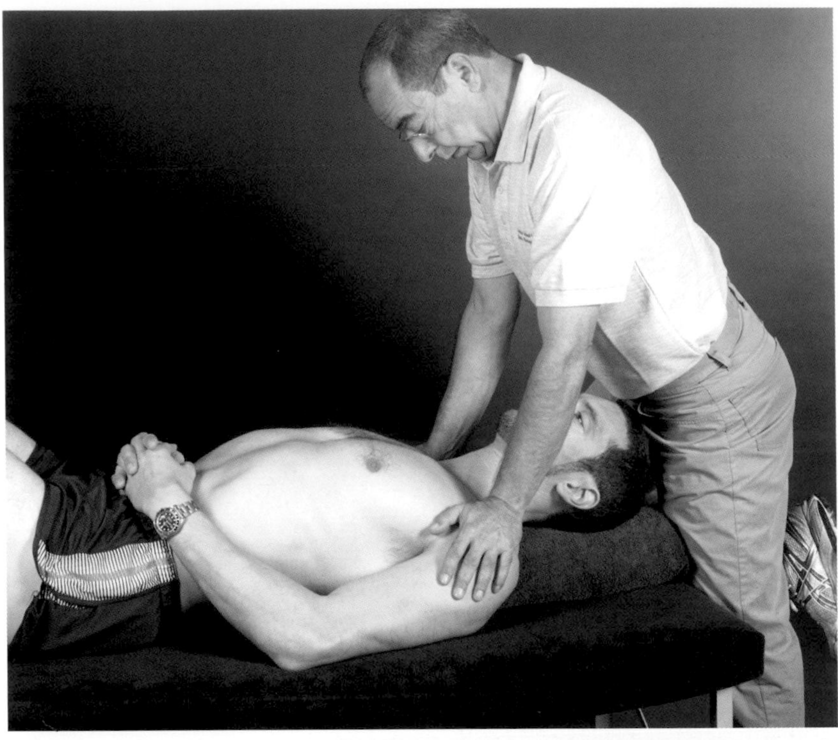

Photo 113. Treating the pectoralis major. With a cushion or bolster under the client's thoracic spine and their fingers linked together on their stomach, the pectoralis major muscles will naturally rest in their Barrier position. From here, the therapist only has to press the shoulders down to perform an MET stretch on both pectoralis major muscles at the same time.

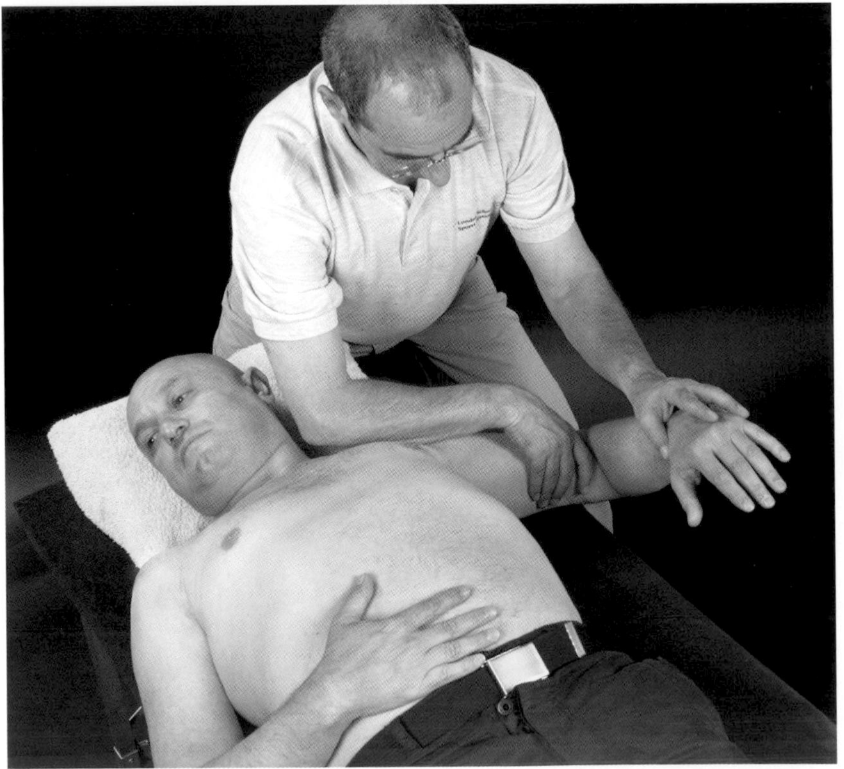

Photo 114. Treating the outward rotators of the shoulder. The therapist uses one arm and hand to fix the shoulder girdle and the degree of shoulder abduction. From here the other hand is used to inwardly rotate the shoulder to apply an MET stretch to the infraspinatus and teres minor. These rotator muscles are relatively small and weak but the arm is a long lever which can apply great force, so this technique must be performed gently to avoid damaging the muscles.

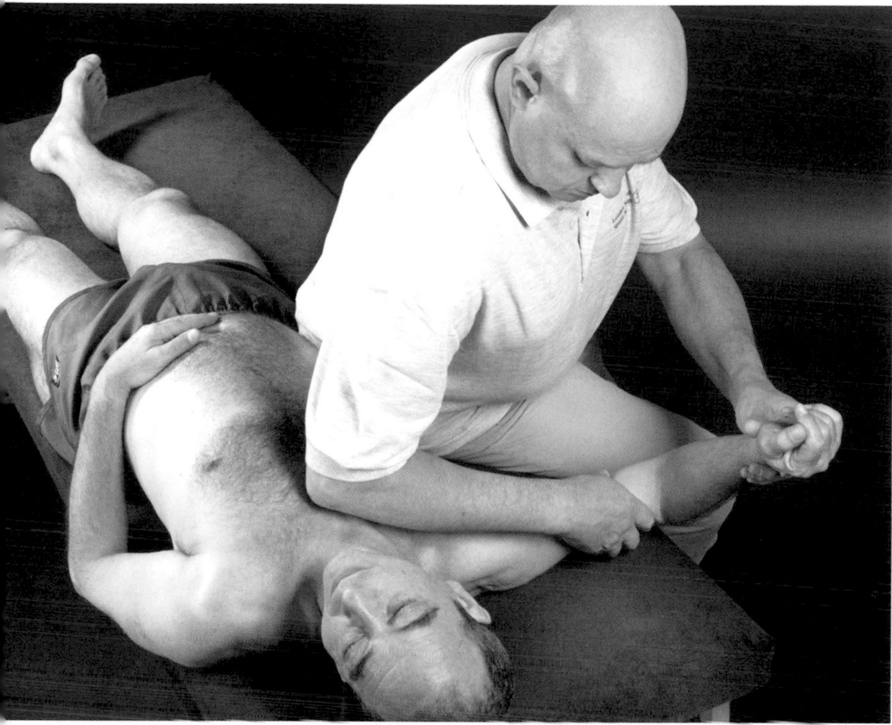

Photo 115. Treating the inward rotators of the shoulder. The therapist uses one arm and hand to fix the shoulder girdle and degree of shoulder abduction. From here, the other hand is used to outwardly rotate the shoulder gently to apply an MET stretch to the subscapularis.

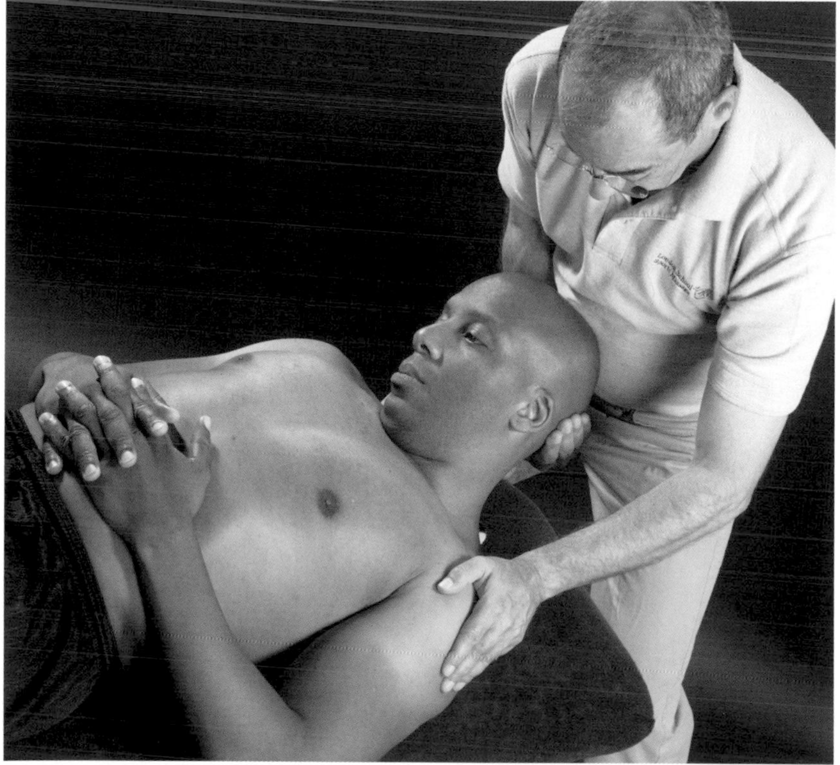

Photo 116. Treating the levator scapula. One hand supports the head in a rotated position, and the other hand presses the shoulder down towards the hip to apply an MET stretch on the levator scapula.

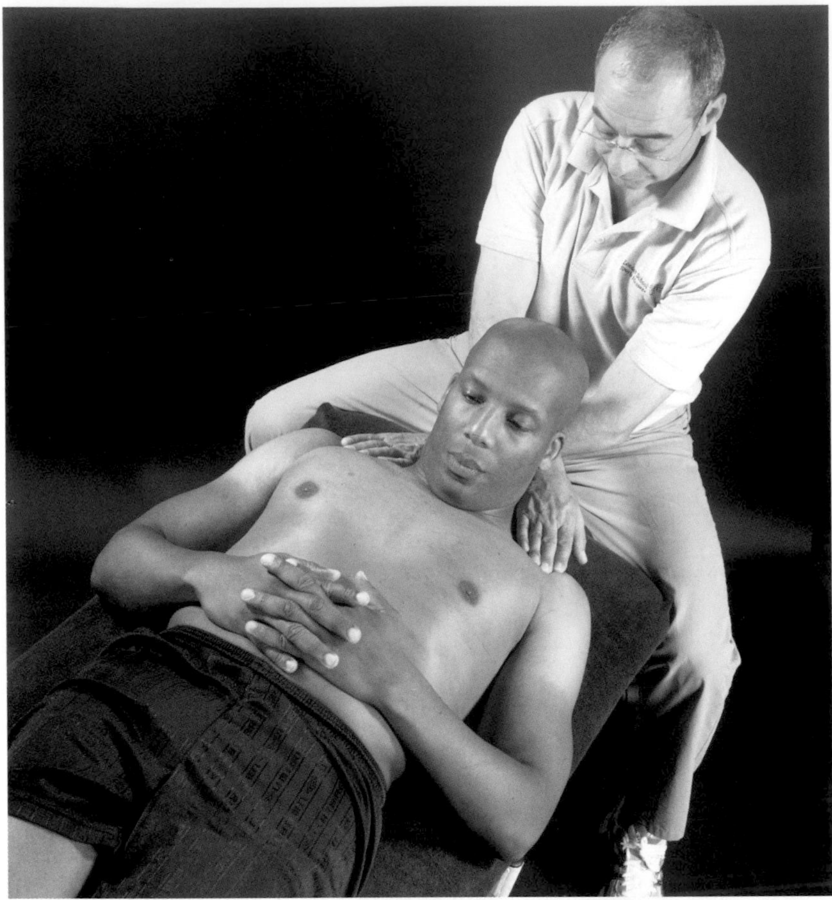

Photo 117. Treating the upper trapezius. With the arms crossed, the hands are placed over the shoulders, and the top forearm lifts the occipital bone up off the couch to apply an MET stretch to the upper trapezius.

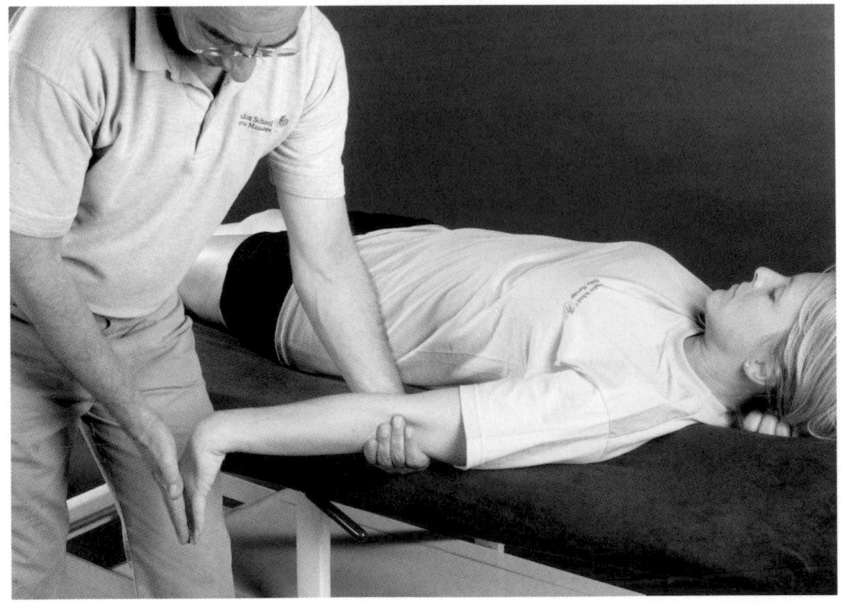

Photo 118. Treating the wrist extensors. As some of these muscles cross the elbow as well as the wrist, it is important to have the elbow fully extended first. The wrist can then be palmer-flexed to apply an MET stretch to the muscles. As these are relatively small and weak muscles, they should be stretched very gently.

9 Soft Tissue Release (STR)

Soft Tissue Release is a name given to this technique in the UK, but the same method is performed in similar ways in other countries under different names like 'Pin & Stretch'. It can also be seen within other traditional therapies like Shiatsu. It is an incredibly versatile technique which can be applied in an infinite variety of ways to release areas of scar tissue and adhesions, and restore elasticity to the muscles. It can be incorporated into a normal massage treatment or used as a stand-alone technique. It can also be applied through clothing, which makes it particularly useful in sports environments like pre- and post-competition.

In essence, the technique is very simple. A strong, focused pressure is used to lock into an area of fibrous adhesions or scarring in the soft tissues. A stretch is then applied away from the lock. This creates a very strong local stretch to the fibres next to the lock, which breaks any adhesive bonds binding them together. It is a very powerful technique and when performed correctly it will cause some pain. It should not be applied directly to recently traumatised tissues which could be re-damaged by the strong forces involved. However, the tissues on the other side of the lock (away from the stretch) remain completely unaffected by the technique. So it can be carefully targeted around an acute area to release secondary tension there without adversely affecting the repairing fibres.

Students start off by thinking about the direction of the lock and the direction of the stretch, but it is also vitally important to accurately feel

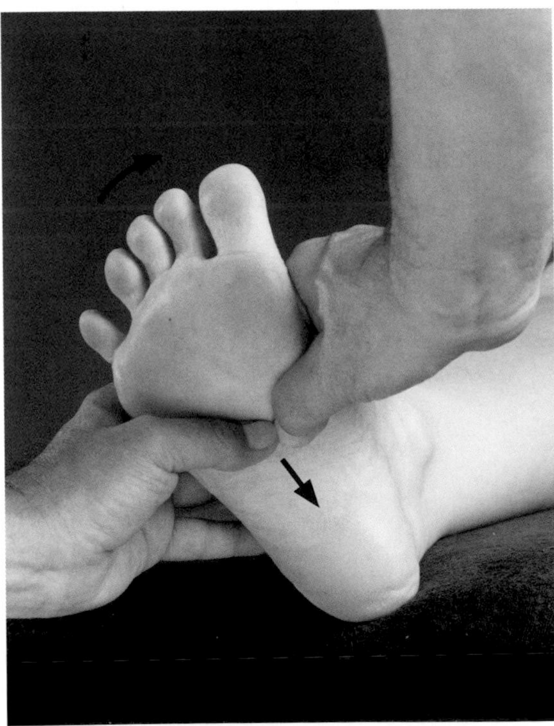

Photo 119. Applying a lock into the planter muscles towards the calcaneum, the client extends their toes to achieve an STR stretch.

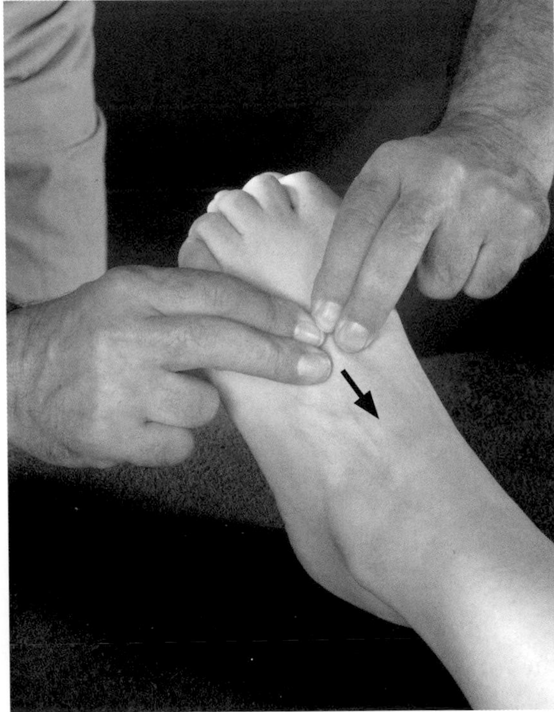

Photo 120. Applying a lock into the dorsal muscles towards the ankle joint, the client flexes their toes to achieve an STR stretch.

where the tissue problem is. A large muscle may be several centimetres thick, and fibrous adhesion could be found anywhere within it. Heavy pressure applied deep into a muscle without care may push past the adhered fibres and squash healthy fibres against underlying bone. This will cause pain, which may give the false impression that the technique is working well, but it may not affect the real problem and may actually cause some tissue damage.

Care must be taken to palpate the tissues at varying depths to find the exact location of the tight or adhered fibres. Then, staying at the same depth, the lock is applied by gliding these tight tissues away from the direction of stretch until they will go no further. When the tissues feel 'locked', the stretch is applied whilst maintaining the lock. This often means that more pressure needs to be used to keep the lock on during the stretch phase and care must be taken to apply this in the right direction rather than just deeper into the tissues.

STR can be a very heavy technique on the therapist's fingers and thumbs, so it is important to protect these, and fists, knuckles or elbows are often used to better effect. This is a painful technique for the client and should not be used on an acute condition, only gently on a post-acute condition, although it can be done quite heavily on chronic conditions. Always start fairly gently and progress with more pressure to find the level that the client can adequately cope with.

STR can be performed passively, with the therapist stretching the tissue by moving the relevant joint. It can also be done actively with the client performing the movement, and this will also add an element of functional rehabilitation to the technique. The active method also means the therapist can use both hands to apply the lock and align their body more efficiently.

To even greater effect, STR can be combined with Muscle Energy Technique by using an active/resisted movement. If the client can forcefully contract the opposing muscle when performing the movement this will reciprocally inhibit (relax) the muscle being treated and will have an even more powerful effect. This can be done by the therapist applying a manual resistance, treating a muscle with the client in a weight-bearing position or moving against the force of gravity.

Application of STR

- Shorten the muscle, actively or passively.
- Palpate to find the area of soft tissue damage or tension.
- Apply extra pressure along the tissues to form a lock on the fibres, without pressing deeper against underlying bones.
- Maintaining the lock whilst the muscle is stretched, actively or passively, away from the lock.
- The lock is released as the muscle is returned to a neutral position.

The technique can be repeated quite rapidly, moving the lock to a new position each time and using a steady rhythm that the client can easily work with. *(See photos 121–132)*

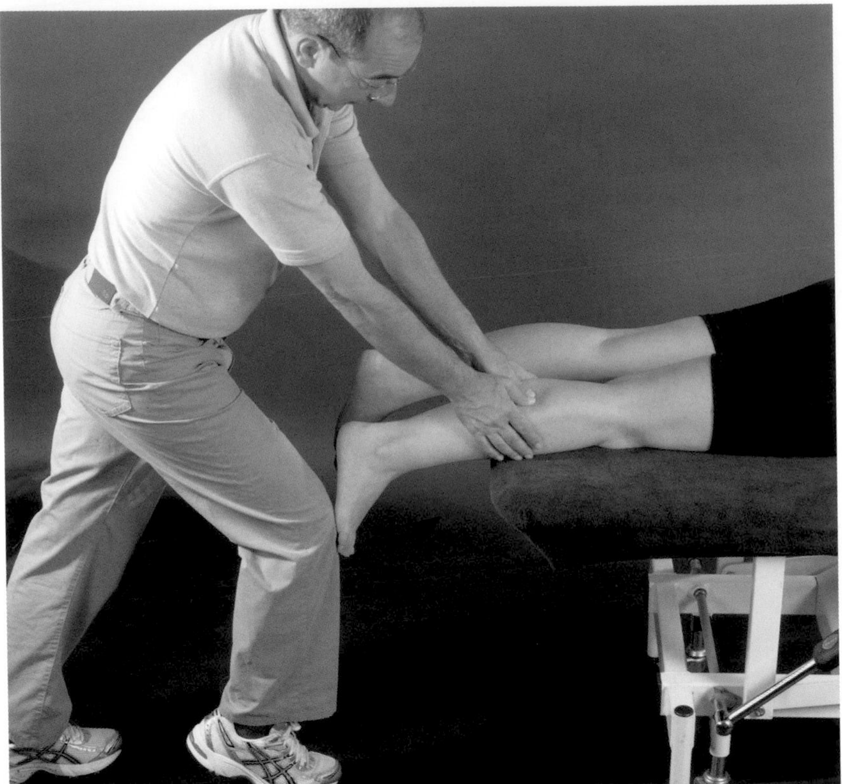

Photo 121. Locking into the calf muscles, the therapist can use their knee to dorsiflex the ankle to apply an STR stretch to the muscles.

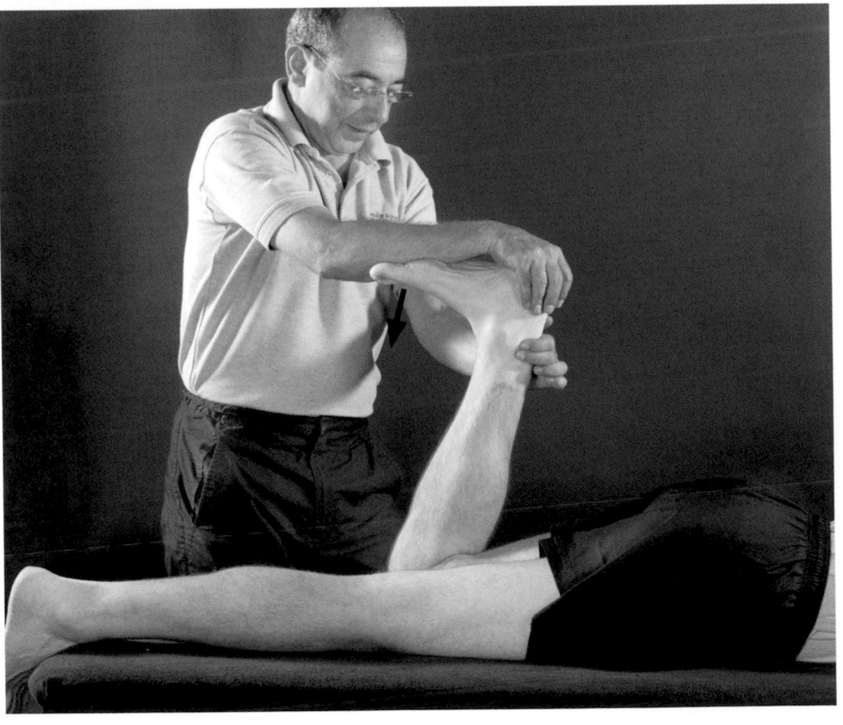

Photo 122. Locking into the Achilles tendon, the therapist can then use the other arm to dorsiflex the ankle and apply an STR stretch.

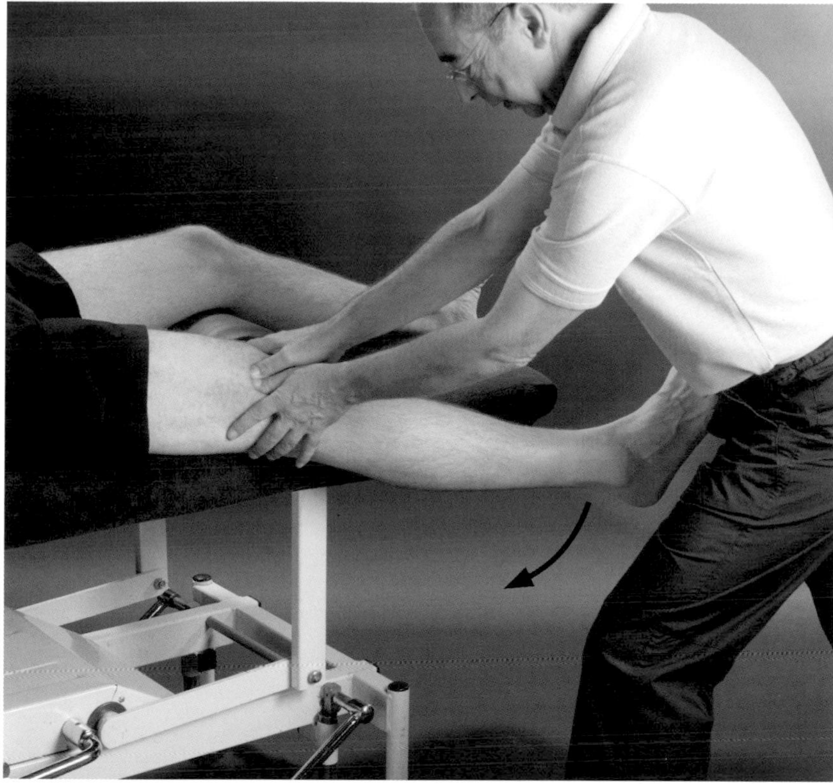

Photo 123. With the client's lower leg extending off the couch, they can first hold their knee in extension whist the therapist locks into the tissues. Then by simply lowering their leg they achieve an STR stretch in the quadriceps.

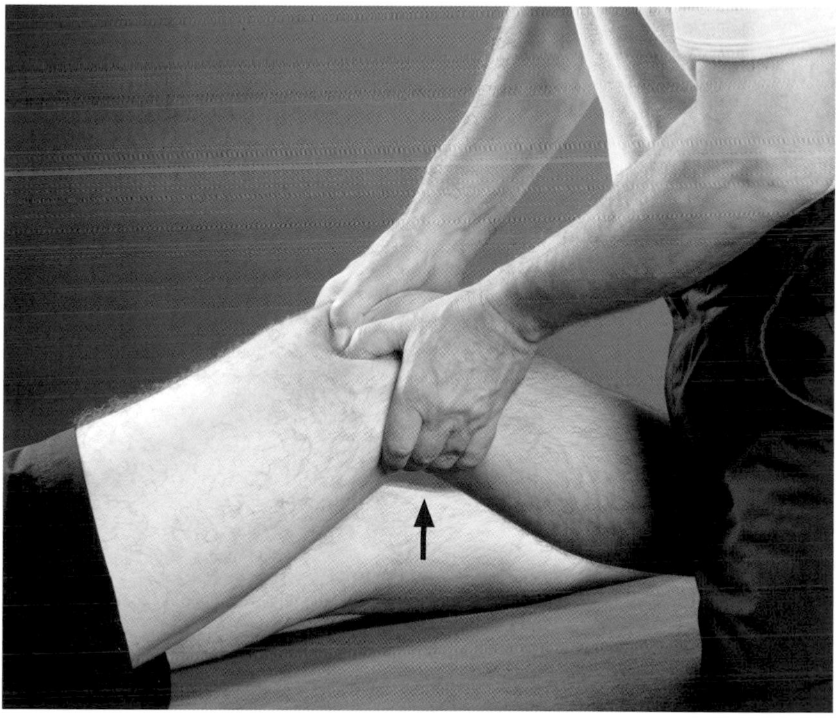

Photo 124. STR can be applied very specifically to the tissue above the patella by locking into the tissues and then lifting the knee up off the couch to achieve knee flexion which applies an STR stretch. If the client pushes the knee up themselves, this adds a functional MET(RI) release at the same time.

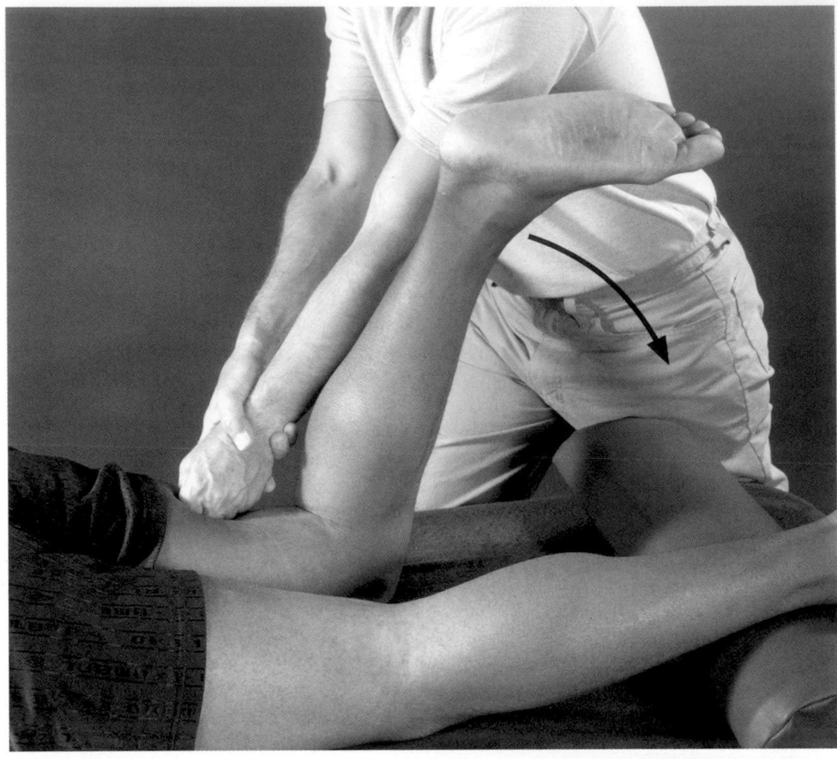

Photo 125. With the client lying prone and holding their knee in flexion, the therapist applies a strong lock into the hamstrings. The client then simply lowers their leg to achieve an STR stretch.

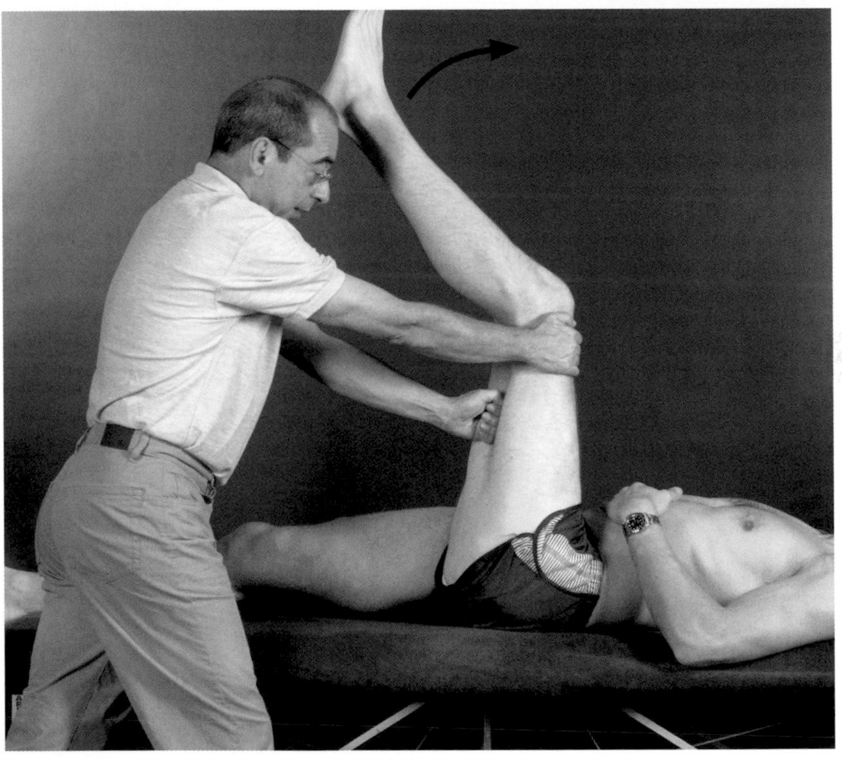

Photo. 126. With the client supine and their hip and knee flexed, the therapist applies a powerful lock into the hamstrings and uses the other hand to pull back on the knee to further strengthen the lock. The client then straightens their leg to extend the knee and achieve an STR stretch to the hamstrings. As the client is contracting their quadriceps at the same time, this adds an MET(RI) release.

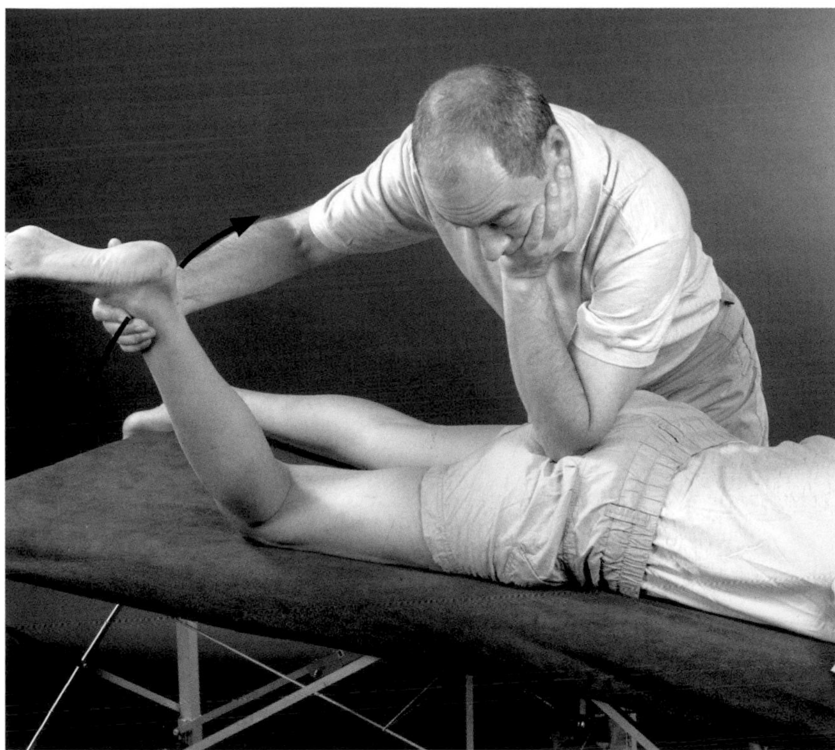

Photo 127. Applying a strong lock into the piriformis and other hip rotators, an STR stretch can be applied by rocking the leg back and forth to rotate the hip.

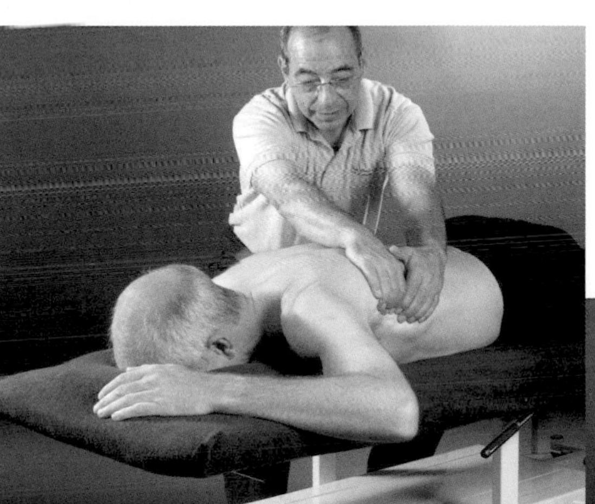

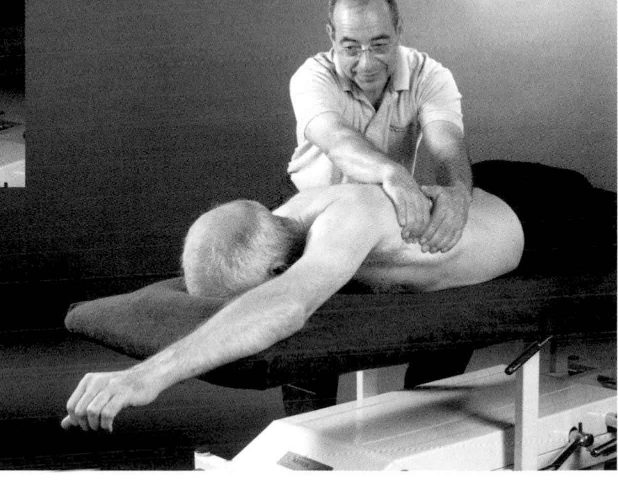

Photos. 128 and 129. Starting with the client's shoulder partially abducted, the therapist can lock into the latissimus dorsi. The client then extends their arm to achieve an STR stretch.

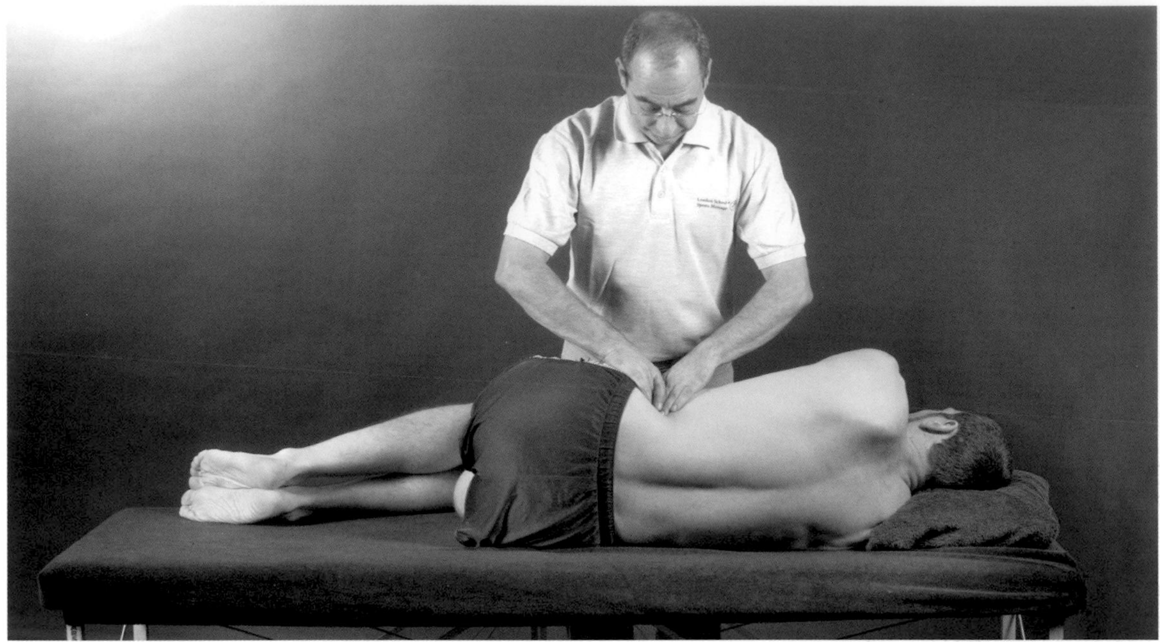

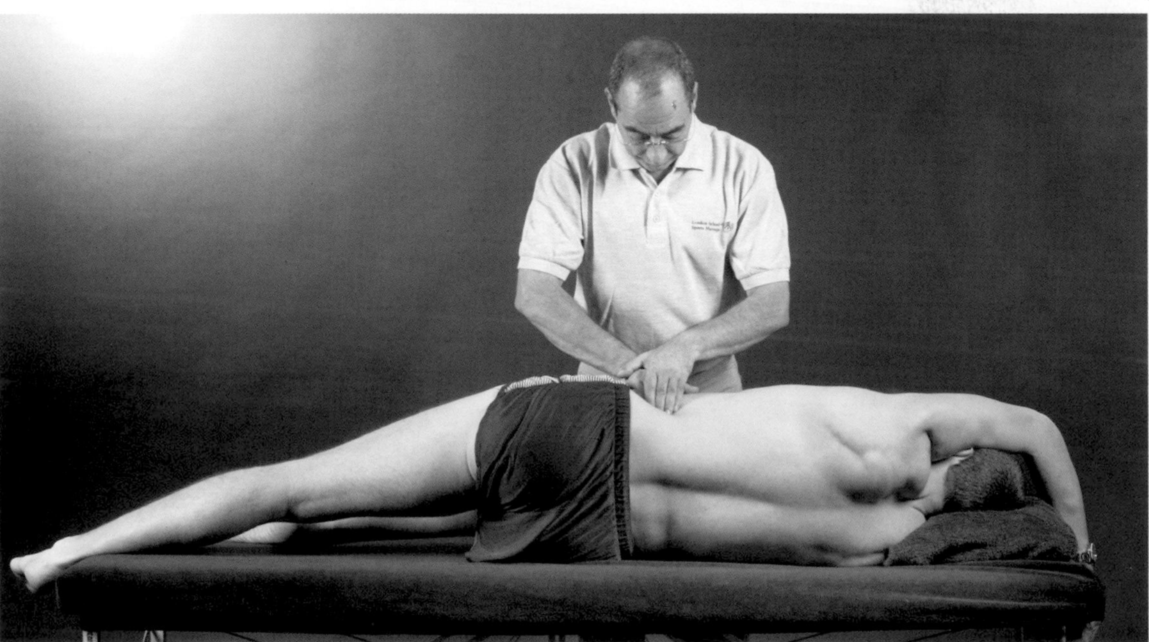

Photos 130 and 131. Starting with the client in a side-lying position with hips and shoulders flexed, the therapist can apply a lock into the lateral part of the quadratus lumborum. The client then extends their leg and arm at the same time to apply a strong STR stretch to the muscle.

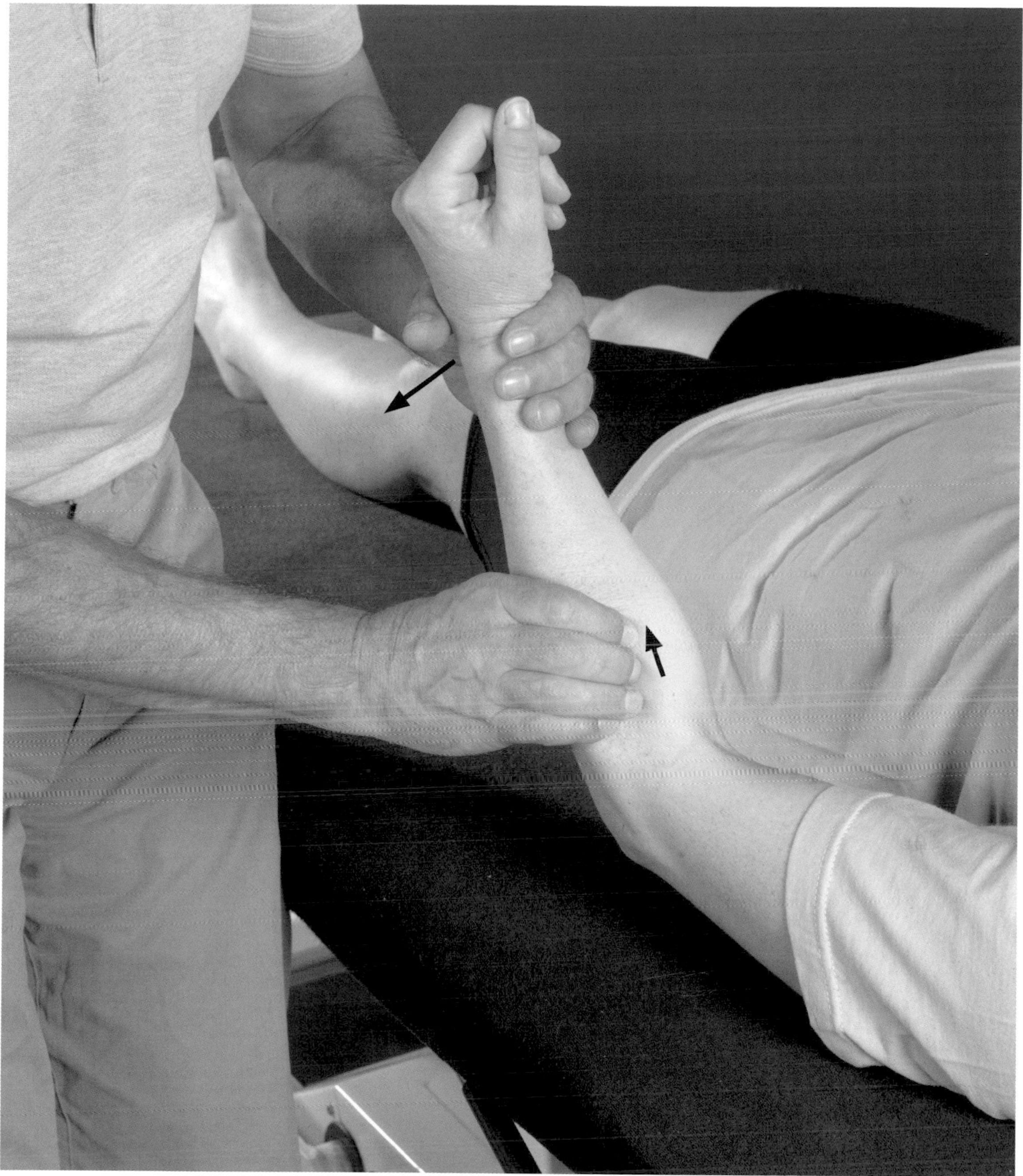

Photo 132. Locking the forearm muscles towards the wrist, an STR stretch can be applied by extending the elbow. Alternatively, locking towards the elbow an STR stretch can be applied by palmer-flexing the wrist.

10 Positional Release Techniques

When treating areas of short, tight and contracted muscle, most soft tissue techniques use a direct force to stretch out the restricted fibres. But Positional Release uses a distinctly different approach and takes the force off the tissues instead to achieve a release. It is also a painless technique, unlike the others which are often quite painful. This makes it especially useful when treating clients who have acute conditions, are in severe pain, sensitive or frail.

The technique seems to have been discovered by accident by an American osteopath, Laurence Jones, who called his technique Strain-Counterstrain. The story goes that a patient arrived with severe lower-back pain and was unable to straighten up. Sitting in the waiting room, he managed to get himself into a comfortable, relaxed and pain-free position and stayed that way for 20 minutes. When asked to stand, he did so very slowly using his hands to push himself up and found that he could stand up straight and all his pain had gone!

How such an amazing phenomenon can occur is hard to imagine, but Jones's theory suggested that it was the particular way the injury had been caused that provided the explanation. (The patient had been bending down to pick something up when his injury occurred.)

The proprioceptive system is constantly sending sensory information from the muscles to the central nervous system (CNS) so it knows what is happening to them. When bending forward, the extensor muscles in the back work eccentrically to control the movement. They lengthen and contract at the same time and this sends out very strong neural messages. The flexor muscles in the abdomen, however, are being shortened and relaxed, and the neural messages coming from these are very greatly diminished. It is believed that in this situation the CNS can 'turn up the volume' from these relaxed muscles so it can still 'hear' what is going on with them.

This should rebalance as the person completes the activity and stands up straight again, but it can go drastically wrong if there is a sudden crisis. For example, if a person bends down to pick up an object they think is going to be light but is actually stuck to the floor, their muscular system will not be prepared for the sudden unexpected forces they are subjected to. In this confusing situation, the extensor muscles in the back and flexors in the abdomen try to balance each other in an effort to stabilise the torso. The flexors need to contract to equalise with the level of activity in the extensor muscles, but they are already fully shortened. A contraction in this situation can make them go into spasm and lock in this position. This reaction will be even stronger if the neural volume is 'turned up'. The extensor muscles in the back then reset their normal resting length in this position also to balance with the abdomen muscles and the whole postural distortion then becomes fixed. Any attempt to straighten up will be met with very strong muscular resistance and pain, but bending down further will be pain free because it takes the tension off the spasm.

The lucky accident for Jones was the way his patient slumped down into a pain-free position which shortened and relaxed the flexor muscle. Staying in this position for a long time allowed the CNS to calm down and the protective spasm in the abdomen muscles could release. But what was even more significant was the way the patient stood up slowly using his hands to push himself up. This meant that he took the muscles passively through the critical position where a trauma had been expected to occur. By passing this point without incident, the CNS remained calm and because there was no actual soft tissue damage the apparent injury was completely resolved.

To reproduce this great outcome, Jones developed his Strain-Counterstrain technique based on the theory of a Positional Release, which certainly explains how it can be so effective with this particular type of injury. In this and similar situations like whiplash, no other soft tissue technique will have much effect and it is the only thing that works well.

But this same method can have the same releasing effect on any area of excessive muscle tension, whatever the cause. Positional Release Technique can be used more generally alongside other soft tissue techniques. It is particularly useful where muscles are tight or in spasm because they are still protecting a past injury. Providing any underlying factors that may have caused this tension in the first place have been resolved, the result should be permanent.

There is also a circulatory factor which can add to the technique's effectiveness. Muscles in spasm have restricted blood flow through them. By shortening and relaxing the tissues, the blood flow increases and helps restore a normal healthy circulation. The fascia also responds very well to Positional Release. (*See p. 235*)

The principles behind the application of PRT are quite simple, but it takes considerable skill in moving and handling the client to be able to perform it effectively.

Tender Points

Tender trigger points develop in hypertonic muscle, and the therapist has to palpate the tissues to find the most tender point within it. A firm and constant pressure must be applied to this point which should cause the client a moderate amount of pain. On a scale of 0 to 10, this should be between 4 and 5. The pressure needs to be maintained evenly throughout the technique, which can take up to 90 seconds. This tender point is used to monitor the technique so it is essential that the pressure remains constant throughout.

Finding the Position of 'Ease'

The therapist then uses the other hand to passively move the client into a position of 'ease', where the client feels a reduction in pain at the tender point, even though the pressure has not been reduced. This normally means shortening the muscle by moving a limb to articulate the joint. This position of ease has to be held still for up to 90 seconds, and the therapist needs to find a comfortable way to do this. When the position has been found, it may be necessary to put the client's limb down and move to another location around the couch to make this easier. It is also possible for the therapist to use their leg or shoulder to support the client; cushions can also be used in some situations. It is important that the client feels that they are well supported so they can relax fully, and the therapist should anticipate this and position themselves carefully.

The position of ease is found when the tissues soften and there is an 80 to 100 per cent reduction in pain felt at the tender point. The joint should be moved through one range to find the position of ease there. From this position, it can be moved in all other directions to try to find even greater ease. *(See photos 133, 134 and 135.)*

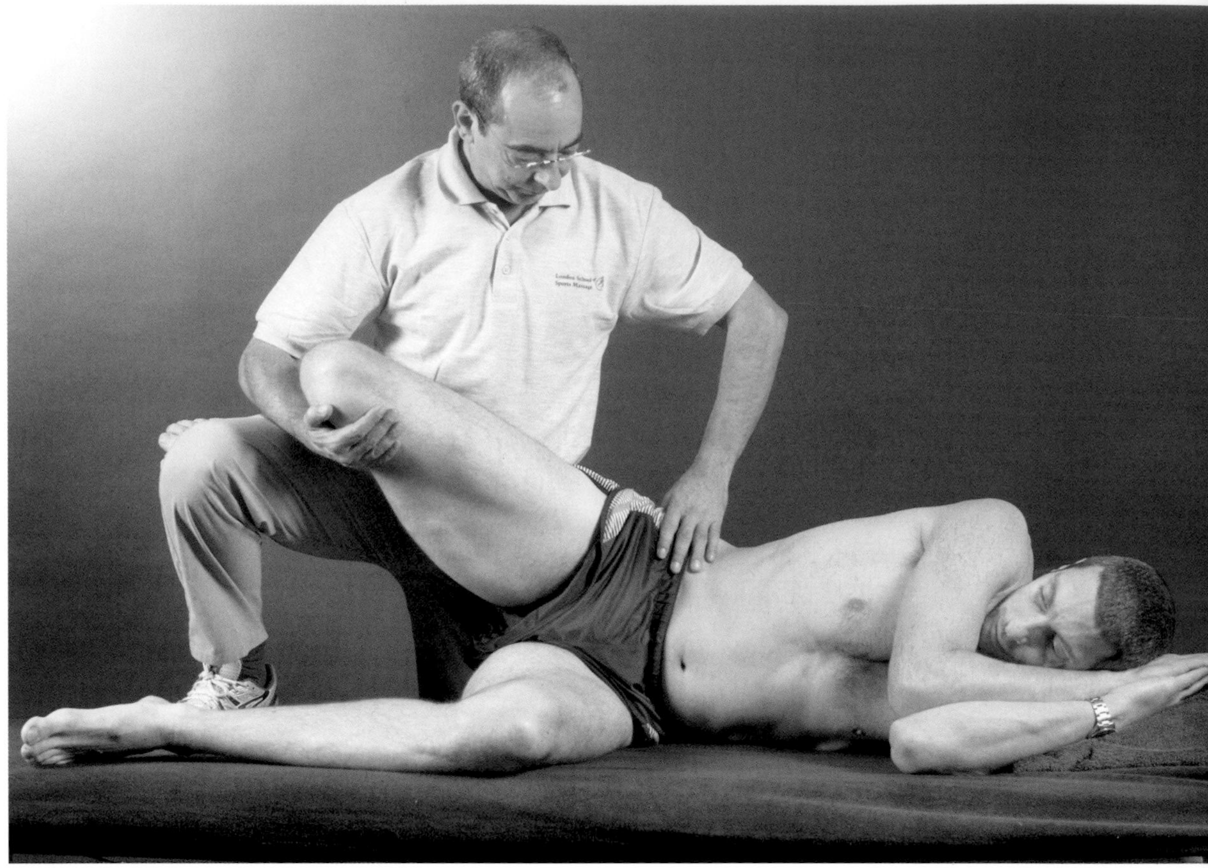

Photo 133. Using a monitoring pressure to a tender point in the hip, the joint is passively moved through abduction, flexion and extension, as well as rotation, to find the greatest 'ease'. The therapist is using his leg to support the weight of the client's leg in this position.

Examples

- **The posterior hip area:** With the client lying prone, the therapist palpates the tender point and then lifts the leg to shorten all the posterior hip muscles and find an initial position of ease. The therapist may then be able to support the weight of the client's leg on their thigh, or a firm cushion, so they can focus their attention better on what they feel at the tender point as they 'fine-tune' the position. From here, the leg can be moved sideways through abduction and adduction to find a position of greater ease, and then through internal and external rotation. Finally the therapist can push the whole leg in towards the torso to further shorten and relax the muscles.
- **The back:** The client should be sitting on a stool or the side of the couch with their arms crossing in front to hold the opposite shoulders. The therapist palpates a tender point in the back with one hand and uses their other arm and torso to move the client. Taking them passively through all the ranges of movement and holding them still in the position of ease can be physically demanding on the therapist, and this may not be possible with very large clients.

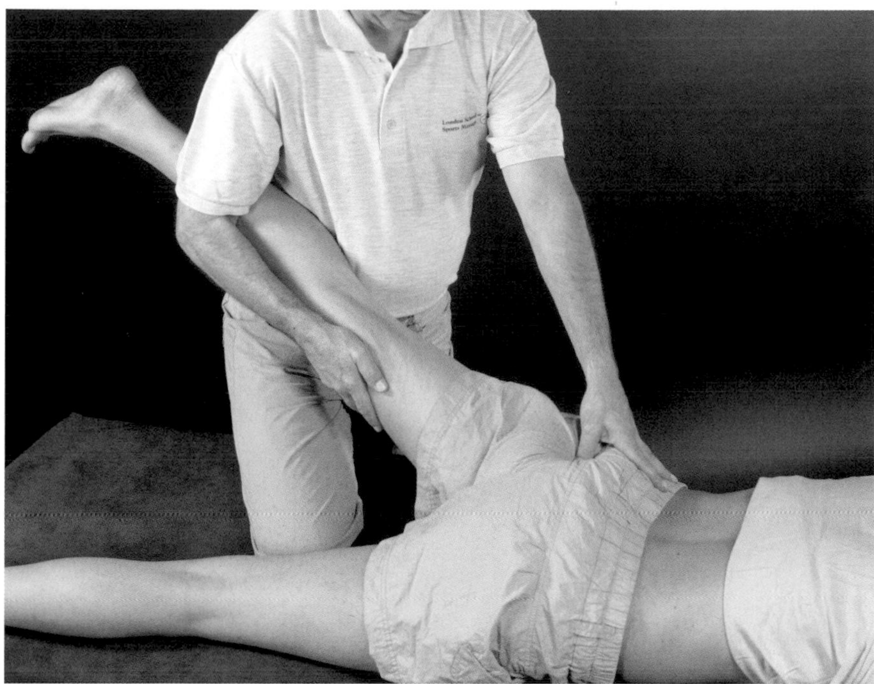

Photo 134. Using a monitoring pressure in the gluteus medius, the hip is moved through extension, abduction and adduction, and rotation, and the whole leg can be pushed in towards the torso to find the greatest 'ease'. The therapist is supporting the weight of the leg on his hip.

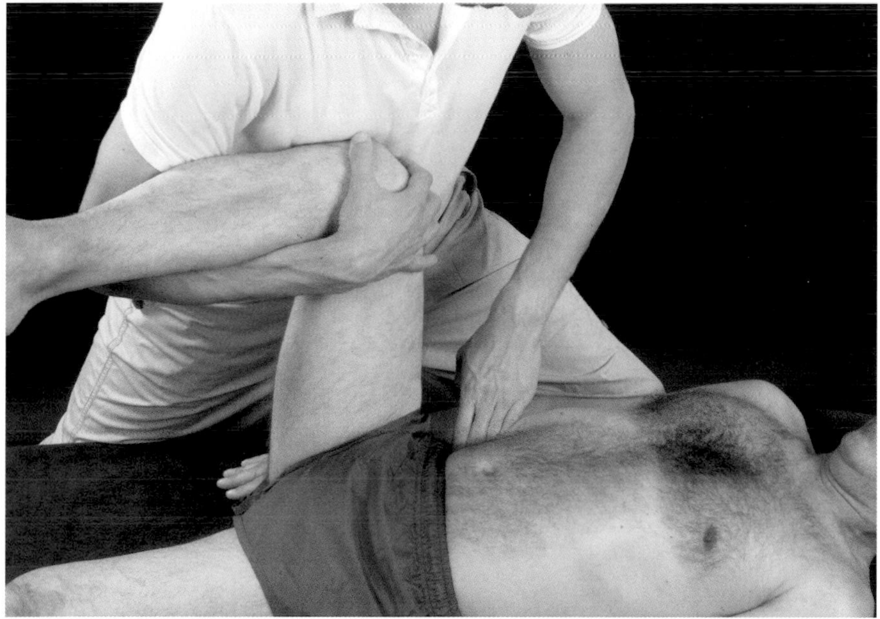

Photo 135. Palpating a tender point in the psoas, the hip is taken through flexion, abduction and adduction, and rotation, to find the greatest position of 'ease'.

Client Feedback

It is essential that the client says when they feel a reduction in pain at the tender point and the position of ease has been found. Relaxation is most important and the client should be encouraged to let go of any tension and breathe deeply. The pain at the tender point should keep reducing until it becomes pain free, and they should eventually feel nothing more than the skin contact from the palpating finger.

With experience, a therapist can feel the tissues release at the tender point and can work intuitively to move the client in all directions to achieve the greatest position of ease without the client telling them anything. But the client's feedback is still important because their focused attention and relaxation helps the technique work better.

After about 90 seconds the tender point should become completely pain free, the client should then be returned very slowly and passively to a neutral position back on the couch. It is essential that the client remains completely relaxed when doing this and they must be encouraged not to assist in any way.

Crowding

The word 'crowding' seems to best describe two very simple variations based on the PRT principle.

Where a small tender point is found, it can be possible to use the other hand to squeeze all the surrounding soft tissues into that point to crowd it in. This can create a very local position of ease in the tissues which can be held for a time and then slowly released to perform the technique.

Larger areas of tight muscle can be treated in a similar way, especially if other techniques do not seem to be working. Without using a tender point as a monitor, the therapist can use both hands placed along the muscle on either side of the tight area. Pressing firmly into the soft muscle, the two ends can be squeezed together and crowd the fibres in towards the area of the tension, and after 90 seconds this can slowly be released. (If lubricant is already on the client's skin it may be necessary to do this through a towel to get a proper grip.)

PRT Combined with Other Techniques

Putting tissues into the release position opens up many possibilities when combined with other techniques. In combination, several techniques together can produce incredible results in just a few minutes.

- **NMT:** Although PRT uses the tender point as a monitor, it is usually also a trigger point which will respond to neuromuscular techniques. So instead of keeping a constant monitoring pressure, a deeper neuromuscular pressure can be applied to combine the two effects.
- **STR:** When releasing the position at the end of PRT, the muscle is already shortened and the therapist is pressing into an area of tension, and this is the perfect starting position for STR. The pressure at the tender point can change into a lock, and the tissues can be stretched away from this when the client is moved back to a neutral position.
- **MET:** At the end of the PRT, the muscle can be taken further to the MET Barrier position. From here, reciprocal inhibition can be used to further lengthen a tight muscle.
- **Fascial release:** See p. 235.

11 Myofascial techniques

Although the fascial system was largely ignored by orthodox medicine, independent manual therapists began to see its importance and developed ways to treat it. Dr Ida Rolf was the first to popularise this, when she found that the application of very considerable force along the fascial layers appeared to result in a change in their density and tension. She believed that the tissues changed from a more dense 'gel' state into a softer and more fluid 'sol' state, and later research on animal fascia proved that these changes do take place.

The strong myofascial strokes move along the layers and break the adhesive bonds that can form between them and restrict their function. As well as this direct mechanical effect, the fascia is also rich in mechanoreceptors which are stimulated by these strong techniques. This has a neurofascial effect which releases tension and also improves the local fluid dynamics with improved hydration.

Myofascial Therapies

The significance of the myofascial system on posture and function is very significant, and therapists need to be able to treat it. The system envelops the whole body as one single unit and any restriction in one part of it can have an effect on the whole system. Pain and dysfunction that appears in one area of the body may be caused by a fascial restriction some way distant from it. Ideally, it is the entire system that needs to be treated to help realign the whole body.

But the fascial network is very complex and it takes in-depth study to fully understand its structure and how to treat all of its parts. Because of this, myofascial therapy has become a treatment modality in itself and is seen as a speciality within physical therapy. This started with *Rolfing*® and since then several other updated variations have evolved. The training courses in these therapies are a great development, and experienced massage therapists should consider further advanced training in this fascinating subject.

It takes a considerable time to train specifically as a myofascial therapist, and it also takes a long time to physically treat the whole system. It is far too extensive to cover it all in a single treatment and it can take up to ten sessions to treat all the fascial bands, with individual sessions often taking more than an hour to complete. This makes it a very expensive form of therapy and, as good as it unquestionably is, unfortunately not too many clients are prepared to make that commitment.

Although it is far better to treat the entire system, it is still possible to get some dramatic results by releasing fascial tension in just the key areas and this can be done within a treatment along with other soft tissue techniques. But it does require very good palpation skills to be able to feel and treat the fascia, and therapists need to develop these skills first through massage before progressing to this more advanced level of work.

The Superficial Fascia

This fascial layer beneath the skin covers the entire body as a single structure and is very influential in the function and dysfunction of movement. Where this fascia has been repetitively held in a shortened position through postural or occupational factors, it gradually becomes set in this tight and restricted position. This needs to be released if any real improvements are going to be made.

When carrying out a postural assessment,

therapists should consider how the fascia could be creating the observed imbalances. If the body is bending to the right, the fascia is very likely to be short and tight along that right side. If the shoulders are protracted forward, the fascia across the front of the chest will be short and restricted. It is necessary to visualise a fascial body stocking and see where the twists and distortion appear to be.

The superficial fascia can be assessed manually by gliding the skin to see how well it moves with the fascial layers below. Because it binds very strongly with the skin on one side and the deep fascia on the other, it will not allow the skin to glide very far if it is restricted.

The therapist applies only a fairly light pressure through a flat hand or pads of the fingers on the client's skin and, without sliding, moves it as far as it will glide in all directions. To ensure a good grip it may be necessary to do this through a towel if a lubricant has already been used. The underlying tissues should allow the skin to glide quite freely with soft elastic feel at the end of its range. This is commonly referred to as the direction or position of 'ease'. But it is often found to do this in only some directions; in others it glides less freely for a shorter distance and comes to a more sharp and sudden stop. This is referred to as the direction or position of 'bind'.

In the upper back, for example, clients who constantly hold their head in a very forward position will usually find the fascia will glide freely (ease) up towards the head but be severely restricted (bind) when being drawn down the back. This is because of the way the fascia adapts to functional misuse from this postural situation.

All massage strokes work through the superficial fascia as they treat the underlying muscles, and this does help improve its hydration and general mobility. But more specific techniques need to be applied to this layer to stretch and release areas that are excessively short and tight. *(See photos 136–148.)*

Short strokes

The same method used to identify a tense area of superficial fascia can be developed into a way of stretching it too. Having moved the skin to the position of 'bind', a short strong stroke can then be applied to force through the restriction. Forcing the layers along in this way breaks the restricting bonds that form between them and this can cause quite considerable pain. But it is very effective and should only be done once and not be repeated on the same tissues in the same session. Doing it more times can over-treat the tissues and cause residual pain for several days afterwards. The fascial release can be instant and long-term providing any other causative factors are dealt with also.

This technique requires considerable skill because it is essential that the therapist does not press any deeper into the tissues but only pushes along it at the same depth. And this needs to be done with considerable force but without sliding on the skin (or burning it with friction from a towel). The client should feel no pain during the initial glide to the point of 'bind' and only the forced stroke beyond this will be painful and the skin will usually redden afterwards because it stimulates the local circulation.

Large areas can be treated this way using the palm of the hand. This is sometimes done best by gliding back and forth a few times to feel where the point of 'bind' is. Then from the position of 'ease' apply a much faster and stronger stroke to break through that 'bind'. Clients should be warned to expect a sudden sharp pain at the end which is a positive sign that it is working effectively. When attempting this

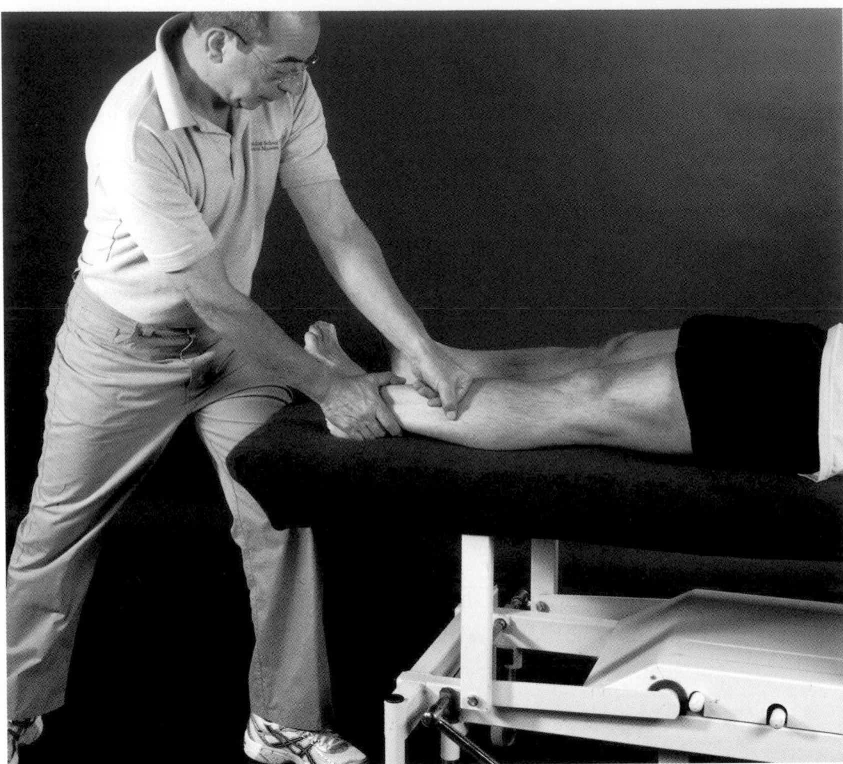

Photo 136. Myofascial stroke with the fist along the surface of the tibialis anterior.

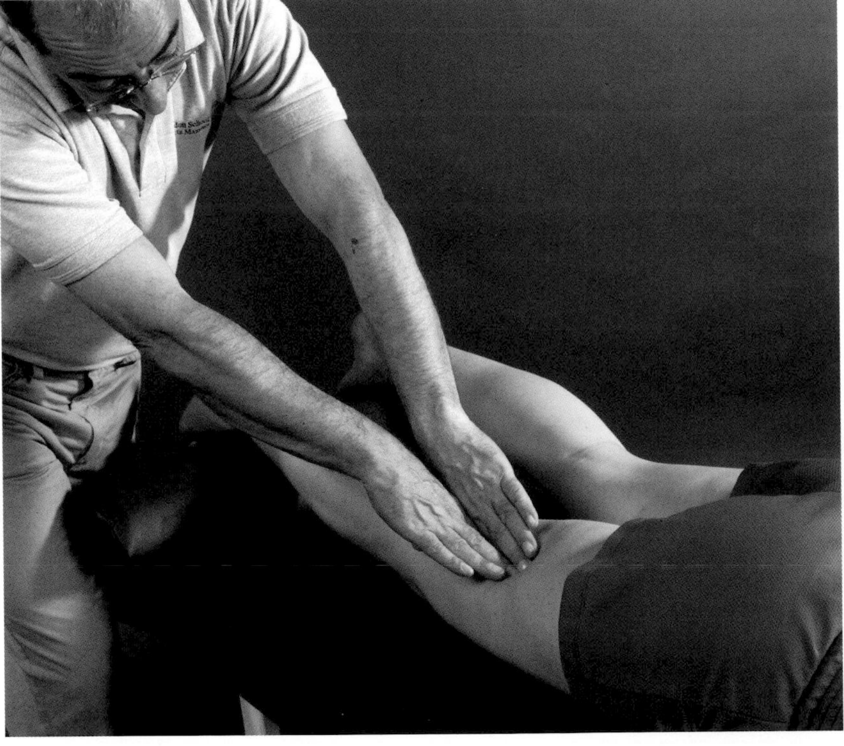

Photo 137. Deep fascial strokes between the hamstrings to release and separate them.

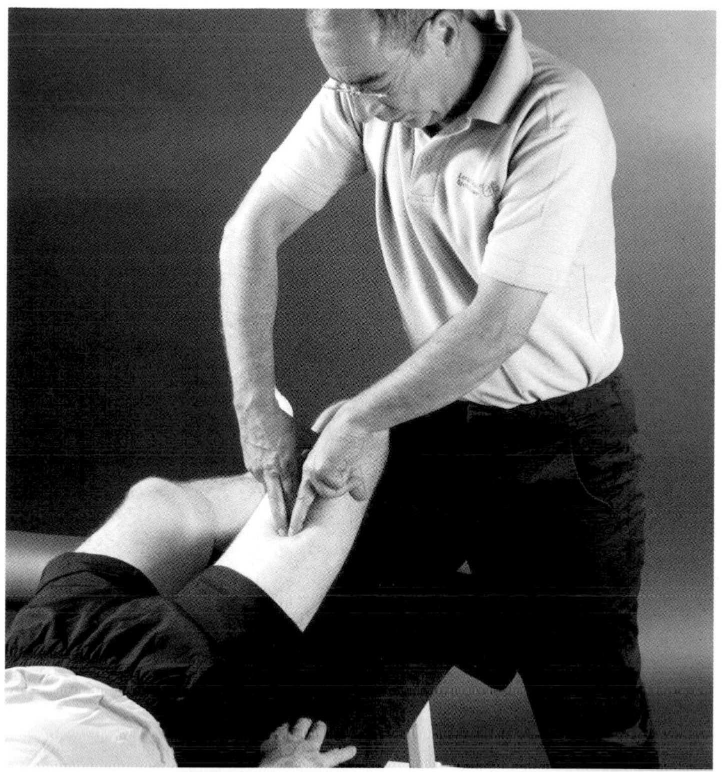

Photo 138. Deep fascial strokes between the adductor muscles to release and separate them.

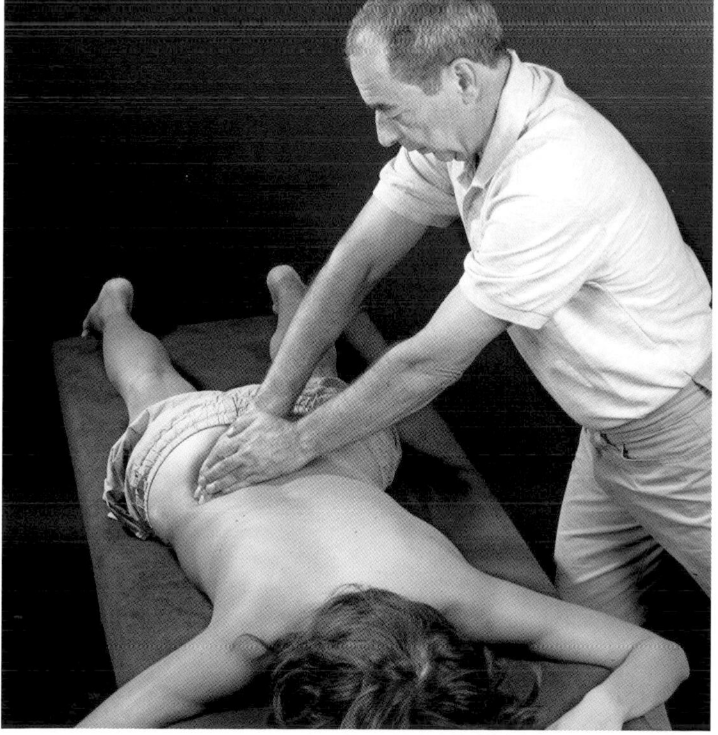

Photo 139. Fascial strokes along the iliac crest.

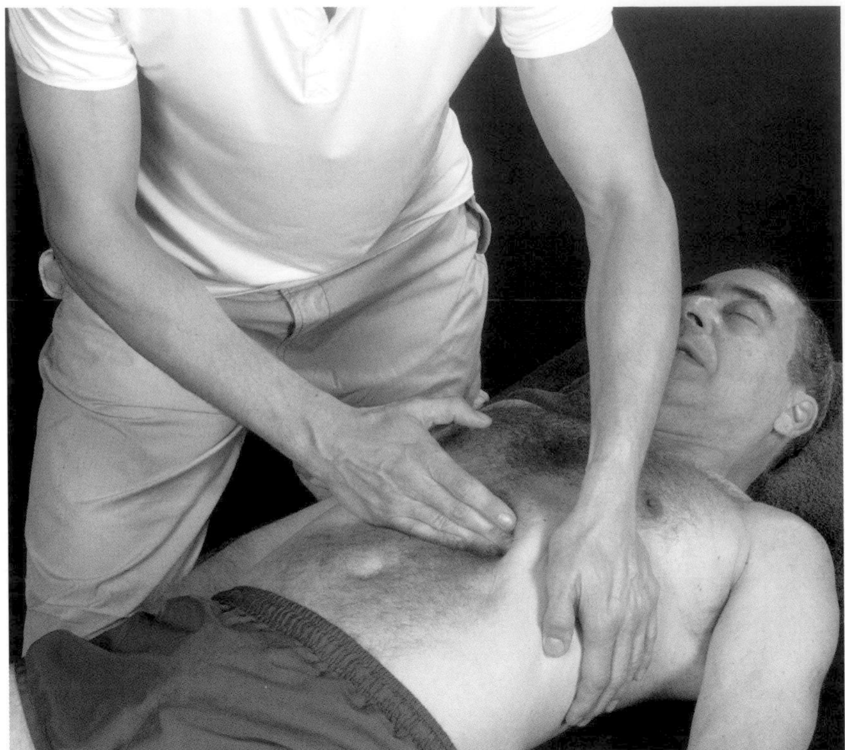

Photo 140. Fascial strokes along the costal border.

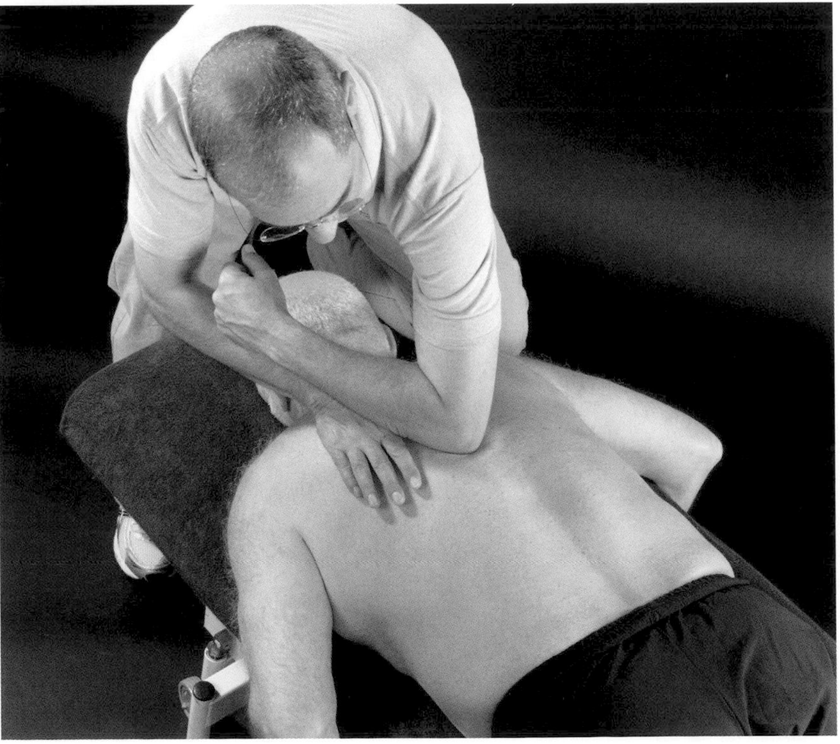

Photo 141. Deep fascial strokes with the elbow along the erector spinae muscles.

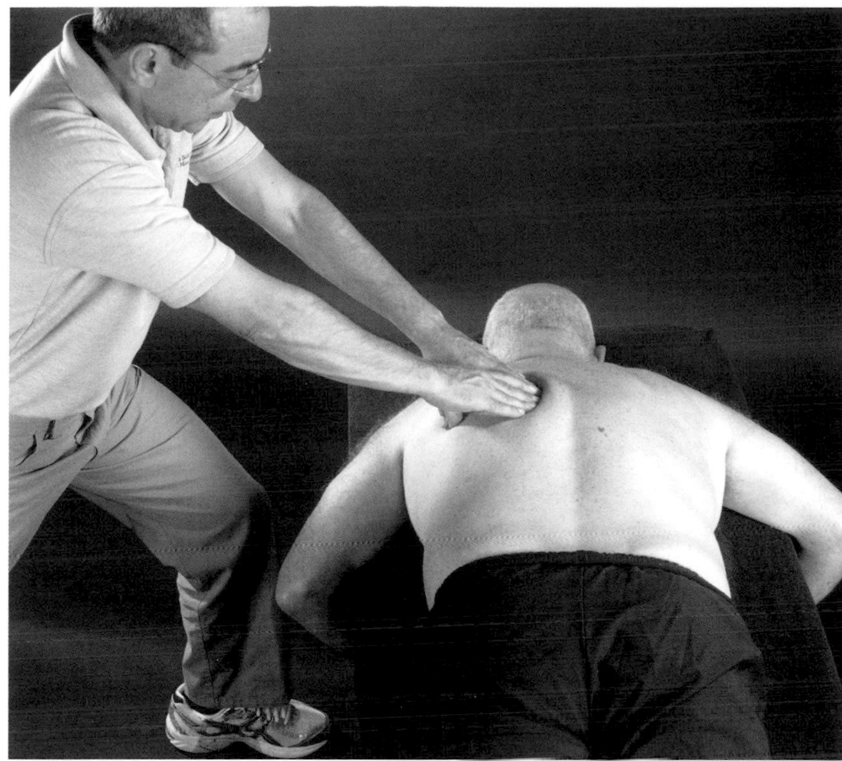

Photo 142. Deep transverse fascial strokes to the lateral border of the erector spinae muscles.

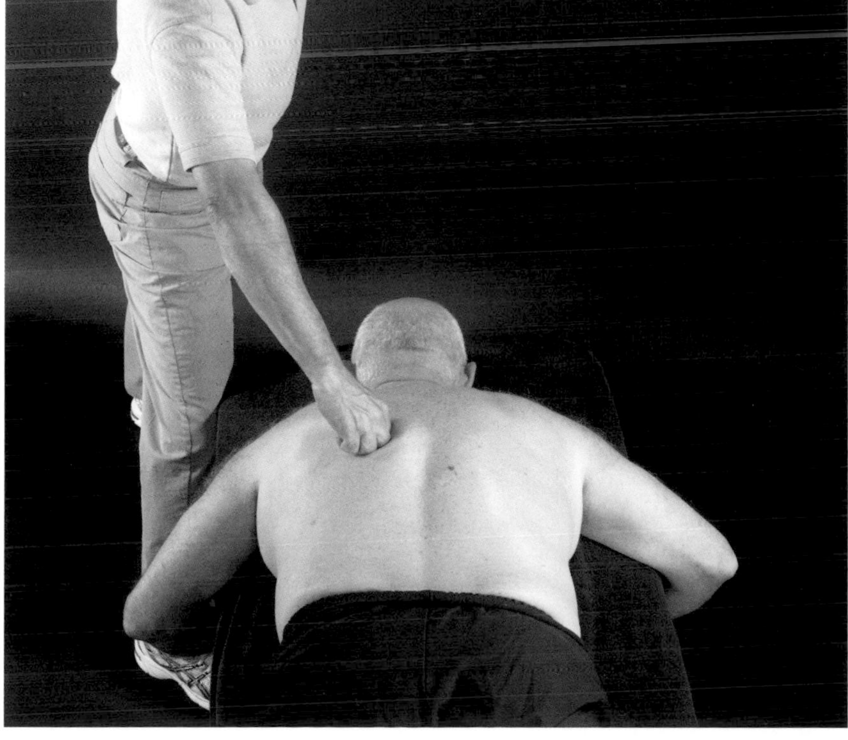

Photo 143. Longitudinal fascial strokes applied with the knuckles down the lateral border of the erector spinae muscles.

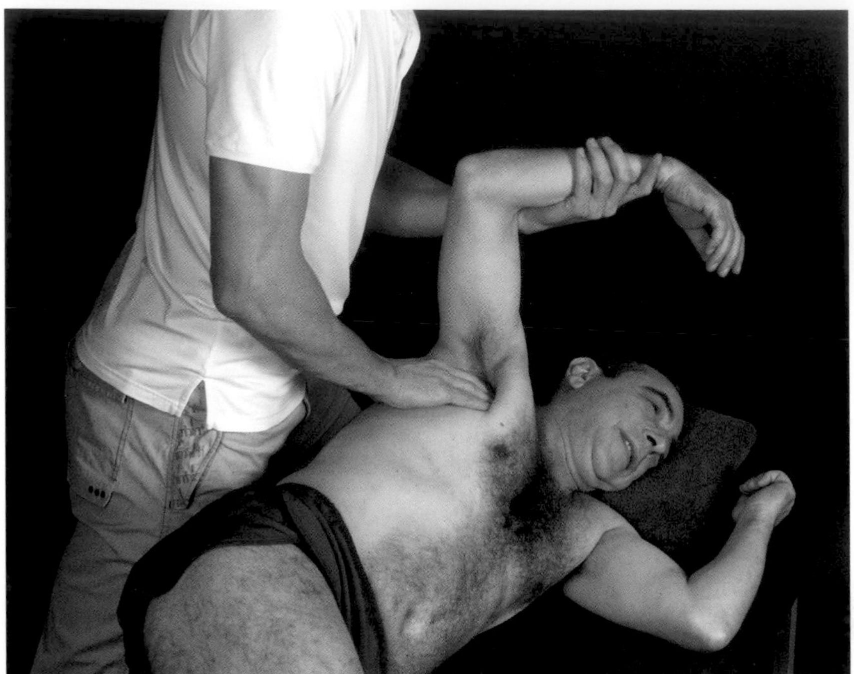

Photo 144. Deep fascial strokes applied to the pectoralis minor.

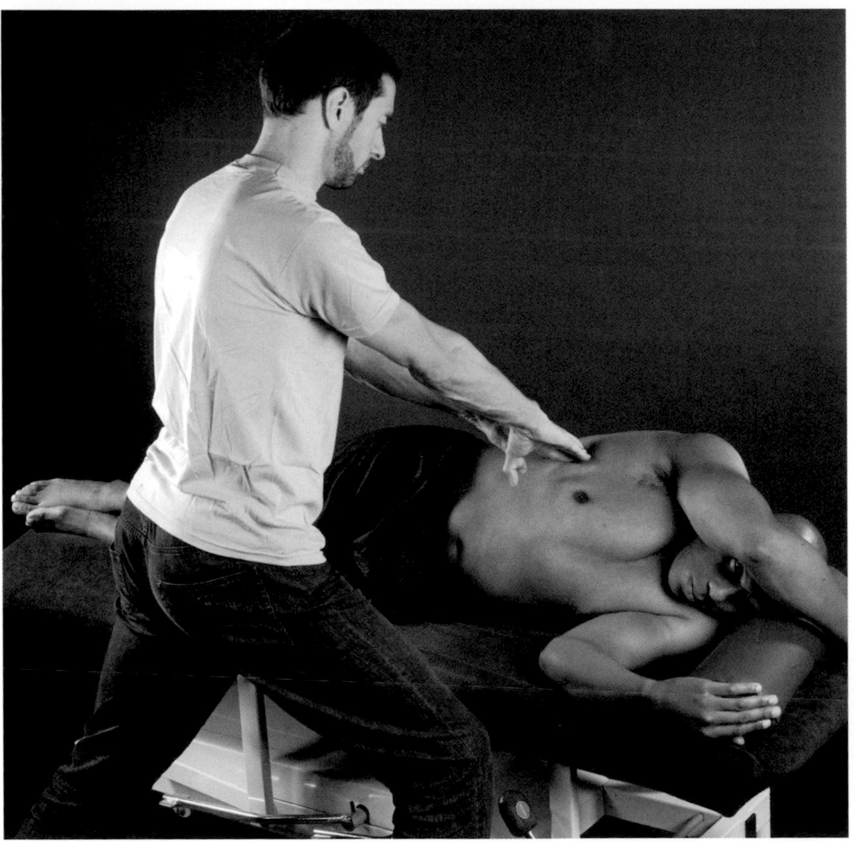

Photo 145. Fascial stroke along the serratus anterior.

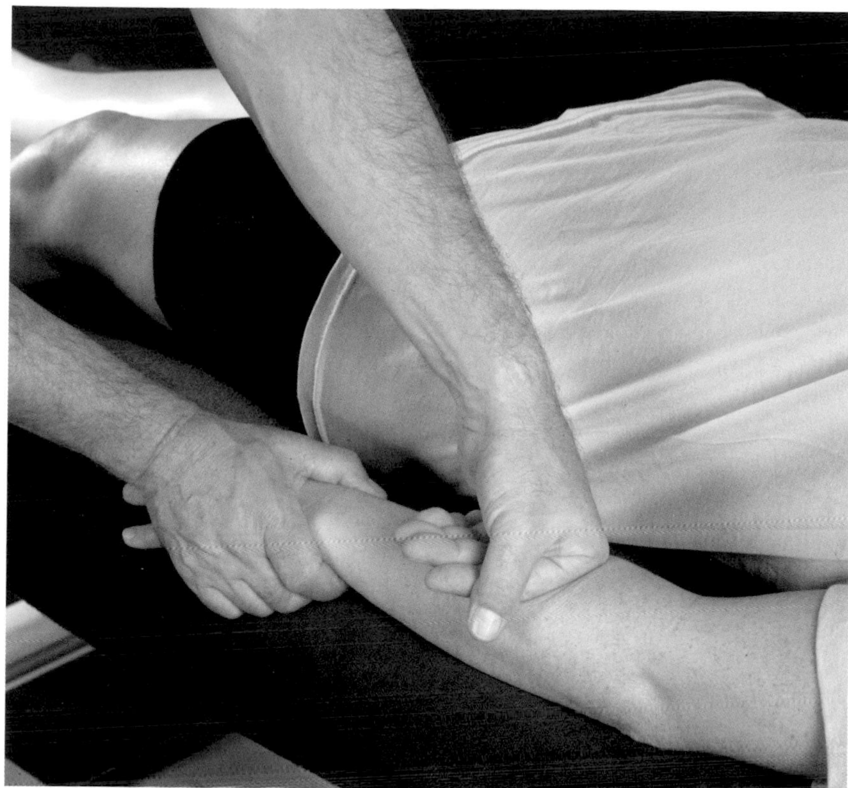

Photo 146. Fascial strokes along the forearm muscles.

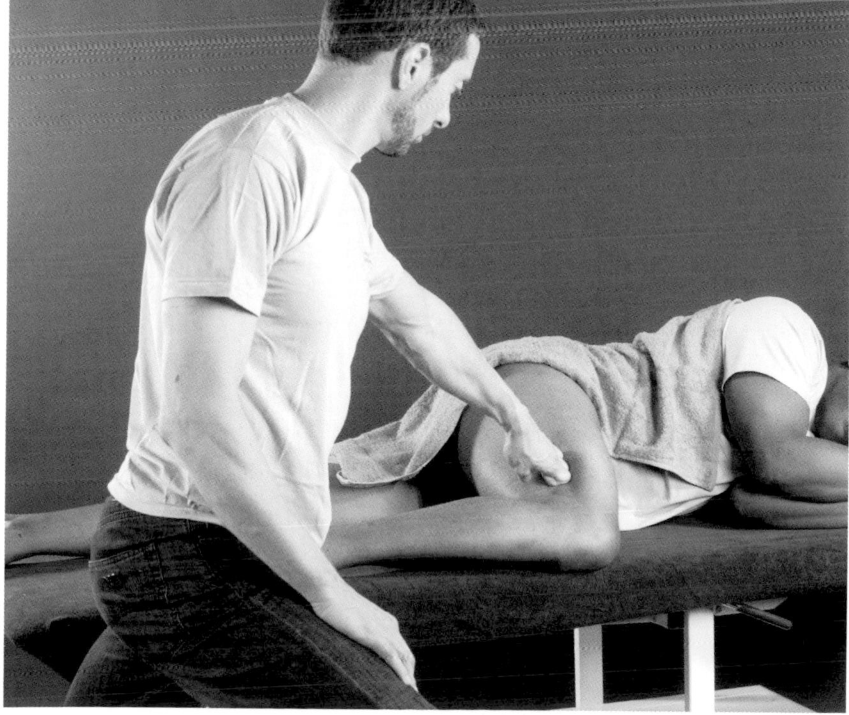

Photo 147. Longitudinal fascial strokes along the posterior border of the iliotibial band.

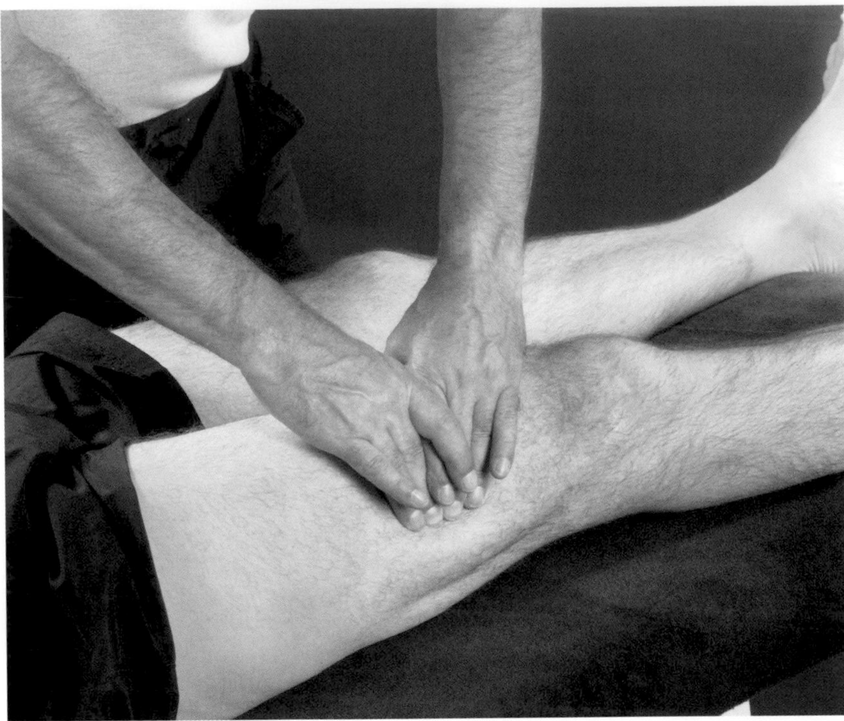

Photo 148. Transverse fascial strokes to the anterior border of the iliotibial band.

technique on healthy mobile fascia, it should cause no pain.

Short strokes can be applied more specifically to smaller areas using fingers or a thumb. As the pressure is more focused, the grip is usually better and the therapist can push through the 'bind' wherever it is found without gliding back and forth first.

Long strokes

The short stroke can be developed into a long stroke by using a very small amount of lubricant. At the end of the short forced stroke, instead of releasing pressure the therapist maintains the stretch on the fascia and keeps pushing along it by allowing the surface of the skin to slowly slide beneath them. These long strokes can be applied over quite long distances with the therapist feeling and following the direction of 'bind'.

This can also be done with the fingers, lifting up and gripping a small area of skin and gliding it to the position of 'bind'. A short stroke is then applied to get an initial stretch on the fascia and turned into a long stroke by using the fingers to walk along the body gathering up the skin ahead.

Sustained stretch

Another way of releasing areas of superficial fascia is by simply maintaining a stretch on it for a sustained period of time. This is done using both hands gliding the skin in opposite directions to reach the position of 'bind'.

Instead of applying a forced stroke, a milder pressure is used to gently stretch the fascia apart. This is held for up to 90 seconds during which time it can be felt to spontaneously release as the therapist's hands slowly drift away from each other.

Using these techniques, the therapist can work quite intuitively all over the body, feeling the glide of the fascia in all directions and treating the areas of 'bind' wherever they occur. As well as using this on soft muscle areas, it is particularly beneficial over more bony areas which are commonly ignored by other soft tissue techniques.

Fascial release strokes across the ribcage and costal cartilage can aid respiration as well as improve posture. The sacroiliac and thoracolumbar areas are also an important area for these techniques. Even the scalp can be treated in this way and can have quite far reaching effects.

Using 'Ease' rather than 'Bind' (Positional Release Technique)

The superficial fascia responds extremely well to a Positional Release Technique, even though it seems to work the opposite way. Normal fascial techniques force through the 'bind' and are painful, but Positional Release uses the position of 'ease' and is pain free, and it can be just as effective.

If the tissues 'bind' in an anterior direction, they should be drawn into the opposite way to a position of 'ease' and held there. From here, the tissues should be glided in medial and lateral directions and held in whichever one achieves the greatest 'ease'. Then the tissues can be rotated in clockwise and anticlockwise directions and held at the position of ease there. This maximum position of ease should then be held for 90 seconds before releasing it. Reassessing the position of 'bind' then often shows a remarkable improvement.

The Deep Fascia

Postural imbalances and dysfunction lead to what we commonly refer to as soft tissue or muscle tension. This is largely caused by fibrous bonds forming between the fascia layers that surround the muscles (perimysium), which restricts their ability to slide freely alongside each other. It also reduces the elasticity of the muscle and impairs its function. The fascia can also become tight and restricted as it extends through the tendon into its attachment and joint ligaments.

To release tension in these deep fascial structures requires good palpation skills, combined with a very detailed knowledge of the musculoskeletal system. The therapist needs to identify each muscle, tendon, ligament and bone separately and work in between them and adjacent structures as well as along their surfaces and borders.

Short strokes

These are applied transversely to the direction of the fibres. The therapist first has to feel the border of the muscle, tendon or ligament and use strong pressure and grip to lock onto its fascial border. The tissues are then pushed transversely to stretch them away from adjacent muscles or bones. Where the fascia is in good condition, it will glide with 'ease' and the client will feel no discomfort at all. But where it is restricted, it will 'bind' and a short strong stroke should then be applied to release it. This will cause considerable pain to the client and is also very hard work on the therapist's fingers. These short strokes should be repeated transversely along all the borders of each individual structure. But, if done well, they should not be repeated more than once on those tissues in a single session.

Long strokes

Starting at one end of the muscle, tendon or bone, the therapist locks onto the fascia along its border and glides it longitudinally to the point of 'bind'. A short strong stroke is applied to force a stretch, and then this is extended into a long stroke following the border as far as possible.

As with all the myofascial techniques, where it is in good condition there is a feeling of 'ease' and the stroke glides along quite freely and painlessly. But where it reaches an area of 'bind' the stroke will slow down considerably, require more force and will cause the client some pain.

These deep long strokes can be very stressful on the therapist's fingers and so many develop the use of their knuckles or elbows to do this instead. These enable even more powerful work to be done on deeper tissues and are particularly effective along bone attachment points like the iliac crest.

Using both long and short strokes, each separate structure can be treated with the therapist focusing on releasing the fascia between each of them. It is important to visualise the anatomy in its three dimensions. As well as working between muscles, it is equally necessary to work underneath them wherever possible to release the underlying structures. As well as working through the area where the client may be suffering painful symptoms these techniques should be continued further, following the fascial network into the adjacent parts of the body.

Myofascial techniques can be combined with functional movements to even greater effect. During both longitudinal and transverse strokes, the client can make functional movements which stretch the area being treated. This helps release the fascia in a direction that best accommodates their movement.

Iliotibial Band (ITB)

One part of the fascial network that requires special consideration is the iliotibial band, which runs down the outside of the hip and thigh. It is unique in the way that the gluteus maximus and tensor fascia lata muscles attach directly into it, and in effect it acts like their tendon. It can become the cause of lateral knee pain and is commonly referred to as being 'tight' in this situation. But that term is misleading because it suggests that it needs to be stretched and made more elastic to solve the problem. The ITB is actually made up of inelastic collagen fibres and is not meant to be elastic.

Certainly if the muscles are tight they will transfer tension into the ITB, so it is important to treat these muscles in connection with any ITB-related knee pain. But rather than think of it as being tight like a muscle, it should be seen as being restricted with the fascial layer and needs releasing that way.

A tight ITB does feel like a separate structure, but it is really just part of a continual sheet of fascia that wraps all the way round the thigh. The collagen fibres stand out clearly from the much more elastic fascia on either side of it, so by gliding transversely through the elastic fascia towards the ITB it can be quite easy to feel its lateral borders.

Rather than press the ITB hard onto the bone, it should be pushed transversely to stretch it within the fascial layer. Short transverse strokes should be repeated all the way along both its anterior and posterior borders. Then long strokes should be applied along these borders from the knee up towards the hip. It requires a lot of force to do this and skill to keep pushing along the fascial layer rather than deeper in towards the bone.

12 Rehabilitation [illegible] and Advice

Rehabilitation of Post-acute Soft Tissue Injuries

The rehabilitation of serious acute injuries should be supervised by an orthopaedic specialist, but people with minor strains and sprains often seek treatment in the private sector, where help can be more readily available.

Rehabilitation should not begin until all signs of inflammation (heat, redness and swelling) have gone from the affected area. Providing it is only a minor soft tissue injury and correct acute procedures have been applied *(see Appendix 2, p. 265)*, this should only take about 48 hours. In practice, however, it often takes longer because clients may not be able to rest the area enough due to lifestyle commitments.

Rest is still very important in the early recovery stage, and remedial exercises must be done gently and carefully. Good treatment and exercise can reduce painful symptoms quickly, but this can fool the client into not resting the area enough. Without sufficient rest, it does not matter how much treatment and remedial exercise is done – the condition may not recover properly.

Ice can still be applied during the early stages of rehabilitation, especially after doing any exercise. This is partly as a precaution in case any fibres have been re-damaged but also for its analgesic effect, which can prevent local muscle spasm.

Compression strapping should still be used in the early stages of rehabilitation, but the client should gradually use it less and less, starting by taking it off when they are at home or sitting at work and only using it when moving about, then using it only when doing any exercise which may overload the area. This also acts as a good reminder still to be careful and not to try to use it fully yet.

Using a support for too long can cause problems. If an area is being artificially supported, the neuromuscular system that should be giving the support becomes less efficient through lack of use. So when the injury has recovered, the client should not keep using it as a precaution unless there is a more serious structural instability that needs protecting.

There can be no set timescale to a client's progress through a rehabilitation programme, because there are just too many variables involved. The simple rule is to progress in small stages and to have a short recovery period after each step up to make sure it is safe to continue at that level.

Muscle and Tendon Strains

In the immediate post-acute phase, the damaged fibres are only just starting to repair and can easily be re-torn. But the longer the area is allowed to remain inactive, the weaker the muscle becomes and fibrous tissue starts to bind up in the area. There is a very thin line between just enough and too much, and there is never an easy answer to this. If the client is not in a desperate hurry, therapists can be more cautious; but with athletes and people who need to recover quickly to get back to work, we have to go much closer to that line.

Active Movements

Initially, the client should just perform concentric contractions with the muscle(s) which oppose the injured muscle/tendon (in the case of a calf/Achilles strain, this would mean dorsiflexing the ankle joint), and stop if they feel anything more than a very mild stretch. This is the safest way to start to gently stretch the damaged area, at the same time releasing tension in it through a reciprocal inhibition. Because the client is doing this actively, if they start to go too far and risk damage, their own neuromuscular system should instantly stop them.

Providing the client is able to do this well, they can then begin to gently contract and shorten the injured muscle as well, within the pain-free range. This should be done slowly and smoothly to maintain and improve the neuromuscular control of the area.

As the injury recovers and strengthens, eccentric contractions can be introduced. These are often more difficult for the client to do smoothly and slowly as they require more subtle neural control. But they need to be practised because eccentric contraction is essential in many normal functional movements.

Passive Movements

These are performed by the therapist moving the client's joint(s) to shorten and lengthen the injured muscle/tendon. This moves the tissue layers and prevents fibrous adhesions forming between them. But this must be done with care and within the pain-free range, otherwise the tissues could be re-torn.

Resisted Movements

As the condition improves, the client can perform movements which both contract to shorten and stretch to lengthen the injured muscle/tendon, with the therapist applying resistance (or equipment such as stretch bands) against this. It is important to encourage the client to go as far as they comfortably can because their neuromuscular system will naturally want to stop short as a natural defence, and this needs to be changed. A variable amount of resistance should be applied at different speeds, and the client needs to move smoothly to further improve the neural control. Taking this even further, they can move an adjacent joint in different directions at the same time.

These exercises are the best way to improve strength and control and are often all that a client needs to be able to start using the area normally. The muscles will then gradually strengthen, in good balance with other muscles, through normal regular use.

Joint Sprains

In the early stage of recovery (post-acute), it is too early to move the joint. Consequently, the lack of activity means the neuromuscular function and muscle strength deteriorates. To try to prevent this, the joint can be fixed in different pain-free positions and the client makes isometric contractions against a fixed resistance in all directions. This helps maintain muscle tone, even though there is no normal functional activity.

Functional Rehabilitation

Clients need to practise normal functional movement carefully before returning to full activity. If only basic muscle strength has been restored it may be enough to get back to normal activities, but poor functional control can lead to other musculoskeletal problems developing later.

Remedial Exercise and Advice

The advice given to clients to help them recover from injury and improve their physical well-being is perhaps the most important aspect of any treatment. Not only does it directly help in the healing process but also makes the client more involved in their recovery and they can use the exercises to monitor their own progress.

We cannot make the client follow advice, and this is often a problem. Treatment may take the pain away, but if they do not carry out some remedial exercise or change the way they misuse their body their condition is most likely to return. The client needs to understand that treatment alone is rarely a full remedy, and they should not think that it is the treatment that has failed if they don't follow the advice given.

If soft tissue treatment alone relieves their pain, they may be inclined to rely on this regularly rather than carry out exercises to try to remedy their problem permanently. This is commonly the case with people who have chronic postural and occupational stress conditions because changing these is difficult, while having regular pain-relieving treatment is easy.

If a client has an injury that causes constant discomfort that prevents them living their normal life, they will be strongly motivated to carry out remedial exercises and will make the time for them. Unfortunately, they often stop as soon as the pain goes away, so the condition never fully recovers and may easily return.

Compliance

To increase the chances of the client carrying out the advice, it must fit in with their lifestyle. Because this will be unique to every client, it is impossible to have a standard list of exercises for particular problems. Instead, therapists have to decide what is most appropriate for that individual.

Not all clients can find the time to exercise at home before and after work, but others can. Someone who is used to doing exercise will be more likely to follow a set programme, but others who don't may be better off with simple exercises that they can easily fit into their daily life. Clients with a sport or dance background may be able to take on quite complex exercises, but others will respond better if given a more practical activity to do which achieves the same thing.

Clients should only be given a few exercises at a time otherwise they may forget some of them or get confused by all of them. And it is always important to explain how and why the exercises will be beneficial, otherwise they are less likely to do them. If they can practise one or two simple exercises and see a real benefit from doing them, they may then be more willing and able to take on more complex exercises as they develop.

It is easy to overestimate a client's understanding of an exercise so it should be demonstrated clearly and practised first under the therapist's guidance. Placing a hand on the tissues that the exercise should be affecting helps the client understand where and how they should feel it working. Then, when they practise this on their own, they can reproduce the feeling rather than just copy the movement. When they come for their next treatment, they should demonstrate how they have been doing the exercise, because they will often not be doing it correctly any more and need to be shown again.

Stretching

Areas of chronic soft tissue tension need to be stretched regularly to continue the effects of their treatment. It takes a good knowledge of anatomy to devise the right stretches for the client, and there is a limitless variety of ways to do them. Therapists need to know a good range of stretching exercises and be able to work out new ones to meet the particular needs of the client when necessary. Therapists also need to practise these techniques themselves so they can demonstrate them well.

To be stretched well, muscles must be relaxed and non-weight-bearing, then passively lengthened to a point of resistance. There are many different views and theories about how strongly the tissues should be stretched and for how long this should be maintained. Therapists should become familiar with a number of stretching methods and decide which best suits the individual client.

If the tissues have been chronically short and tight for a long time, a strong stretch for a sustained period is usually best. This allows time for the fascia to release and for the neuromuscular system to adapt to the new lengthened position. But a muscle which is short and tight following a trauma should be stretched more gently for much shorter periods. Ballistic stretching which involves heavy bouncing actions can cause tissue damage and should normally be avoided. But if the client needs to be able to perform this type of action in their job or sport then they must carefully train the muscle to do this.

Occasionally a client stretches too much, and this can cause problems with over-lengthening and weakening. They may continue to do the stretch after an injury has recovered and, although this can be a good preventative measure, it is not always appropriate.

Clients can also be shown how to use Muscle Energy Techniques to enhance the effectiveness of the stretch.

Example: To stretch the upper trapezius and levator scapulae muscles when sitting at a desk, the client should first sit up straight with their chin in line with their forehead, which corrects the cervical spine alignment. They then turn the head about 45 degrees to one side and look down towards that hip. They stop at the position where they feel a mild stretch in the upper trapezius muscle (the Barrier position) over the other shoulder. Then, keeping their head and neck still, they should press this other shoulder down to stretch the muscles. This uses reciprocal inhibition, which stretches and also relaxes the muscles on a neural level.

Strengthening

Muscles that are held in a lengthened position, weakened through underuse or following a trauma, need to be strengthened. Although gym-type exercises can be easy to describe, they may not be practical for the client to do. Using a client's own body-weight and gravity, plus everyday objects, much can be achieved with a little initiative. Standing on one leg and doing slow squatting movements and forward lunges are good easy examples, which clients can do within their normal life.

With athletes and those who need to regain full strength quickly, it is often necessary to use strong resistance training to speed up their recovery and return to normal fitness. Although these can make muscles and tendons stronger, they do have limitations in terms of real function. There is a tendency to perform concentric contractions and only work through the mid-range of movement where a muscle has its greatest strength. This can make the muscle develop too short and so be more vulnerable to injury when trying to work in the lengthened position. Also, if a muscle has to perform eccentric contractions to control movement in normal activities, developing strength only through concentric contraction will not help. Ideally, the client should do resistance exercises through the full range in a way that most closely resembles normal movements or the specific action of their sport or job.

Too Much Strength Can Be a Bad Thing

Although weak muscles can lead to injury and need to be strengthened this does not mean that all muscles should be strengthened to prevent injury. Some people think they have to have very strong abdominal muscles, but in normal life these muscles have to work subtly at low levels to control posture and stability and do not require great strength. Too much strengthening can make them hypertonic, increasing visceral pressure which restricts the diaphragm and respiration.

Some women do strong pelvic floor exercises after childbirth to strengthen and restore its normal function. But the pelvic floor should naturally recover through normal use without extra strong exercising just as it has done for billions of women over many thousands of years. Some moderate exercise to help recovery is very important in the early stage but excessive strong exercises for too long can lead to hypertonicity. This can raise the pelvic floor, which compresses the bladder and can lead to incontinence issues. Women may then do even more strengthening exercise, thinking this will help improve their bladder control, but this could actually make it worse.

Proprioception Exercises for the Lower Limb

These build a client's confidence to start using their leg normally and stop poor postural habits developing.

For the ankle

The client should stand on one leg (preferably barefoot), with their arms hanging relaxed by their sides and with their eyes closed. To maintain balance in this position, the client's proprioceptive system has to make rapid instant adjustments at the ankle joint, and this is a simple and effective way of exercising this. The client may need to start with their eyes open using their arms to help their balance and should then gradually progress as they improve. The traditional 'wobble board' is usually too drastic for ankle rehabilitation in the early stage. Because the joint is very weak, the muscles have to hold it rigidly still and the client has to use the rest of their body to maintain balance instead, so it does little to improve proprioception in the ankle.

For the hip, knee and ankle together

The client stands upright on one leg with their arms hanging relaxed by their sides and tries to keep balance as they perform short, slow, smooth squatting movements.

For the knee

The client takes a step forward and then lunges forward to flex the knee, trying to maintain balance with the knee moving smoothly forward in a straight line over the foot. Then they have to push back through the knee to return to an upright position again. They can start with a small step and gradually increase this as they develop their strength and control.

Functional Movement Patterns

Through injury and postural imbalances, people often have a poor quality of movement in a particular area of their body, often without realising it. For example, instead of turning their head round fully, they may rotate their upper back more to assist it. Or instead of fully abducting their shoulder joint, they elevate their shoulder girdle to achieve the same task. They may be unaware of the rigidity in their lumbar spine because they are overusing their hips and upper back when bending forward.

To improve this situation, the client needs to become more animated in their movements in the area with each joint playing a full and balanced role. This can only be done through practice, and they need to regularly perform movements at each joint separately through its full range.

For example, a client with poor movement in their neck and shoulders should sit (facing a mirror if possible) with their hands palm-up on their lap. It is essential that they keep everything else still and relaxed as they slowly and smoothly raise and lower just their shoulder girdle on one side as far as they can. Then they should take it backwards and forwards, and circle it in both directions. They can then repeat the procedure moving just the neck only, taking it slowly through its ranges of movement with everything else remaining relaxed and still.

Although clients usually find this fairly easy to do quickly, when they try to do it slowly the poor quality of movement becomes more apparent. They often make jerky movements and can find some ranges almost impossible to do. To help them do it properly, it is important to stress that movements must be slow, smooth, to the fullest range and with nothing else moving.

Their neuromuscular system will naturally stop short of the end of their capable range, and the client needs to be encouraged to keep pushing this further to break through any restricting holding pattern. To help get them started, the therapist can use light finger pressure or gently tap them above, below, in front or behind the shoulder joint. This gives them something to press against and initiate the movement. Verbal encouragement to keep pushing until they can go no further also helps.

For the shoulder joint (glenohumeral), the client can bring one arm across the front of their body to hold down the shoulder girdle on the other side to prevent it moving. Then slowly and smoothly move the joint through all its ranges of movement, taking it to its fullest pain-free limits.

For poor mobility in the lower back, the client can perform 'cat and dog' type movements, arching the back up and down, but concentrating the movement in the lumbar spine to improve the mobility there. When sitting at work, they can also practise this by rocking their pelvis back and forth on their sitting bone (ischial tuberosity) to move just their lumbar spine whilst keeping the upper back still. The client can also do mild abdominal contractions to assist the lumbar flexion to get even more benefit from the exercise.

These are just some common examples, but wherever there is an area of dysfunction the same principles can be applied. Isolate the restriction and have the client practise good quality movements at that joint only and without assistance from any other areas.

Postural Improvement

Postural problems develop because of the way people use their bodies in their normal daily life. Setting aside time to do exercises to stretch the tight areas and strengthen the weak ones does very little to actually change this. Although formal exercises can help they are not the full answer.

There are some excellent disciplines – Pilates, the Feldenkrais method, the Alexander technique and others – which specifically aim to improve posture, and they can all be very effective. But some people seem to think quite wrongly that doing a Pilates class once a week is an easy 'pill' that will give them good posture, and they do not need to do anything about it the rest of the time. There is also the inherent problem that in any group situation one individual may not get exactly the help they need.

The best way to achieve postural improvement is through simple ideas and strategies that the client can easily and regularly incorporate into their normal daily life.

When standing and walking, they can imagine that there is a high fence in front of them and they have to peer over it to see where they are going. Keeping their eyes in a horizontal alignment, they should see how much higher they can go. To get this extra height they will find that they have to lower their tailbone and slightly contract their abdominal muscles as well as straighten their neck. The client should be made aware of these changes and get used to how this feels so they can keep repeating it as often as possible.

A similar method can be used when sitting at a desk in front of a computer. The client should remember to keep their chin in line with their forehead. To maintain this simple position, they have to straighten their neck and upper thorax. Although they may only remember to do this for a few moments at a time, it is much better than not doing it at all. If they keep it up, real improvements will result over time.

Trunk Stability

Modern lifestyles can lead to poor tone and function in the stability muscles of the abdominal wall and pelvic floor. Most people with sedentary jobs would benefit from doing some regular exercise to keep these key muscles in good efficient condition. There are formal training methods like Pilates and similar exercises done in gyms and studios which may be ideal, but many clients will not be able to fit this into their lifestyle. So the therapist should also recommend some very simple and basic exercises that the client can do at home.

Exercise

The client lies supine on the floor with a small cushion under their head for comfort, hips and knees flexed with the feet flat on the floor at a comfortable distance.

First the client has to learn how to engage their core muscles, and this can be very difficult to start with. They should breathe in first and then, as they breathe out, attempt to squeeze in their abdomen using only about 30 per cent of their strength. To help the client do this, the therapist can spread their fingers along either side of the abdomen and with light pressure gently draw the fingers towards the centre. This encourages them to squeeze, and the therapist can monitor how the muscles are contracting. It can also be helpful to put a hand under the small of the client's back and have them attempt to gently press against this at the same time.

Initially they should relax as they breathe in again, but once they are able to apply this mild abdominal contraction with some ease they should keep holding it as they take a few slow breaths in and out before relaxing.

Once they are able to engage these muscles well, they can progress with more specific exercises for the lower part of the abdomen. They should hold the contraction when they inhale and then when they exhale they lift just their tailbone (sacrum/coccyx) off the floor. This must be done with the abdominal muscles only and not by pushing through the legs and contracting the gluteal muscles. This position should be held as they inhale; they slowly lower their pelvis as they exhale again. They can then repeat this, lifting the tailbone and fifth lumbar vertebra, and gradually add each of the other vertebrae along the lumbar spine. Eventually, they should aim to be able to control their core whilst curling up and down through their pelvis and lumbar spine using only their abdominal muscles. This exercise must be done slowly without rushing and it can take several sessions before the client can do it well.

It is important to make sure the client does not use their gluteus maximus and hamstrings to assist the action, and the therapist and/or client can use their hands to feel the muscles and ensure they stay soft and relaxed. They should also keep their chest and upper body completely relaxed when doing these exercises. To monitor how well they are doing the exercise, the client should place one hand on their stomach to feel the activity in the muscles and the other on their chest to feel any movement there.

The same method can then be used to exercise the upper part of the abdomen. The client puts their hands behind their head with their elbows resting out to the sides. With the core muscles engaged first, they then raise their head by tucking their chin into the chest, and lower it again without using their arms to assist. This can gradually be increased to include the whole thoracic spine, but this must be done vertebra by vertebra in a curling movement. There should be no attempt to raise the lumbar spine in a 'sit-up' action because this will start to engage the psoas and hip flexor muscles. To focus these exercises more into the oblique muscles, the client can curl up in an angle towards one hip and then the other.

It is common to find that a client can contract part of the abdominal wall more strongly than the rest, or that one part appears weaker than the rest. To try to correct this, the therapist needs good palpation and verbal skills to get them to contract or relax just parts of the muscle group, but with time, patience and practice it can be achieved.

Respiration

Poor breathing patterns are frequently an underlying factor in injury situations, and this is not just a problem for those with respiratory conditions. People with high levels of stress and anxiety often develop shallow breathing patterns in their upper chest. A similar thing can also happen in people suffering with any chronic painful disorder. Hypertonic abdominal muscles which increase visceral pressures and restrict the diaphragm will also result in a poor upper-chest breathing pattern.

This can be observed when the client is relaxed in a supine position on the couch. In this situation, their diaphragm should be the only muscle actively involved in breathing, and the abdomen needs to distend outwards to give it the space to move down when they breathe in. So only the abdomen should be seen slowly and smoothly moving up and down whilst the chest remains completely still.

It is easy to see when the chest is moving and the abdomen is not, and the client needs to be made aware of this. As the diaphragm is controlled by the autonomic nervous system, it is very difficult to directly exercise it to improve its function. Instead, the client should focus their attention on the abdomen, pushing it out as they breathe in because this makes them effectively work their diaphragm. Pressing lightly on their abdomen to give them something to push against can be very helpful at the start. Placing the other hand on the upper chest and gently rocking it will also help them learn to keep this area as relaxed as it should be.

The client can then practise this themselves as a home exercise using one hand on the stomach and the other on their chest to monitor how well they do it.

Relaxation

Stress, anxiety or psycho-emotional issues can be an important factor behind some injury conditions. Massage can be a good way of relieving some of the physical symptoms of these stresses and many people find it very helpful. Some clients may benefit from advice on relaxation exercises or seeking other professional help in this area.

Sport

People should be encouraged and helped to live active healthy lifestyles, and the massage therapist may be the only 'authority' many people have on this subject. When people try to become more physically active, they are likely to suffer a few initial aches and pains at the start. This is a critical time because without the right help and support they are likely to give up at this point. People tend to start a new fitness regime with too much enthusiasm and this has to be controlled.

For example, a 40-year-old man may take up an aerobic activity like running, but if he is a little overweight with postural imbalances he may soon get an injury. As well as treating his injury, the therapist needs to give him sound advice so he can overcome these early difficulties, recommending, for example, that he go for brisk walks to start with and introduce running gradually as he gets fitter, or join a gym and do low-impact exercises to improve fitness more safely first, and to stretch and rest between days with exercise.

Although therapists may concentrate on the musculoskeletal system, it is important to remember that the single most important muscle in the body is the heart, and sedentary lifestyles do little to help keep this fit and healthy. Clients often want to know what the best aerobic exercise is to help them improve their cardiovascular fitness, and this must be the one they enjoy doing. But then it is also important that they have a good technique when they do it. Swimming for example is thought to be a very good exercise, but poor technique can cause injury, and postural imbalances can be no less a problem in the water than they are on dry land.

For people with sedentary occupations, any sport they do should be good for them because it will involve normal functional movements. In life, we run, walk, throw, jump, etc. Sport takes these normal daily activities and challenges people to see how far or fast they can go with them, or how skilled they can become. Top competitive athletes have the highest expectations and want to be as good as they possibly can be. But pushing themselves to the maximum makes injury almost inevitable. Most recreational competitors may still have high expectations but prefer to maintain a good standard for many years without risking injury by training for absolute maximum performance. For elite athletes, their sport is their most important goal in life, but for everyone else it is just part of their life and it has to fit in with other goals too. A very competitive amateur athlete may do 10 hours of hard training a week, but he could also spend 35 hours a week sitting behind a desk at work, and this cannot be ignored.

You can have too much of any good thing, so it is important that the client does not overtrain, and that they give themselves enough time to recover before doing more hard exercise. Because occupations do not always help good recovery, it can be more necessary to do regular exercises such as stretching to aid the process. Recreational athletes may also have poor technique and it is sometimes worth recommending some proper, sport-specific coaching to correct any basic problems.

Although sport resembles life by involving normal movement patterns, this is not what we always see in the Fitness Industry. At the modern gym, people often perform strong exercises on machines that do not match normal daily actions: when flexing the elbow to pick up an object, people do not normally sit on a chair and rest their elbow so only their arm muscles have to do the work. In normal life, their elbow flexion is just part of an action that involves muscles all over the body which have to adjust to the changes in force and balance. These machines may make a muscle 'strong', but the exercise requires no skill or control. In normal daily activities we rarely need maximum strength but we always need skill and control. They may be better than no exercise but they have great limitations, and clients should not rely on them alone to make them properly fit for life.

13

Remedial massage may be associated mostly with treating musculoskeletal conditions, but its uses and benefits can be applied to a much wider variety of other medical conditions, too.

It can often be used in a complementary role alongside other medical procedures to help alleviate the soft tissue symptoms associated with the condition. The effects of massage on blood circulation can help generally in the healing process, and its relaxing qualities can have great benefits too. As well as the physiological effects, the holistic way the therapist is able to treat and support their client can help them in many ways to overcome or cope better with their condition.

There is a vast number of medical conditions, and nobody can know them all. To be confident in applying the most appropriate treatment for a client with a known condition, therapists used to have to refer to large clinical medicine books, but modern information technology has now made this less necessary. Those books provide very good information about the conditions and the orthodox medical procedures used to treat them, but they rarely mention any complementary soft tissue therapy to support this.

Modern internet searches can now not only show details of the conditions but also sometimes give good accounts of how massage and soft tissue therapy can be used to help. All the same skills are used when treating clients with medical conditions; it is only the aims and objectives that are different. Muscles and joints may not be injured through physical activity, but they can suffer due to inactivity and the physical stresses brought on by the condition.

Therapists rarely have access to full medical records and have to rely on the information given to them by the client. This may not always be as accurate as it should be and can depend on their level of understanding more than the medical facts. If a therapist has any doubts about the true nature of a client's condition, they should not consider treating them until it has been clarified.

Many medical conditions include the suffix *-itis* in their name, which usually means inflammation and might suggest a contraindication. This is correct if there is any inflammation present at the time, but many medical conditions go through chronic or remission phases and soft tissue treatment can be used safely then.

If a client is currently undergoing medical treatment for a condition then the therapist should ideally have approval from their medical practitioner, but this is not always essential. Often the client has musculoskeletal symptoms which are secondary effects of their condition. In this situation soft tissue treatment is very unlikely to cause any negative effects, and it should be quite safe to proceed. The general health benefits of massage are such that it can help almost anyone with any condition in some way.

This section covers a few common conditions which affect some of the main systems of the body and is only a general guide to what can be done with other similar conditions.

Conditions Affecting the Digestive System

- **Irritable Bowel Syndrome** (IBS, or Spastic Colon) is a motility disorder often associated with anxiety, stress or depression. The condition is often long term and continually fluctuates between periods of inflammation and remission. When it is safe to treat – and providing the client is willing – deep abdominal massage can be of great benefit. It not only improves motility through the digestive tract but can also improve their levels of stress and anxiety. People with IBS often hold tension in the abdomen and are very protective of it. They have to be able to fully relax and trust the therapist to allow the treatment to be carried out, and this 'letting go' can have a profound effect on them.

- **Crohn's disease** is an inflammatory bowel condition which causes multiple lesions anywhere along the gastrointestinal tract. These cause scar tissue to build up and thicken the walls of the bowel and other tissues. Abdominal massage can be done during periods of remission when there is no current inflammation. As well as trying to improve digestive motility, it may be possible to release fibrous scar tissue and adhesions by carefully using friction and connective tissue techniques.
- **Constipation** is a common condition, and massage has been used to treat this for many centuries. Where a hard blockage is felt in the colon, gentle circular strokes can be applied to try to soften it. This must be followed by slow smooth strokes in a clockwise direction away from the blockage to aid its passage towards the bowel. It is important that strokes are not applied along the colon towards the blockage as this could compact it further and make the problem worse.

Abdominal massage should always be done with great care, especially when a medical condition exists there. Very deep techniques can be applied if done slowly and with sensitivity to avoid causing excessive pain or damaging the delicate tissues there.

Conditions Affecting the Visceral Organs

There are many medical conditions which affect visceral organs, and although manual therapy is rarely considered it can sometimes be very influential. The organs are all surrounded by fascia which performs several functions. It acts as a filter and barrier which controls the flow of fluids through the organ, and it also maintains its shape and holds it in position. This fascia is an integral part of the whole fascial network and can become tight and restricted through stress, anxiety and postural imbalance. The function of the organ will suffer if the fascia is restricted and manual therapy can be the only way to improve this.

Visceral manipulation techniques can be used to release fascial tension around the organs, but they require specialist advanced training. It takes the highest level of palpatory skill to safely treat these deep structures and should only be attempted by very experienced therapists with specific training.

Conditions Affecting the Respiratory System

- **Bronchitis:** Inflammation of bronchial passages.
- **Emphysema:** Enlargement of the airways, with damage to the alveoli in the lungs.
- **Asthma:** Chronic inflammation and narrowing of the airways.

Although these conditions are very different, they all involve laboured breathing and excessive coughing. This puts great stress on the respiratory muscles and surrounding fascia, which in the long term leads to adverse postural changes.

People suffering these conditions often have hunched-up and protracted shoulders with a hollow chest. This posture further reduces their lung capacity, which compounds the problem. With poor respiration, sufferers often have very sedentary lifestyles and find exercise difficult. This adds to their problems and often leads to other health issues, with hypertension being a common side effect.

Although massage may not be able to treat the conditions, it can address the associated musculoskeletal issues, and that can improve respiratory function and reduce symptomatic discomfort. All the respiratory muscles should

Respiratory Muscles

INHALATION	
Primary muscles	
Diaphragm	Drawn downwards to create a vacuum in the chest which sucks air into the lungs
External intercostals	Make the ribs draw outwards to create the space for the lungs to expand
Accessory muscles	
Scalenes	Raise the upper two ribs
Trapezius	Draws back the shoulders to open the chest
Rhomboids	
Levator scapulae	Raise the scapula with the upper ribs
Serratus posterior, superior and inferior	Raise upper ribs and pull down lower ribs
Pectoralis minor	Raises upper ribs
EXHALATION	
Primary muscles	
Diaphragm	Primary muscle only in relaxed breathing through natural recoil into its raised position
Internal intercostals	Draw the ribcage inwards
Accessory muscles	
Abdominal muscles	Most important muscle in forced exhalation, increasing visceral pressure to push the diaphragm up and expel air quickly
Serratus anterior	Draw scapula forward as the ribcage closes
Pectoralis major	
Quadratus lumborum	Pulls ribcage down as diaphragm is forced up

be assessed and treated with soft tissue techniques, and tight muscles need to be stretched. The thoracic spine also tends to become rigid through coughing and laboured breathing, so this area needs to be treated as well.

Fascial tension is an important factor and the whole chest and thoracic area should be treated with myofascial techniques. This is particularly effective around the ribs, costal cartilage and upper abdomen area.

Emotional stress and anxiety are often a contributing factor with respiratory conditions, especially asthma, so the relaxing effects of general massage should also be considered. Remedial exercises should be encouraged to improve muscle function and posture along with advice on improving relevant lifestyle factors.

Conditions Affecting the Circulatory System

- **Hypertension** (high blood pressure) is usually a side effect of other health issues and/or lifestyle factors like smoking, alcohol intake, emotional or occupational stress. Although any other health issues need to be considered, massage does usually have a good effect on lowering blood pressure by assisting blood flow and generally relaxing the client.

It is important to ensure that all massage strokes assist in venous return by working towards the heart. The abdomen is an important area to treat because on a physical level it has a high concentration of blood vessels and on a neurological level can have a very relaxing effect.

Any lowering of blood pressure as a result of a single treatment may be only temporary but if done regularly in conjunction with improved lifestyle it can play a significant part in improving the condition.

- Clients with **heart conditions** can also benefit indirectly from regular massage treatment. If performed with care and caution, massage will have no adverse effect and, by assisting circulation and relaxation, its effects are usually very positive.

Following heart surgery, clients often develop a protective holding pattern by protracting their shoulders and they have an inherent fear of opening out their chest. This is a good safety strategy immediately following surgery, but after a few weeks this needs to be discouraged as it may become permanent and possibly lead to a respiratory restriction. Techniques to gently release muscle and fascial tension across the chest with exercise advice to improve posture and function should be safe to do after about six weeks.

In the case of bypass surgery, clients will have scars down their legs where the veins have been removed. These often cause them considerable discomfort which can discourage them from starting to safely exercise and improve their cardiovascular fitness. Techniques should be used to improve the recovery of these scars as soon as possible along with support and encouragement to exercise.

Treating Surgical Scars or Puncture Wounds

Providing there are no longer any medical problems to consider, soft tissue techniques can be applied to aid the recovery of the scar. It is important to prevent the formation of scar

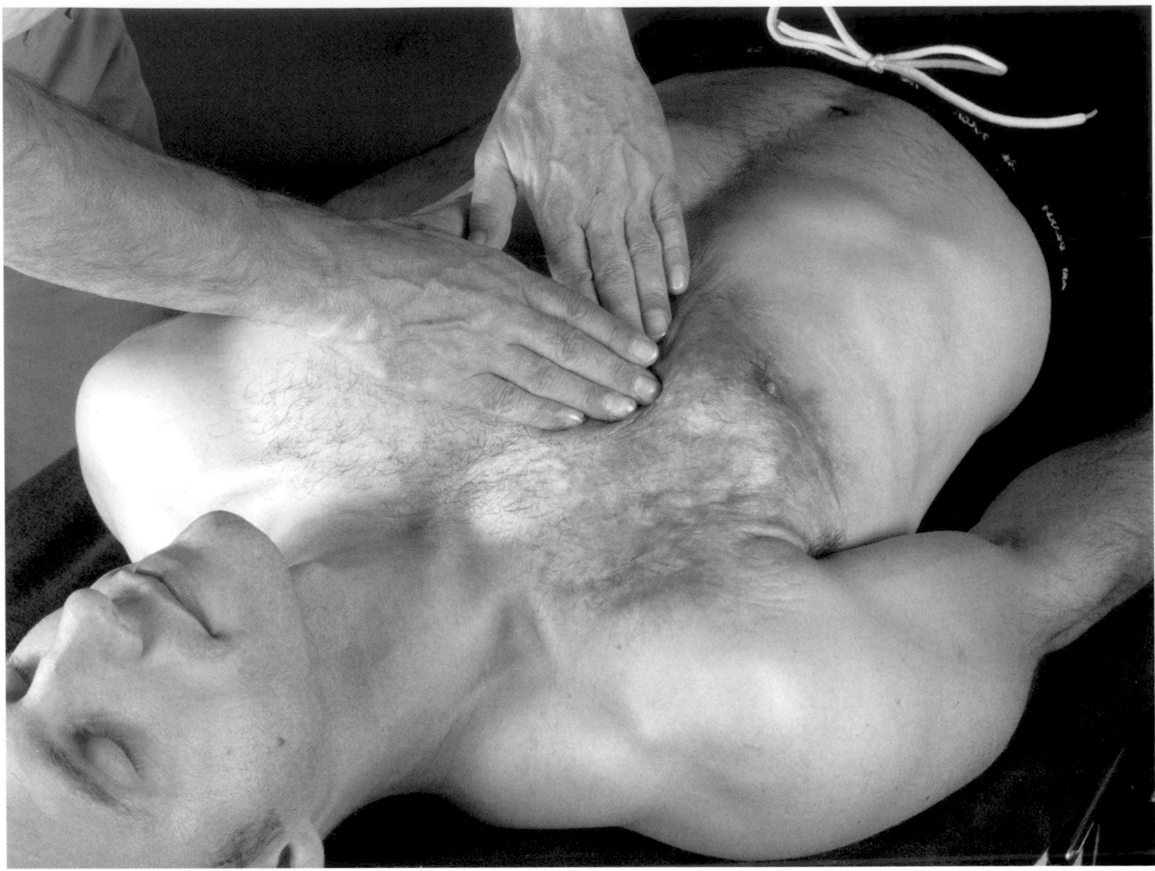

Photo 149. Fascial release strokes applied to large areas of scarring on the skin.

tissue which stick (adhere) the fascial layers together and restrict movement.

Incisions usually close within a few days and can hold together with normal movement after a week. Treatment should not begin if sutures (stitches) are still present, and it is always necessary to make sure the skin has joined together well with no sign of weeping or inflammation. No lubricant which could soften the scar should be used, and great care must be taken in the early stage to make sure that treatment causes no sharp pain.

The therapist should gently press their fingers into the skin on either side of the scar and hold the two edges of it together. Then, without releasing this, the hand can be used to glide the underlying superficial fascia back and forth in a transverse direction to the scar. This can be done with greater pressure as the scar recovers over time. Eventually the scar can be pushed out of the way and quite deep friction applied to the underlying tissues. When the scar becomes paler and matches the colour of the normal skin, short transverse strokes in opposite directions can be applied across the scar itself.

All these techniques are aimed at preventing adhesions forming in the fascia beneath the skin and help the new collagen fibres bind the skin in an integrated and uniform way. *(See photos 149, 150 and 151.)*

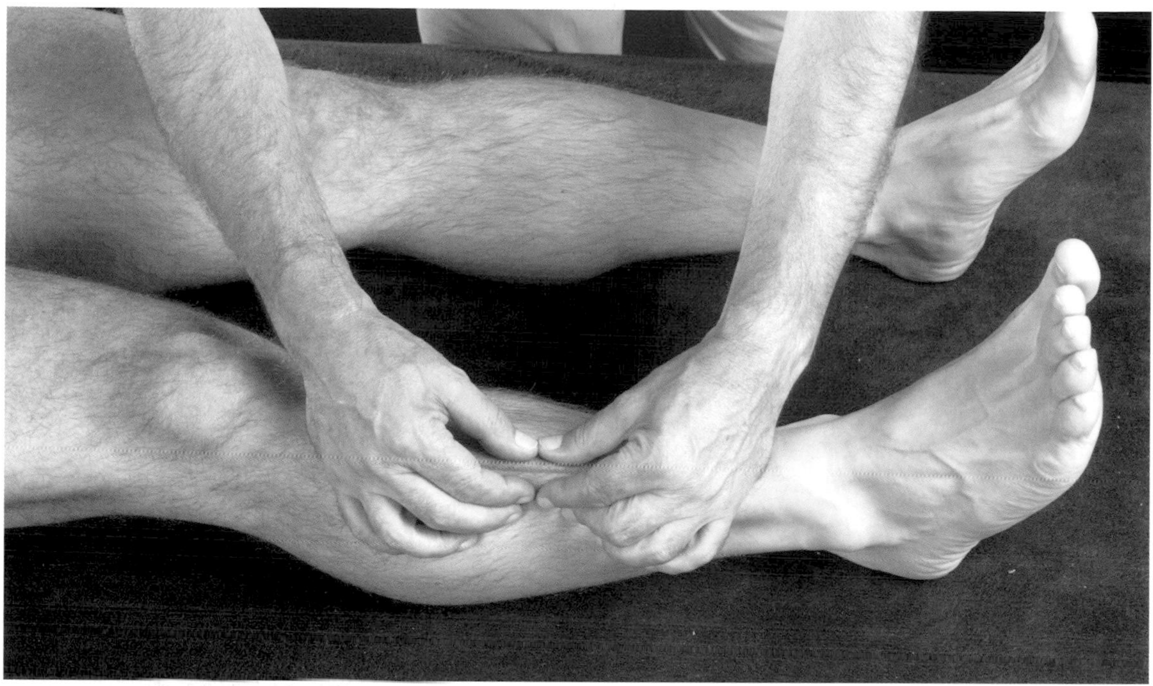

Photo 150. Holding the sides of the scar together, transverse strokes can be applied to prevent scar tissue formation in the underlying tissues.

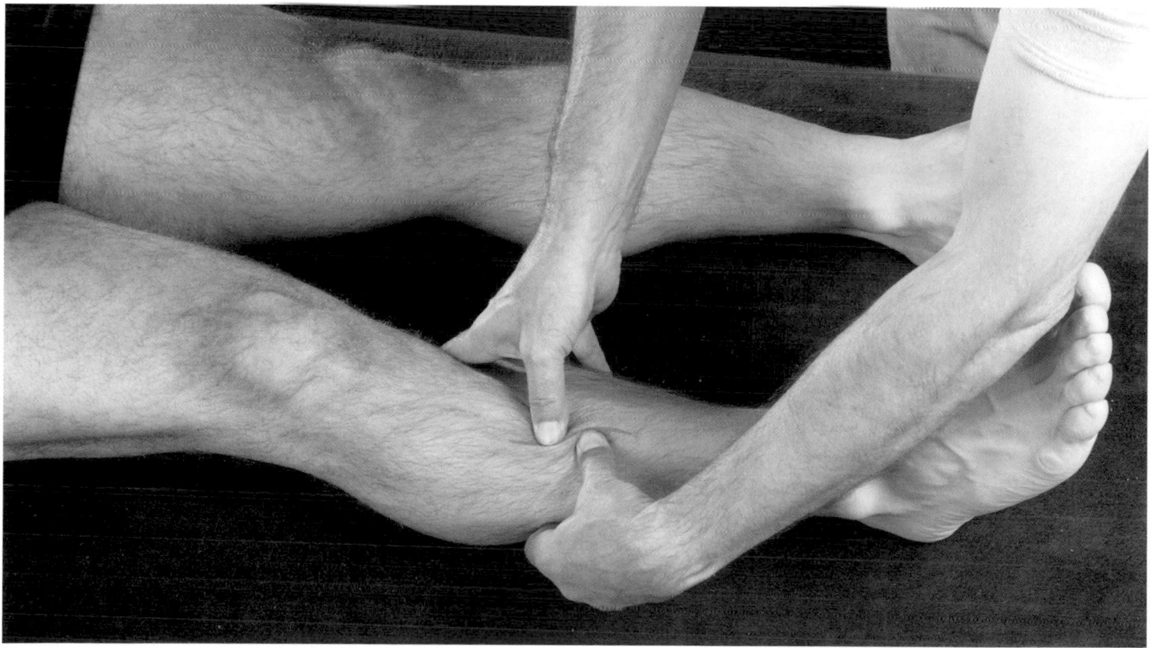

Photo 151. Opposite transverse strokes applied to the skin to improve scar repair in the later stage of recovery.

Conditions Affecting the Peripheral Nervous System

- **Nerve lesions** can occur through traumatic incidents which cause physical damage to a peripheral nerve. This leads to a very severe loss of motor and/or sensory function away from the damaged site along the limb. The condition often improves very slowly as the nerve regenerates but some permanent neural dysfunction may result. Massage can do little to help this other than maintain tissue health in immobile muscles, and the sensory stimulation may help encourage neural improvement.
- **Nerve compression** can happen where a nerve gets trapped as it passes through other tissues. This is more likely to occur at a joint where the nerve has to glide smoothly round the articulating structures. Joint misalignment and local scar tissue can restrict the nerve and cause a degree of motor and/or sensory loss along the limb. Some positions may be pain free, with symptoms only occurring in some positions or movements which stretch the nerve. Symptoms may only appear in a distal area with no apparent pain in the area where the compression is.

Common sites of nerve compression

- Lower back: **Sciatica.** The nerve is compressed between the lumbar vertebrae, leading to symptoms running along one or both legs. Soft tissue techniques to release muscle tension along the lumbar spine can alleviate some symptoms in minor situations, but postural improvement to release the pressure from the nerve is the only realistic solution.
- Neck: **Thoracic outlet syndrome.** Postural misalignment in the neck and shoulders with severe cervical lordosis can compress the nerves between the cervical vertebrae. Chronic muscle tension in the neck and shoulders can also compress the nerves (and blood vessels), adding to the problem. Neural symptoms occur along the brachial nerve plexes into the arm. Soft tissue techniques can relieve symptoms to some extent but postural improvement is essential.
- Wrist: **Carpal tunnel syndrome.** The nerves can get trapped as they pass through the carpal tunnel in the wrist if it becomes restricted with scar tissue or compressed with soft tissue tension. Friction techniques and stretching across the wrist on the palmer side can help relieve symptoms but in severe cases surgical repair may be the best option.
- Forefoot: **Mortens neuroma.** Dropped transverse arch closes the toe joints together, compressing the nerves passing between them and causing pain in the forefoot. Treatment approach is the same as carpal tunnel syndrome.
- Hip: **Piriformis syndrome.** In some people the sciatic nerve passes through the belly of the piriformis muscle, and if this is chronically tight it can compress the nerve and lead to sciatic symptoms. Soft tissue treatment of the muscle can be very effective.

Conditions Affecting the Central Nervous System

- **Parkinson's disease*** is a progressive disorder that affects the part of the brain that produces dopamine, and this slows down the neural messages to the muscles. The main symptoms are slow hesitant movements, tremors and shaking. Massage has no direct effect on this condition, but massage treatment to promote relaxation and support general health can help a sufferer's quality of life.

- **Multiple Sclerosis*** is a progressive disease that causes inflammation of the myelin sheath which surrounds the nerve fibres in the brain and spinal cord. During periods of remission, there is some recovery of these cells but over the longer term there is progressive and permanent nerve damage. Symptoms vary from person to person but typically involve a loss of muscle control. Some muscles become excessively tight whilst others become weak and massage therapy can be used to try to address both of these wherever they occur. Techniques can be tried to release tense areas and exercise advice to try to strengthen those that are weakening. Although this will not reverse the neural damage, it can slow down the functional deterioration. All sufferers will be different, and techniques that work well in some cases may not be so effective with others. The therapist has to be versatile and ask the client about the techniques they like and what they feel is helping them.
- **Cerebral Palsy*** is a general term covering a number of disorders caused by brain damage which is present from birth. It normally involves spasticity of muscles and/or mental retardation and can vary enormously between individuals ranging from very minor to extremely profound. It is not progressive, but secondary conditions and complications often develop in later life. Massage and soft tissue techniques can be used to improve the musculoskeletal symptoms and can help sufferers deal with their condition.
- **Spinal Cord injuries*** can occur as a result of major traumatic accidents and cause severe paralysis to large areas of the body. Once the damage has been done, there is no further progression of the paralysis although secondary medical complications may develop in later life.

With any **paralysis**, the general health of the immobile tissues can deteriorate through poor circulation and massage can improve this. With lack of movement, the fascia will tighten and this leads to the joints going into **contractures**. Passive stretching techniques can be used to try to prevent this.

To help cope with their lives, people with paralysis in one area often have to overuse other parts of their body. It is very important to pay attention to these areas to prevent any injury problems occurring there.

Conditions Affecting the Muscular System

- **Rheumatoid arthritis** and **Osteoarthritis:** *See Inflammatory Joint Conditions, p. 141.*
- **Duchenne muscular dystrophy*** is a progressive hereditary disease which causes the muscles to weaken; eventually they lose all their functional ability. Massage can do nothing to stop the degeneration but can help improve the client's quality of life to some extent. As they become less able to move themselves, they feel the stiffness and discomfort which massage can temporarily relieve. Because sufferers often sit in a slumped position which compresses their abdomen, they can suffer with constipation which massage can help alleviate.

Special Care for Clients with Severe and Terminal Diseases*

When treating clients with severe conditions like multiple sclerosis or muscular dystrophy, the therapist should consider much more than just the physical effects of treatment. If the client is severely disabled, the only time they may get physical contact from another person is when they are being dressed, put in a wheelchair, being washed or put on a commode. These are not experiences they can enjoy and may be uncomfortable or even embarrassing. But massage is something they can enjoy, and this can be more important to them than any of the musculoskeletal benefits.

Everything possible should be done to make treatment as pleasant an experience as possible. This may mean treating them on their bed or in a wheelchair and working through their clothes rather than getting them to undress. This may be more uncomfortable and difficult for the therapist, but this is a small price to pay compared to the client's disability.

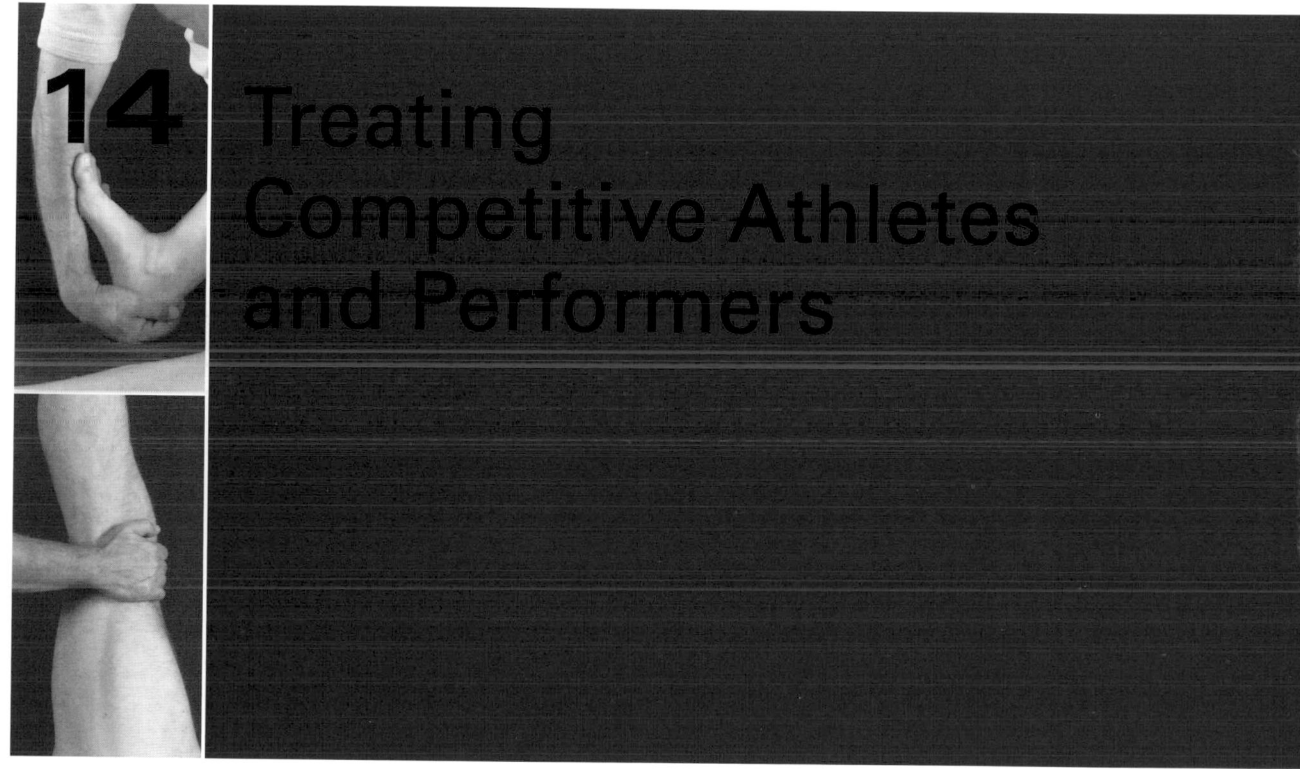

14 Treating Competitive Athletes and Performers

Sports Massage is not a therapy in itself because it is not possible to massage a sport, only a person. We treat people who live complex and varied lives which involve far more than just the sport they do. For serious athletes and performers who have the highest competitive goals, remedial massage and soft tissue techniques can be used specifically to help them achieve these. But it has to be accepted that most athletes aim to be better than they ever will be and test themselves to the limit, which makes injury an almost inevitable consequence.

Overtraining is a major risk because they naturally want to do as much quality training as they can to reach their highest potential. Injuries can easily develop if they train too hard before they have fully recovered from the previous session. The secret of good performance ultimately has as much to do with how well an athlete recovers between sessions as it has to do with how hard they train.

It takes time for the tissues to recover from hard exercise. As well as the need for any micro-trauma to repair, it takes time for the blood flowing through the area to flush out any accumulated muscle waste and to replenish the nutritional stores. By pumping blood more forcefully through the micro-circulation, basic massage strokes can greatly speed up both of these processes. If an athlete can recover more quickly, they can then train more intensively and with less risk of overuse injury. For this reason alone, massage should always be an integral part of any hard training programme. The best time to have a general massage to aid this recovery is as soon as possible after the athlete's hardest training sessions.

Many overuse injuries develop slowly over a period of time as micro-trauma gradually builds up in small areas of tissue. They usually remain unnoticed in the early stage because the neuromuscular system can adapt to the very minimal changes in the tissue's function. But eventually it can reach a critical level, the symptoms become apparent, and the athlete thinks they have only just sustained the injury.

When performing deep general massage strokes, the therapist can feel these small areas of tissue damage before they develop into noticeable injuries. Direct treatment can be instantly applied to resolve these potential problems at this early stage and the athlete can continue to train safely without the interruption of an injury. Soft Tissue Release (STR) applied with active movements is a very good way of dealing with these small local issues. Not only does it release the scar tissue, but also the active movement helps realign the fibres correctly, whilst at the same time activating the neuromuscular system.

The therapist can feel the problem, but the deep techniques create some pain for the athlete, too, so they also become aware of the potential problem and can take early preventative action. Because they have felt its exact location, they can adjust their stretching techniques more accurately to target those affected tissues. They can also try to improve their technique and training methods to avoid the overuse factor in the first place.

However well an athlete's training programme has been devised, its effectiveness can only be judged by results. If it is not ideal and the athlete goes on to perform poorly or gets injured, it is usually too late to correct the training problem. But regular massage can identify how well the tissues are responding to training, and so adjustments can be made along the way. If overuse tension is building up, the athlete could take a short break from hard training to allow better recovery, or increase their training if they are recovering very well. Similarly, the programme of massage treatment can be planned around the training programme so they receive more treatment when their training is most intense.

Many sports require a good range of movement and flexibility, but hard training and poor stretching often result in muscle tightness. Advanced stretching techniques like MET are an excellent way of dealing with this, and athletes can be shown how to perform these themselves.

Pre-event

In the final build-up to a competition, the main objective is to achieve the fullest recovery from training so the athlete is free to perform at their very best. This requires good, thorough massage which will identify and treat any areas of adverse tension in the soft tissues. During the last 24 hours, all soft tissue issues should hopefully have been resolved and the main focus is then on mental preparation. This is both sports-specific and unique to the athlete. If they appear overexcited, they may require more calming and relaxing massage, but otherwise a fast light and stimulating massage might be more appropriate. It is important that the therapist knows what best suits both the athlete and the sport and treats each individual athlete accordingly.

Post-event

The main focus is recovery, and massage should be given as soon as possible using flowing techniques which flush blood through the micro-circulation. Deep pressure should be avoided over areas that may be injured and massage can be applied around an ice pack if necessary. Gentle passive stretching can also be very effective, providing there is no acute injury.

Appendixes

Appendix 1

Common Contraindications for Massage and Soft Tissue Therapy

- **Acute inflammation:** When tissue fibres are torn as a result of a trauma, they bleed. This blood causes the skin to feel hotter and appear reddened as well as swollen. Massage at this stage will further aggravate the torn fibres, causing them more damage and increasing the bleeding.
- **Open Wounds:** Massage strokes over an open wound could increase the damage and encourage infection into the wound.
- **Bone fractures:** The pressure caused by manual techniques will aggravate the fracture and cause further damage as well as a great deal of pain. If there is any possibility of a fracture, this must be assessed first by X-ray.
- **Joint dislocations:** Traumatic incidents can lead to joint dislocation, particularly the shoulder. There will be a huge amount of pain, movement will be drastically restricted and the joint will appear deformed. Although there will be a large amount of soft tissue damage with this injury, the joint must first be assessed and treated by an orthopaedic specialist.
- **Deep Vein Thrombosis (DVT):** A blood clot can form in a vein, usually in the calf. Massage would be very likely to dislodge this and it will then travel with the blood being pumped towards the heart. The veins get larger as they converge towards the heart, so there is nothing to impede the blood clot and it will pass through the ventricles of the heart and enter the pulmonary circulation. Here the blood vessels reduce in size as they branch out and the blood clot will eventually get blocked and stop the blood flowing to an area of the lung. If the blood cannot reach the alveoli in the lungs it cannot take on the vital oxygen the body needs and this can have fatal consequences in a very short time.
  DVT is more likely in elderly people with sedentary lifestyles, who usually have other medical conditions also, but it can occur on rare occasions to apparently fit, young, healthy people. The client will report having a fairly sudden onset of pain without there being any obvious musculoskeletal cause. There will be a small specific area of swelling, and the skin may appear shiny as it is locally stretched. The client will normally also feel generally unwell as there is restricted blood flow round the body. Any suspected DVT must be referred to a hospital immediately.
- **Varicose veins:** This occurs, usually in the posterior lower leg, when the non-return valves in the vein break down. The vein becomes enlarged and the walls become brittle. Massage strokes are perfectly safe, except to the actual site of the problem because it could easily damage the fragile vein and cause severe bleeding.
- **Bleeding disorders:** Conditions like haemophilia prevent the blood from clotting properly when bleeding occurs. Deep massage techniques may possibly cause slight trauma and bleeding, so this must be avoided in these conditions.

Appendix 2

Treatment Procedure for Acute Inflammation

When the soft tissues are acutely inflamed following a trauma, massage and other manual techniques are contraindicated. Normally, the client will describe a recent musculoskeletal incident, and the bleeding will cause heat, redness and swelling, along with pain and dysfunction.

Rest

It is essential the client rests the affected area. Any activity will keep opening the damaged fibres and prevent them from starting to repair. It will also increase bleeding, which adds to the swelling and scar tissue formation.

Ice

Applying ice will slow blood flow to the area and so reduce the amount of bleeding immediately following the trauma. But if the area is rested well the damaged fibres will start to knit together fairly quickly, and the bleeding should then stop. But ice also has a great analgesic effect, and reducing pain prevents protective muscle spasm occurring in the area. Ice should be applied as part of recovery so long as the client has painful symptoms.

Ice should not be applied for too long in the early acute stage. Although it slows blood flow, eventually the nervous system responds to the risk of the skin freezing and to prevent this sends more blood to the area instead. This increase in blood flow could cause more bleeding from the torn fibres.

How long ice should be applied for will depend on the area. Initially the skin should appear paler when ice is applied, but it then becomes more reddened if kept on for too long. A large area such as the gluteal muscles will allow ice to be applied for much longer than a smaller area like the wrist.

Compression

Compressing the injured area will squash the blood vessels, reduce blood flow and slow down the bleeding. It is important that only the local injury site is compressed and blood flow is not restricted to other areas. Pressure also has a pain-relieving effect.

Elevation

Whenever there is swelling in the soft tissues, elevation will help. If the area can be supported above the height of the torso, it allows gravity to drain excess fluid from the area.

Appendix 3

Example of a Client Record Card

Based on the information given here the therapist can then ask the client more detailed questions about any factors that could be relevant to the condition they are seeking treatment for.

Name: ____________________

Address and contact details: ____________________

Date of birth: ____________________

Gender: ____________________

Occupation: ____________________

Sport and leisure activities: ____________________

Have you had any of the following? ____________________

High/low blood pressure	Surgery		Cancer	
Heart condition	Metal/plastic implants		Skin conditions	
Thrombosis	Haemophilia		Any other conditions:	
Varicose veins	Diabetes			

Are you taking any medication? ____________________

Appendix 4

How I Got Into Massage

I am often asked how I got into massage and some of my colleagues who know the story have said I should put it in this book. So here it is tucked away at the back in case anyone wants to read it.

I got a degree in Business Studies in 1975 which was supposed to prepare me for a career in management, wearing a tie! But the student lifestyle in the 1970s had turned me into a hippie instead and a 'proper' job was not what I wanted. After some time travelling I opened a second-hand furniture shop which was fun for a few years but it was not very fulfilling.

Then in 1981 I watched the first London Marathon and it inspired me to start running. But unlike other fads I had tried and given up after a few weeks I found that this was something I was actually quite good at and I kept on going. In my late 20's I was running sub-3-hour marathons (my PB was 2:48) and took up triathlon when it very first started.

One Wednesday night in mid-winter 1984, having just finished a 14-mile training run, I was sitting in my kitchen eating and reading a magazine article about massage written by an osteopath/runner called Guy Ogden. I was about to take a shower anyway so I thought I may as well give it a try first. I took a bottle of salad oil out of the cupboard and did some stroking and squeezing techniques up my left leg. Before moving on to my right leg I felt the call of nature and it was the short walk through my flat to the toilet that was the turning point of my life (a friend has suggested that I should title this 'It started with a piss!'). I could not believe how different my two legs felt and I was soon massaging the right one to even them up.

Then in the shower, with my legs feeling so much better than they normally would, I started to think about it. All the guys I run with could do with this, and what about normal people with everyday aches and pains, massage has got to be good for them too.

But in those days massage was not at all well recognised or respected; in fact it hardly existed outside the sex industry. So I had this burning desire to become a massage therapist even though they didn't really exist yet. I told some fellow athletes about massaging my own legs and a few of them started to do it as well, and also felt the benefits. But I was not yet brave enough to say, 'Hey, can I massage your legs' and so it remained a secret desire.

Then one day I went to a running shop in Camden Town and was chatting to the owner Chris who was a fellow athlete from Highgate Harriers. I think he could tell that I was not happy in my job but I was really passionate about running. He also knew Guy Ogden who had written the article. He suddenly said, 'Have you ever thought of doing massage?' and I said, 'Yes!' before he even finished the sentence.

At the time I was sharing a flat with a final year medical student who was also a keen sportsman. When I got home I asked Mark what he thought of me doing massage for athletes and he too was full of enthusiasm for it. Suddenly this was not such a crazy idea anymore.

The only proper massage course I could find was based in Blackpool (a coastal resort in the North of England) and coincidentally that was where my flatmate came from. I could get some free accommodation there by swapping with his friends who could visit London and stay at my place. Mark continued to be a big help because I had access to all his medical books and he even sneaked me into some lectures at his medical school.

So one Sunday morning running across Hampstead Heath I was chatting to a club-mate called Anthony and told him I wouldn't be there next week because I was starting my massage training.

Sitting in a classroom on the first day of the course I realised that apart from doing my own legs I had never actually had a massage in my life, so what was I doing there? After a demonstration by the tutor it was time to find out and full of confidence I walked up to the biggest guy in the class and said, 'Okay, I'll start on you.' Now this is where it gets almost spiritual because I can remember every detail of the exact moment I applied my first massage stroke on another person. The way the light shone through the window, the smell, the noise of the traffic outside and the background chatter in the room, and the overwhelming feeling that I had somehow been doing this all my life. I felt completely 'at home'.

Back in London a week later and the phone rang. It was Anthony asking if I was now doing massage because he thought he would like to have a treatment. I had only done my first four days of training and desperately wanted some practice so I eagerly agreed. I told him I didn't want any payment because I was just learning and sensing my enthusiasm he asked if I could treat his girlfriend as well, and of course I agreed. He then told me that she was a soloist in the Royal Ballet at Covent Garden and a shudder went through my self-confidence.

A week later my new couch arrived and off I went to see Anthony and his girlfriend, my first clients. Back in my car a few hours later I was looking at the £10 note they had insisted on giving me, but it was much better than that. Genisia, the ballerina, had given me such great feedback, encouraging me to work deeper where necessary and helped me locate the problem areas she had. But the very best thing of all was, 'Can you come back next week and can I bring a couple of other Royal Ballet dancers as well?' I was in business and getting the best possible practice on some of the top dancers in the world. This later led me to work with the Prima ballerina Sylvie Guillem for over 10 years, accompanying her on many tours around the world. It's amazing what can result from a chance conversation.

It was a financial struggle to build a viable practice in the first few years. I had never been so poor but at the same time so positive about the future. And then it just got better and better.

I learned my craft from the clients I treated and was lucky to get such a wide variety of experiences. I started with a few athletes and dancers who mentioned me to others and word spread in directions I had not expected. One day a lady called saying she had Multiple Sclerosis and wondered if I could help her. This led me on to discover how massage could also be used to help people suffering with a wide range of other medical conditions too. I treated her one morning and then went to treat a world heavyweight boxer (Frank Bruno) and then on to treat Sylvie the ballerina; now that was an interesting day's work! When I started I only thought I would treat athletes and watch them win, I never expected that one day I would treat a client in a hospice the day before she passed away. They have all helped make me the therapist I am and I am equally grateful to them all.

My Learning Adventure

My original training in 1985 taught massage on a very superficial level and the ancient skills of remedial massage had almost died out. Physiotherapy had begun in the early 1900s and at the time was based solely on remedial massage and exercise. But because this had clinical limitations the new profession looked for ways to overcome these and widen its scope of treatment. This led to great new developments in their techniques and methods, but along the way massage became a smaller and smaller part, until eventually it almost disappeared from physiotherapy training altogether. What massage was being taught elsewhere was aimed primarily at the luxury, leisure and beauty sectors where more advanced remedial skills were not required.

But I got into massage because of my involvement in sport and the superficial techniques I was taught were not up to the job I was facing, so I started to discover more effective methods myself. Initially this focused on developing the basic massage skills but I then discovered that there were more advanced soft tissue techniques being used by osteopaths which could take me further.

Manual therapy techniques are not discovered by clever scientists, they come about because therapists combine their experience, skill and knowledge to discover the ways that achieve the greatest results. Science then tries to catch up with this by finding a theory to explain it and then gives it a name. I may have thought these were 'new' techniques at the time but when you look at older traditional forms of manual therapy they can be seen there too in one form or another. The intuitive skills of the therapist today are no different than they were thousands of years ago, and the tissues we treat and the injuries they can suffer have also not changed. I believe that all the techniques we use today have probably been done before and there is nothing that is really new.

It was perhaps good fortune that I could not afford to do an osteopathy degree at the time because it meant I had to work these techniques out for myself. I bought books and although I struggled to understand them at first I gradually began to integrate these soft tissue techniques into my work. In this way they evolved within a more massage-based structure, with greater versatility that could adapt to the more extreme limits of the athletes and dancers I treated.

Other modalities like Shiatsu, the Feldenkrais method, Pilates and the Alexander technique, to name just a few, also had a lot to offer me. Again I couldn't afford to do all these courses but managed to develop long-term 'swapping' arrangements with therapists from a variety of different disciplines which have all influenced the way I work.

In recent years I have had the good fortune to do a number of cadaver and dissection classes at a teaching hospital in London. These have increased my understanding of the human body to a new level and I am very grateful to have this great opportunity.

Index

Note: page numbers in **bold** refer to diagrams and photographs, page numbers in *italics* refer to information contained in tables.